TEXTBOOK OF AN
UPPER LIMB AND THORAX

MW00764191

TEXTBOOK OF ANATOMY
UPPER LIMB AND THORAX

Volume I

Second Edition

Vishram Singh, MS, PhD
Professor and Head, Department of Anatomy
Professor-in-Charge, Medical Education Unit
Santosh Medical College, Ghaziabad
Editor-in-Chief, Journal of the Anatomical Society of India
Member, Academic Council and Core Committee PhD Course, Santosh University
Member, Editorial Board, Indian Journal of Otology
Medicolegal Advisor, ICPS, India
Consulting Editor, ABI, North Carolina, USA

Formerly at: GSVM Medical College, Kanpur
King George's Medical College, Lucknow
Al-Arab Medical University, Benghazi (Libya)
All India Institute of Medical Sciences, New Delhi

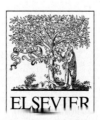

ELSEVIER

ELSEVIER
A division of
Reed Elsevier India Private Limited

PARAS MEDICAL BOOKS PVT. LTD.
D.No. 6-3-866/A, 101, 1st Floor,
Mekins Maheswari Mayank Plaza,
Opp. Green Park Hotel,
Above Deccan Pen Stores, Hyderabad-500 016.
Tel: 040-66785613, 32995825
e-mail: parasameerpetshowroom@parasmedicalbooks.com

Textbook of Anatomy: Upper Limb and Thorax, Volume I, 2e
Vishram Singh

© 2014 Reed Elsevier India Private Limited

First edition 2010
Second edition 2014

All rights reserved. No part of this publication may be reproduced or transmitted in any form or by any means, electronic or mechanical, including photocopying, recording, or any information storage and retrieval system, without permission in writing from the Publisher.

This book and the individual contributions contained in it are protected under copyright by the Publisher (other than as may be noted herein).

ISBN: 978-81-312-3729-8
e-book ISBN: 978-81-312-3625-3

Notices

Knowledge and best practice in this field are constantly changing. As new research and experience broaden our understanding, changes in research methods, professional practices, or medical treatment may become necessary.

Practitioners and researchers must always rely on their own experience and knowledge in evaluating and using any information, methods, compounds, or experiments described herein. In using such information or methods they should be mindful of their own safety and the safety of others, including parties for whom they have a professional responsibility.

With respect to any drug or pharmaceutical products identified, readers are advised to check the most current information provided (i) on procedures featured or (ii) by the manufacturer of each product to be administered, to verify the recommended dose or formula, the method and duration of administration, and contraindications. It is the responsibility of practitioners, relying on their own experience and knowledge of their patients, to make diagnoses, to determine dosages and the best treatment for each individual patient, and to take all appropriate safety precautions.

To the fullest extent of the law, neither the Publisher nor the authors, contributors, or editors, assume any liability for any injury and/or damage to persons or property as a matter of products liability, negligence or otherwise, or from any use or operation of any methods, products, instructions, or ideas contained in the material herein.

Please consult full prescribing information before issuing prescription for any product mentioned in this publication.

The Publisher

Published by Reed Elsevier India Private Limited
Registered Office: 305, Rohit House, 3 Tolstoy Marg, New Delhi-110 001
Corporate Office: 14th Floor, Building No. 10B, DLF Cyber City, Phase II, Gurgaon-122 002, Haryana, India

Senior Project Manager-Education Solutions: Shabina Nasim
Content Strategist: Dr Renu Rawat
Project Coordinator: Goldy Bhatnagar
Copy Editor: Shrayosee Dutta
Senior Operations Manager: Sunil Kumar
Production Manager: NC Pant
Sr. Production Executive: Ravinder Sharma
Sr. Graphic Designer: Milind Majgaonkar

Typeset by Chitra Computers, New Delhi

Printed and bound at Thomson Press India Ltd., Faridabad, Haryana

Dedicated to

My Mother
Late Smt Ganga Devi Singh Rajput
an ever guiding force in my life for achieving knowledge through education

My Wife
Mrs Manorama Rani Singh
for tolerating my preoccupation happily during the preparation of this book

My Children
Dr Rashi Singh and **Dr Gaurav Singh**
for helping me in preparing the manuscript

My Teachers
Late Professor (Dr) AC Das
for inspiring me to be multifaceted and innovative in life
Professor (Dr) A Halim
for imparting to me the art of good teaching

My Students, Past and Present
for appreciating my approach to teaching anatomy and
transmitting the knowledge through this book

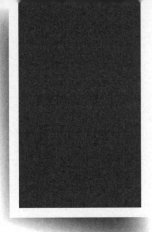

Preface to the Second Edition

It is with great pleasure that I express my gratitude to all students and teachers who appreciated, used, and recommended the first edition of this book. It is because of their support that the book was reprinted three times since its first publication in 2009.

The huge success of this book reflects appeal of its clear, unclustered presentation of the anatomical text supplemented by perfect simple line diagrams, which could be easily drawn by students in the exam and clinical correlations providing the anatomical, embryological, and genetic basis of clinical conditions seen in day-to-day life in clinical practice.

Based on a large number of suggestions from students and fellow academicians, the text has been extensively revised. Many new line diagrams and halftone figures have been added and earlier diagrams have been updated.

I greatly appreciate the constructive suggestions that I received from past and present students and colleagues for improvement of the content of this book. I do not claim to absolute originality of the text and figures other than the new mode of presentation and expression.

Once again, I whole heartedly thank students, teachers, and fellow anatomists for inspiring me to carry out the revision. I sincerely hope that they will find this edition more interesting and useful than the previous one. I would highly appreciate comments and suggestions from students and teachers for further improvement of this book.

*"To learn from previous experience and change
accordingly, makes you a successful man."*

Vishram Singh

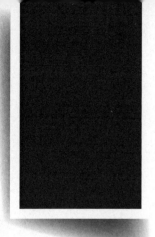

Preface to the First Edition

This textbook on upper limb and thorax has been carefully planned for the first year MBBS students. It follows the revised anatomy curriculum of the Medical Council of India. Following the current trends of clinically-oriented study of Anatomy, I have adopted a parallel approach – that of imparting basic anatomical knowledge to students and simultaneously providing them its applied aspects.

To help students score high in examinations the text is written in simple language. It is arranged in easily understandable small sections. While anatomical details of little clinical relevance, phylogenetic discussions and comparative analogies have been omitted, all clinically important topics are described in detail. Brief accounts of histological features and developmental aspects have been given only where they aid in understanding of gross form and function of organs and appearance of common congenital anomalies. The tables and flowcharts summarize important and complex information into digestible knowledge capsules. Multiple choice questions have been given chapter-by-chapter at the end of the book to test the level of understanding and memory recall of the students. The numerous simple 4-color illustrations further assist in fast comprehension and retention of complicated information. All the illustrations are drawn by the author himself to ensure accuracy.

Throughout the preparation of this book one thing I have kept in mind is that anatomical knowledge is required by clinicians and surgeons for physical examination, diagnostic tests, and surgical procedures. Therefore, topographical anatomy relevant to diagnostic and surgical procedures is clinically correlated throughout the text. Further, Clinical Case Study is provided at the end of each chapter for problem-based learning (PBL) so that the students could use their anatomical knowledge in clinical situations. Moreover, the information is arranged regionally since while assessing lesions and performing surgical procedures, the clinicians encounter region-based anatomical features. Due to propensity of fractures, dislocations and peripheral nerve lesions in the upper limb there is in-depth discussion on joints and peripheral nerves.

As a teacher, I have tried my best to make the book easy to understand and interesting to read. For further improvement of this book I would greatly welcome comments and suggestions from the readers.

Vishram Singh

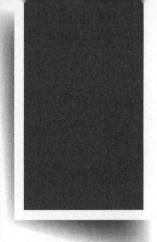

Acknowledgments

At the outset, I express my gratitude to Dr P Mahalingam, CMD; Dr Sharmila Anand, DMD; and Dr Ashwyn Anand, CEO, Santosh University, Ghaziabad, for providing an appropriate academic atmosphere in the university and encouragement which helped me in preparing this book.

I am also thankful to Dr Usha Dhar, Dean Santosh Medical College for her cooperation. I highly appreciate the good gesture shown by Dr PK Verma, Dr Ruchira Sethi, Dr Deepa Singh, and Dr Preeti Srivastava for checking the final proofs.

I sincerely thank my colleagues in the Department, especially Professor Nisha Kaul and Dr Ruchira Sethi for their assistance. I gratefully acknowledge the feedback and support of fellow colleagues in Anatomy, particularly,

- Professors AK Srivastava (Head of the Department) and PK Sharma, and Dr Punita Manik, King George's Medical College, Lucknow.
- Professor NC Goel (Head of the Department), Hind Institute of Medical Sciences, Barabanki, Lucknow.
- Professor Kuldeep Singh Sood (Head of the Department), SGT Medical College, Budhera, Gurgaon, Haryana.
- Professor Poonam Kharb, Sharda Medical College, Greater Noida, UP.
- Professor TC Singel (Head of the Department), MP Shah Medical College, Jamnagar, Gujarat.
- Professor TS Roy (Head of the Department), AIIMS, New Delhi.
- Professors RK Suri (Head of the Department), Gayatri Rath, and Dr Hitendra Loh, Vardhman Mahavir Medical College and Safdarjang Hospital, New Delhi.
- Professor Veena Bharihoke (Head of the Department), Rama Medical College, Hapur, Ghaziabad.
- Professors SL Jethani (Dean and Head of the Department), and RK Rohtagi, Dr Deepa Singh and Dr Akshya Dubey, Himalayan Institute of Medical Sciences, Jolly Grant, Dehradun.
- Professors Anita Tuli (Head of the Department), Shipra Paul, and Shashi Raheja, Lady Harding Medical College, New Delhi.
- Professor SD Joshi (Dean and Head of the Department), Sri Aurobindo Institute of Medical Sciences, Indore, MP.

Lastly, I eulogize the patience of my wife Mrs Manorama Rani Singh, daughter Dr Rashi Singh, and son Dr Gaurav Singh for helping me in the preparation of this manuscript.

I would also like to acknowledge with gratitude and pay my regards to my teachers Prof AC Das and Prof A Halim and other renowned anatomists of India, viz. Prof Shamer Singh, Prof Inderbir Singh, Prof Mahdi Hasan, Prof AK Dutta, Prof Inder Bhargava, etc. who inspired me during my student life.

I gratefully acknowledge the help and cooperation received from the staff of Elsevier, a division of Reed Elsevier India Pvt. Ltd., especially Ganesh Venkatesan (Director Editorial and Publishing Operations), Shabina Nasim (Senior Project Manager-Education Solutions), Goldy Bhatnagar (Project Coordinator), and Shrayosee Dutta (Copy Editor).

Vishram Singh

Contents

Introduction to the Upper Limb

The upper limb is the organ of the body, responsible for manual activities. It is freely movable, especially its distal segment—the hand, which is adapted for grasping and manipulating the objects.

A brief description of comparative anatomy of the limbs would facilitate understanding of their structure and function.

All the terrestrial vertebrates possess four limbs—a pair of forelimbs and a pair of hindlimbs. In quadrupeds such as dogs and buffaloes, both forelimbs and hindlimbs are evolved for transmission of body weight and locomotion. In human beings, due to evolution of erect posture, the function of weight bearing and locomotion is performed only by the hind limbs (lower limbs), while upper limbs are spared for prehensile/manipulative activities, such as grasping, holding, picking, etc. (Fig. 1.1).

There are three types of grips: (a) power grip, (b) hook grip, and (c) precision grip. The power and hook grips are primitive in nature, hence found in higher primates. The precision grip is characteristic of human beings hence only humans can properly hold a pen, pencil, needles, instruments, etc. As a result, human beings could make advancements in arts, craft, and technology, of course, with the help of intelligence.

To suit the prehensile activities, the following changes took place in the upper limbs of humans during evolution:

1. Appearance of joints permitting rotatory movements of the forearm, viz. supination and pronation.
2. Addition of clavicle to act as a strut and keep upper limb away from the body for prehension.
3. Rotation of thumb to 90° for opposition.
4. Suitable changes for free mobility of the fingers and hand.

N.B. The human hand with its digits can perform complex skilled movements under the control of the brain. Hence man is considered as the *master mechanic of the animal world*. The disabling effects of an injury to the upper limb, particularly

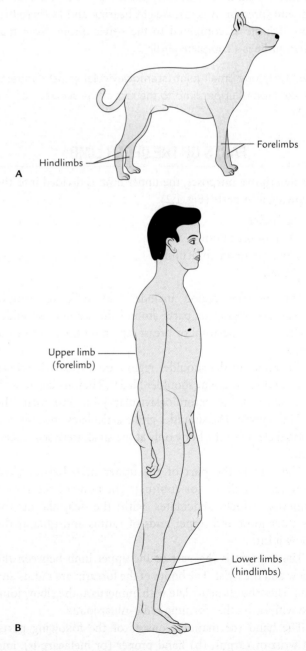

Fig. 1.1 Position of limbs: A, in quadrupeds; B, in humans.

that of hand is far more than the extent of an injury. Therefore, a sound understanding of its structure and functions is of great clinical significance—the ultimate aim of treating any ailment of the upper limb being to restore its function.

The upper limbs are connected to the trunk by a pectoral girdle. The limb girdle is defined as the bones which connect the limbs to the axial skeleton. The **pectoral girdle** is composed of two bones – scapula and clavicle. The scapula is connected to the clavicle by the acromioclavicular joint, and the clavicle is attached to the axial skeleton by the sternoclavicular joint. The pectoral girdle is not a complete girdle because it is attached to the axial skeleton only anteriorly. The primary function of the pectoral girdle is to provide attachment to numerous muscles, which move the arm and forearm. It is not weight bearing and is, therefore, more delicate as compared to the pelvic girdle. Note that pelvic girdle is a complete girdle.

N.B. Only one small joint (**sternoclavicular joint**) connects the skeleton of upper limb to the rest of the skeleton of the body.

PARTS OF THE UPPER LIMB

For descriptive purposes, the upper limb is divided into the following four parts (Fig. 1.2):

1. Shoulder.
2. Arm or brachium.
3. Forearm or antebrachium.
4. Hand.

The shoulder region includes: (a) axilla or armpit, (b) scapular region or parts around the scapula (shoulder blade), and (c) pectoral or breast region on the front of the chest.

The bones of the shoulder region are the clavicle (collar bone) and the scapula (shoulder blade). They articulate with each other at the acromioclavicular joint and form the shoulder girdle. The shoulder girdle articulates with the rest of the skeleton of the body only at the small sternoclavicular joint.

The arm is the part of the upper limb between the shoulder and elbow (or cubitus). The bone of the arm is humerus, which articulates with the scapula at the shoulder joint and upper ends of radius and ulna at the elbow joint.

The forearm is the part of the upper limb between the elbow and the wrist. The bones of the forearm are radius and ulna. These bones articulate with humerus at the elbow joint and with each other forming radio-ulnar joints.

The hand (or manus) consists of the following parts: (a) wrist or carpus, (b) hand proper (or metacarpus), and (c) digits (thumb and fingers).

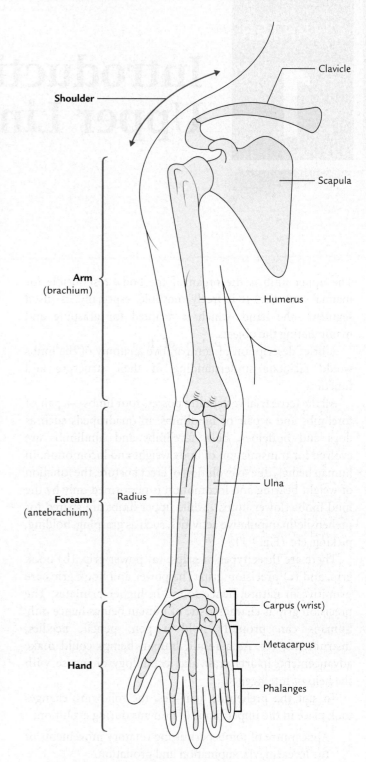

Fig. 1.2 Parts of the upper limb.

The wrist consists of eight carpal bones arranged in two rows, each consisting of four bones. The carpal bones articulate (a) with each other at intercarpal joints, (b) proximally with radius forming radio-carpal wrist joint, and (c) distally with metacarpal bones at carpometacarpal joints.

Table 1.1 Parts of the upper limb

Part	Subdivisions	Bones	Joints
Shoulder region	• Pectoral region • Axilla • Scapular region	• Clavicle • Scapula	• Sternoclavicular • Acromioclavicular
Arm	—	Humerus	Shoulder
Forearm	—	• Radius • Ulna	• Elbow • Radio-ulnar
Hand	• Wrist (carpus) • Hand proper (metacarpus) • Digits	• Carpal bones • Metacarpal bones • Phalanges	– Wrist/radio-carpal – Intercarpal – Carpometacarpal – Intermetacarpal – Metacarpophalangeal – Proximal and distal interphalangeal

The *hand proper* consists of five metacarpal bones numbered one to five from lateral to medial side in anatomical position. They articulate (a) proximally with distal row of carpal bones forming carpometacarpal joints, (b) with each other forming intermetacarpal joints, and (c) distally with proximal phalanges forming metacarpophalangeal joints.

The *digits* are five and numbered 1 to 5 from lateral to medial side. The first digit is called *thumb* and remaining four digits are *fingers*. Each digit is supported by three short long bones—the phalanges except thumb, which is supported by only two phalanges. The phalanges form metacarpophalangeal joints with metacarpals and interphalangeal joints with one another. The first carpometacarpal joint has a separate joint cavity hence movements of thumb are much more free than that of any digit/finger.

N.B. The functional value of thumb is immense. For example, in grasping, the functional value of thumb is equal to other four digits/fingers. Therefore, loss of thumb alone is as disabling as the loss of all four fingers.

The subdivisions, bones and joints of different parts of the upper limb are summarized in Table 1.1.

COMPARISON AND CONTRAST BETWEEN THE UPPER AND LOWER LIMBS

Both the upper and lower limbs are built on the same basic principle. Each limb is made up of two portions: proximal and distal.

The proximal part is called *limb girdle* and attaches the limb to the trunk. The distal part is free and consists of proximal, middle, and distal segments, which are referred to as arm, forearm, and hand respectively in the upper limb, and thigh, leg, and foot respectively in the lower limb. The homologous parts of the upper and lower limbs are enumerated in Table 1.2.

A short account of the development of the limbs further makes it easier to understand the differences between the upper and lower limbs (Fig. 1.3).

The development of upper and lower limbs begins in the 4th week of intrauterine life (IUL). A pair of small elevations appears on the ventrolateral aspect of the embryo called *limb buds*. The anterior pair of the upper limb buds appears opposite the lower cervical segments. The posterior pair of lower limb buds appears 3 or 4 days later at the level of lumbar and upper sacral segments. Thus during an early stage of development all the four limbs appear as paired limb buds. First they are simple flipper-like appendages so that the upper and lower limbs are similar in their appearance. Each has dorsal and ventral surfaces, and preaxial and postaxial borders. The preaxial border faces towards the head. Later in

Table 1.2 Homologous parts of the upper and lower limbs

Upper limb	Lower limb
Shoulder/pectoral girdle	Hip girdle/pelvic girdle
Shoulder joint	Hip joint
Arm	Thigh
Elbow joint	Knee joint
Forearm	Leg
Wrist joint	Ankle joint
Hand (a) Carpus (b) Metacarpus (c) Fingers*	Foot (a) Tarsus (b) Metatarsus (c) Toes*

*First digit in hand is termed *thumb* and first digit in foot is termed *great toe*.

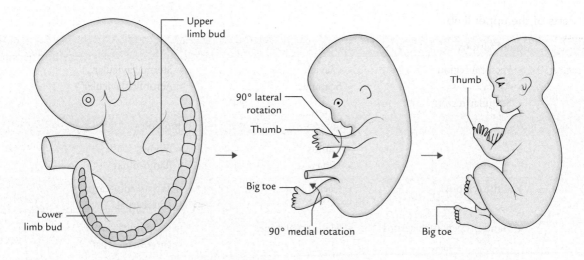

Fig. 1.3 Development of the limbs.

Table 1.3 Differences between the upper and lower limbs

	Upper limb	Lower limb
Function	Prehension (i.e., manipulation of objects by grasping)	Locomotion and transmission of weight
Bones	Smaller and weaker	Larger and stronger
Joints	Smaller and less stable	Larger and more stable
Muscles	• Smaller and attached to smaller bony areas • Antigravity muscles less developed	• Larger and attached to larger bony areas • Antigravity muscles more developed
Girdle	Pectoral girdle (a) Made up of two bones, clavicle and scapula (b) No articulation with vertebral column (c) Articulation with axial skeleton is very small through sternoclavicular joint	Pelvic girdle (a) Made up of single bone, the hip bone* (b) Articulates with vertebral column (c) Articulation with axial skeleton is large, through sacroiliac joint
Preaxial border	Faces laterally	Faces medially

*The hip bone essentially consists of three components: ilium, ischium, and pubis, which later fuse to form a single bone.

the development, the ends of limb buds become expanded and flattened to form the hand and foot plates in which the digits develop. The digits nearest to the preaxial border are thumb and big toe in the upper and lower limbs, respectively. The limbs then rotate.

The lower limb buds rotate medially through 90° so that their preaxial border faces medially and their extensor surface faces forwards. The upper limb buds on the other hand rotate laterally through 90° so that their preaxial border faces laterally their extensor surface faces backwards.

The differences between the upper and lower limbs are listed in Table 1.3.

TRANSMISSION OF FORCE IN THE UPPER LIMB (Fig. 1.4)

The pectoral girdle on each side consists of two bones: clavicle and scapula, only clavicle is attached to the rest of skeleton by a small joint—the sternoclavicular joint. The two bones of girdle are joined together by even smaller joint, the acromioclavicular joint. The clavicle is attached to the scapula by a strong coracoclavicular ligament (strongest ligament in the upper limb), and the clavicle is anchored to the 1st costal cartilage by the costoclavicular ligament.

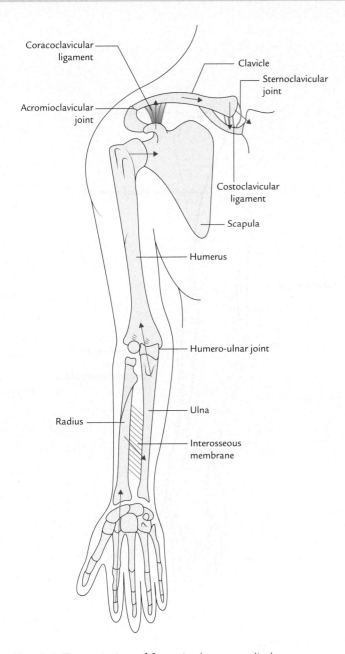

Coracoclavicular ligament

Clavicle

Sternoclavicular joint

Acromioclavicular joint

Costoclavicular ligament

Scapula

Humerus

Humero-ulnar joint

Ulna

Radius

Interosseous membrane

Fig. 1.4 Transmission of force in the upper limb.

Forces of the upper limb are transmitted to the axial skeleton by clavicle through costoclavicular ligament and sternoclavicular joint. The lines of force transmission in the upper limb are shown in Flowchart 1.1.

BONES OF THE UPPER LIMB

They are already described with parts of the upper limb (for details see Page 2).

MUSCLES OF THE UPPER LIMB

The muscles of upper limb include (a) the muscles that attach the limb and girdle to the body and (b) the muscles of arm, forearm, and hand. The deltoid muscle covers the shoulder like a hood and is commonly used for intramuscular injections.

The arm and forearm are invested in the deep fascia like a sleeve and are divided into anterior and posterior compartments by intermuscular septa. The muscles of anterior and posterior compartments mainly act synergistically to carry out specific functions. The muscles of anterior compartment are mainly flexors and those of posterior compartment extensors.

The muscles of hand are responsible for its various skilled movements such as grasping, etc.

NERVES OF THE UPPER LIMB (Fig. 1.5)

The nerve supply to the upper limb is derived from the brachial plexus (formed by ventral rami of C5 to C8 and T1 spinal nerves). The five main branches of brachial plexus are axillary, musculocutaneous, median, ulnar, and radial nerves.

- The *axillary nerve* supplies the deltoid and teres minor muscles.

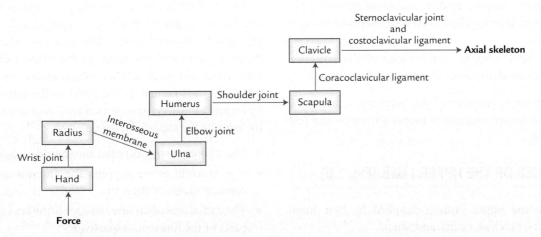

Flowchart 1.1 Lines of force transmission in the upper limb.

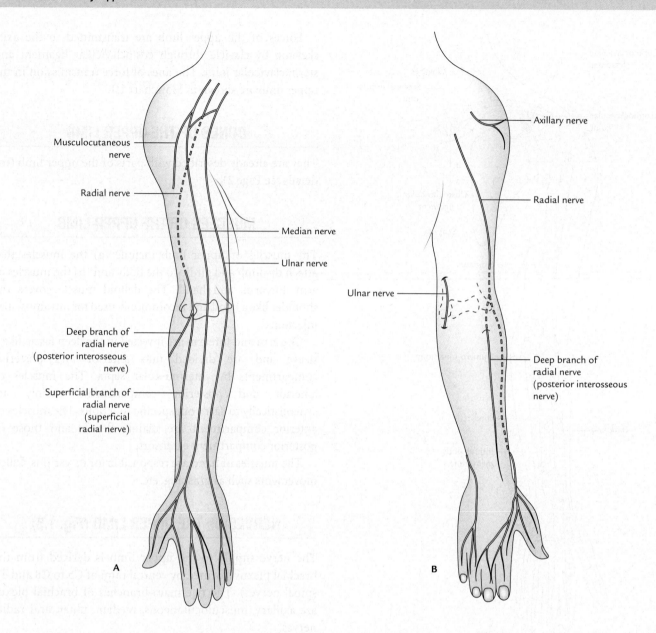

Fig. 1.5 Main nerves of the upper limb. **A,** anterior aspect; **B,** posterior aspect.

- The *musculocutaneous, median,* and *ulnar nerves* supply the muscles of anterior (flexor) compartments of the arm and forearm.
- The *radial nerve* supplies the muscles of the posterior (extensor) compartments of the arm and forearm.

N.B. All the intrinsic muscles of the hand are supplied by the ulnar nerve except muscles of thenar eminence and first two lumbricals.

ARTERIES OF THE UPPER LIMB (Fig. 1.6)

The blood to the upper limb is supplied by four main arteries: axillary, brachial, radial, and ulnar.

The axillary is the continuation of subclavian artery. At the lower border of the teres major muscle its name is changed to brachial artery. The brachial artery continues down the arm and just distal to the elbow joint, it divides into radial and ulnar arteries, which follow the bones, after which they are named. In the hand, radial artery terminates by forming the deep palmar arch and ulnar artery terminates by forming the superficial palmar arch.

- The *axillary artery* supplies the shoulder region.
- The *brachial artery* supplies the anterior and posterior compartments of the arm.
- The *radial and ulnar arteries* supply the lateral and medial parts of the forearm, respectively.

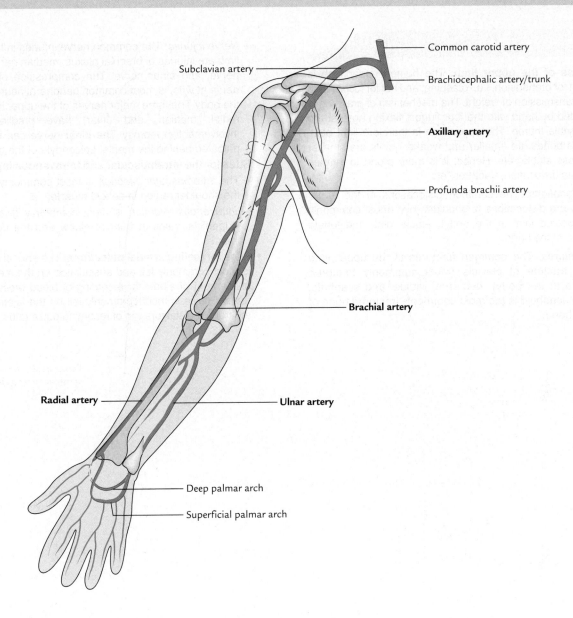

Common carotid artery

Subclavian artery

Brachiocephalic artery/trunk

Axillary artery

Profunda brachii artery

Brachial artery

Radial artery

Ulnar artery

Deep palmar arch

Superficial palmar arch

Fig. 1.6 Arteries of the upper limb.

VEINS OF THE UPPER LIMB

The deep veins of the upper limb follow the arteries and run superiorly towards the axilla, where axillary vein travels superiorly and becomes subclavian vein at the outer border of the 1st rib. The subclavian vein continues towards the root of the neck where it joins the internal jugular vein to form the brachiocephalic vein. The two brachiocephalic veins (right and left) join each other to form superior vena cava, which drains into the heart.

The superficial veins of the upper limb originate from the dorsal venous arch of the hand. The lateral end of the dorsal venous arch forms the cephalic vein, which runs along the lateral aspect of the upper limb and terminates into the axillary vein in the axilla. The medial end of the dorsal venous arch forms the basilic vein, which ascends along the medial aspect of the upper limb and empties into the axillary vein as well. Anterior to the elbow, the cephalic vein is connected to the basilic vein via the median cubital vein.

LYMPHATICS OF THE UPPER LIMB

The lymphatics of the upper limb originate in the hand. The superficial lymph vessels follow the superficial veins. The deep lymph vessels follow the deep arteries (viz. radial, ulnar, and brachial) and pass superiorly to the axilla where they drain into the axillary lymph nodes.

Clinical correlation

- **Injuries of the upper limb:** The human upper limb is meant for prehension, i.e., grasping, and not for locomotion and transmission of weight. The mechanism of grasping is provided by hand with the four fingers flexing against the opposable thumb. The upper limb is therefore light built, i.e., its bones are smaller and weaker, joints are smaller and less stable, etc. Hence, it is more prone to injuries such as dislocation, fractures, etc.
  - *Dislocations:* The common dislocations in the upper limb are dislocations of shoulder joint (most commonly dislocated joint in the body), elbow joint, and lunate bone of the hand.
  - *Fractures:* The common fractures in the upper limb are fracture of clavicle (most commonly fractured bone in the body), humerus, radius, and scaphoid. The scaphoid is the most commonly fractured bone of the hand.
  - *Nerve injuries:* The common nerve injuries in the upper limb are injuries of brachial plexus, median nerve, radial nerve, and ulnar nerve. The compression of median nerve at wrist is most common peripheral neuropathy in the body. The three major nerves of the upper limb (e.g., radial, median, and ulnar) have predilection of involvement in leprosy. The ulnar nerve can be easily palpated behind the medial epicondyle of the humerus.
- **Sites for the intramuscular and intravenous injections:**
  - The *intramuscular injection* is most commonly given in the shoulder region in deltoid muscle;
  - *intravenous injection* is most commonly given in the superficial veins in front of elbow and the dorsum of hand.
- **Sites for feeling arterial pulsations:** The arterial pulsation is most commonly felt and auscultated on the medial side of the front of elbow for recording of blood pressure. The arterial pulse is most commonly felt on the lateral side of the front of distal forearm of recording pulse rate.

Golden Facts to Remember

▶ Most important function of hand	Prehension (i.e., grasping)
▶ Most important feature of human hand	Opposition of thumb and precision grip
▶ Only point of bony contact between the upper limb and chest	Sternoclavicular joint
▶ Part of the upper limb having largest representation in the brain	Hand
▶ Most important digit of the hand	Thumb

Bones of the Upper Limb

The study of bones of the upper limb is important to understand the general topography of the upper limb and the attachment of various muscles and ligaments. The students must read the features and attachments of the bones before undertaking the study of the upper limb.

The study of bones also helps to understand the position of various articulations, wide range of the movements executed by the upper limb and the genesis of various fractures, which are common in the upper limb bones.

Each upper limb contains 32 bones (Fig. 2.1), viz.

- **Scapula,** the shoulder blade (1). } Bones of the pectoral
- **Clavicle,** the collar bone (1). } girdle
- **Humerus,** the bone of arm (1).
- **Radius and ulna,** the bones of forearm (2).
- **Carpal bones,** the bones of wrist (8).
- **Metacarpals,** the bones of hand (5).
- **Phalanges,** the bones of digits (fingers) (14).

CLAVICLE

The clavicle (L. clavicle = key) or collar bone is the long bone, with a slight S-shaped curve. It is located horizontally on the anterior aspect of the body at the junction of root of the neck and trunk. It articulates medially with the sternum and 1st rib cartilage and laterally with the acromion process of the scapula. It is subcutaneous and hence it can be palpated through its entire extent. It is the only bony attachment between the trunk and upper limb.

FUNCTIONS

The functions of the clavicle are as follows:
1. It acts as a strut for holding the upper limb far from the trunk so that it can move freely. This allows free swing of the upper limb for various prehensile acts such as holding, catching, etc.

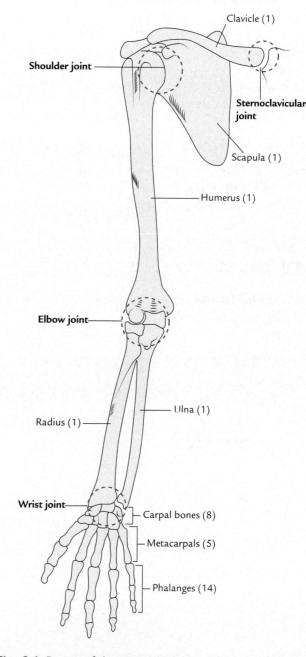

Fig. 2.1 Bones of the upper limb.

2. It transmits forces from the upper limb to the axial skeleton (sternum).
3. It provides an area for the attachment of muscles.

PECULIARITIES

The peculiar features of the clavicle are as follows:

1. It is the only long bone which lies horizontally.
2. It has no medullary cavity.
3. It is subcutaneous throughout its extent.
4. It is the first bone to start ossifying (between the fifth and sixth week of intrauterine life) and last bone to complete its ossification (at 25 years).
5. It is the only long bone which ossifies by two primary centers.
6. It is the only long bone which ossifies in membrane except for its medial end (cf. long bones ossify in cartilage).
7. It may be pierced through and through by cutaneous nerve (intermediate supraclavicular nerve).

PARTS

The clavicle consists of three parts: two ends (medial and lateral) and a shaft (Fig. 2.2):

Ends

1. The **lateral (acromial) end** is flattened above downwards and articulates with medial margin of the acromion process.
2. The **medial (sternal) end** is enlarged and quadrilateral. It articulates with the clavicular notch of the manubrium sterni.

Shaft

The **shaft** is curved. Its medial two-third is round and convex forwards, and its lateral one-third is flattened and concave forwards. The inferior surface of the shaft possesses a small longitudinal groove in its middle third.

ANATOMICAL POSITION AND SIDE DETERMINATION

The side of clavicle can be determined by holding the bone horizontally in such a way that its flattened end is on the lateral side and its enlarged quadrilateral end is on the medial side. The convexity of its medial two-third and concavity of its lateral one-third face forwards with longitudinal groove in the middle third of shaft facing inferiorly.

FEATURES AND ATTACHMENTS (Fig. 2.3)

Lateral End/Acromial End

It is flattened above downwards. An oval facet on this end articulates with the facet on the medial margin of the acromion to form **acromioclavicular joint**. The lateral end provides attachment to fibrous capsule of acromioclavicular joint.

Medial End/Sternal End

The enlarged medial end has a saddle-shaped articular surface, which articulates with the clavicular notch of manubrium sterni to form **sternoclavicular joint**. It provides attachment to (a) fibrous capsule (b) articular disc, and (c) interclavicular ligament.

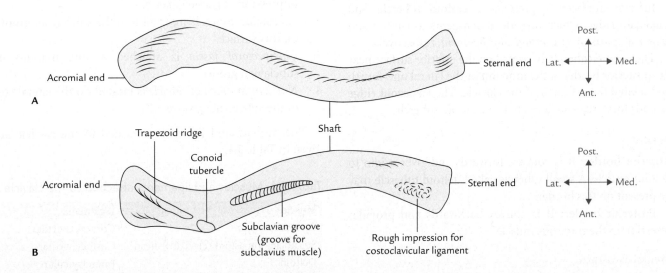

Fig. 2.2 Right clavicle: **A**, superior aspect; **B**, inferior aspect.

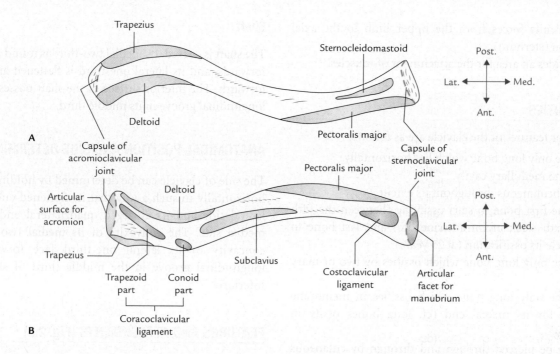

Fig. 2.3 Right clavicle showing attachments of the muscles and ligaments: **A**, superior surface; **B**, inferior surface.

Shaft

The shaft of the clavicle is divided into two parts: lateral one-third and medial two-third. The medial two-third of shaft is convex forward and lateral one-third is concave forward.

Lateral One-third

It is flattened from above downwards. It has two surfaces, i.e., superior and inferior, and two borders, i.e., anterior and posterior.

Surfaces

Superior surface: It is subcutaneous between the attachments of deltoid and trapezius.

Inferior surface: It presents a **conoid tubercle** and **trapezoid ridge,** which provide attachments to conoid and trapezoid parts of *coracoclavicular ligament*, respectively.

The **conoid tubercle** is located on the inferior surface near the posterior border at the junction of the lateral one-fourth and medial three-fourth of the clavicle. The **trapezoid ridge** extends forwards and laterally from conoid tubercle.

Borders

Anterior border: It is concave forwards and gives origin to deltoid muscle. A small tubercle called **deltoid tubercle** may be present on this border.

Posterior border: It is convex backwards and provides insertion to the trapezius muscle.

Medial Two-third

It is cylindrical in shape and presents four surfaces: anterior, posterior, superior, and inferior.

Anterior surface: It is convex forwards and gives origin to clavicular head of pectoralis major.

Posterior surface: It is concave backwards and gives origin to sternohyoid muscle near its medial end. The lateral part of this surface forms the anterior boundary of cervico-axillary canal and is related to the following structures:

1. Trunks of brachial plexus.
2. Third part of subclavian artery.

Superior surface: The clavicular head of sternocleido-mastoid muscle originates from medial half of this surface.

Inferior surface: It presents the following features:

1. Costoclavicular ligament is attached to an oval impression at its medial end.
2. *Subclavius muscle* is inserted into the subclavian groove on this surface.
3. *Clavipectoral fascia* is attached to the margins of subclavian groove.
4. *Nutrient foramen of clavicle* is located on the lateral end of the subclavian groove.

The muscles and ligaments attached to the clavicle are given in Table 2.1.

Table 2.1 Muscles and ligaments attached to the clavicle

Muscles	Ligaments
Pectoralis major	Coracoclavicular
Sternocleidomastoid (clavicular head)	Costoclavicular
Deltoid	Interclavicular
Trapezius	
Subclavius	

Clinical correlation

Fracture of clavicle (Fig. 2.4): The clavicle is the most commonly fractured bone in the body. It commonly fractures at the junction of its lateral one-third and medial two-third due to blows to the shoulder or indirect forces, usually as a result of strong impact on the hand or shoulder, when person falls on the outstretched hand or the shoulder. When fracture occurs, the lateral fragment is displaced downward by the weight of the upper limb because trapezius alone is unable to support the weight of the upper limb. In addition, the lateral fragment is drawn medially by shoulder adductors viz. teres major, etc. The medial fragment is slightly elevated by the sternocleidomastoid muscle. The characteristic clinical picture of the patient with fractured clavicle is that of a man/woman supporting his sagging upper limb with the opposite hand. The fracture at the junction of lateral one-third and medial two-third occurs because:

(a) This is the weakest site.
(b) Two curvatures of clavicle meet at this site.
(c) The transmission of forces (due to impact) from the clavicle to scapula occur at this site through coracoclavicular ligament.

N.B.

- The clavicle is absent in animals in which the upper limbs are used only for walking and weight transmission, and not for grasping such as horse, etc.
- One of the two primary centers of clavicle is regarded as *precoracoid element of reptilian shoulder girdle.*

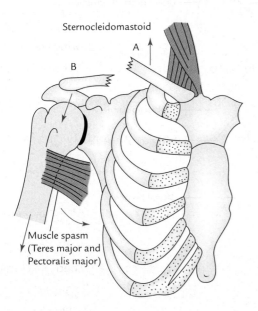

Fig. 2.4 Clavicle fracture: **A**, medial fragment; **B**, lateral fragment. (*Source:* Fig. 2.1, Page 51, *Clinical and Surgical Anatomy*, 2e, Vishram Singh. Copyright Elsevier 2007, All rights reserved.)

Table 2.2 Ossification centers of the clavicle

Site of appearance	Time of appearance	Time of fusion
Two primary centres (medial and lateral) in the shaft	5–6 weeks of intrauterine life (IUL)	45th day of IUL
Secondary centre at sternal end	19–20 years (2 years earlier in female)	25th year
Secondary centre at the acromial end (occasional)	20th year	Fuses immediately

OSSIFICATION (Fig. 2.5)

The ossification of clavicle is **membranocartilaginous.** Whole of it ossifies in the membrane except its medial end which ossifies in the cartilage. The clavicle begins to ossify before any other bone in the body. It ossifies by four ossification centres – two primary centres for shaft and two secondary centres, one for each end.

The site of appearance, time of appearance, and time of fusion of various centres is given in the Table 2.2.

N.B. *Growing end of clavicle:* The sternal end of clavicle is its growing end, because epiphysis at this end appears at the age of 19–20 years and unites with the shaft at the age of 25 years. It is the last of all the epiphyses in the body to fuse with the shaft. The radiological appearance of this epiphysis in females confirms their bone age for legal consent to marriage.

Clinical correlation

Congenital anomalies:
- **Clavicular dysostosis:** It is a clinical condition in which medial and lateral parts of clavicle remain separate due to nonunion of two primary centers of ossification.
- **Cleidocranial dysostosis:** It is a clinical condition characterized by partial or complete absence of clavicle associated with defective ossification of the skull bones.

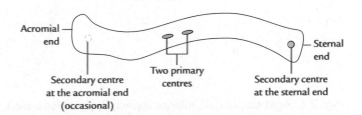

Fig. 2.5 Ossification of the clavicle.

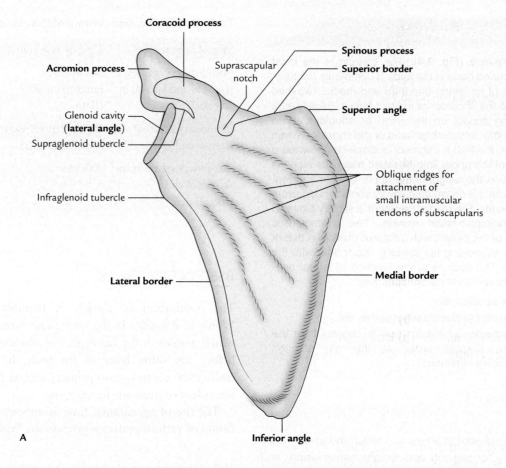

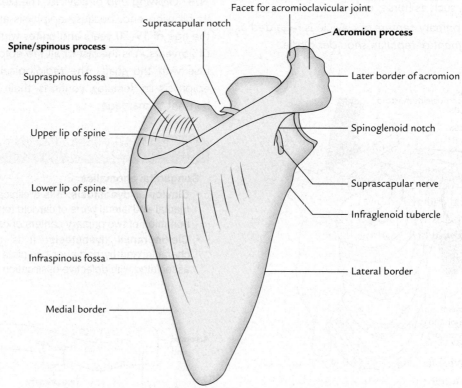

Fig. 2.6 Right scapula: A, anterior aspect; B, posterior aspect.

SCAPULA

The scapula (**shoulder blade**) is a large, flattened, and triangular bone located on the upper part of the posterolateral aspect of the thorax, against 2nd to 7th ribs.

PARTS (Fig. 2.6)

The scapula is highly mobile and consists of four parts: a body and three processes—spinous, acromion, and coracoid.

N.B. Some authorities divide scapula into three parts, viz. head, neck, and body.

Body

The body is triangular, thin, and transparent. It presents the following features:

1. Two surfaces: (a) costal and (b) dorsal.
2. Three borders: (a) superior, (b) lateral, and (c) medial.
3. Three angles: (a) inferior, (b) superior, and (c) lateral.

The **dorsal surface** presents a shelf-like projection on its upper part called **spinous process.**

The **lateral angle** is truncated to form an articular surface—the **glenoid cavity.**

The lateral angle is thickened and called **head of the scapula,** which is connected to the plate-like body by an inconspicuous **neck.**

Processes

There are three processes. These are as follows:

1. Spinous process.
2. Acromion process.
3. Coracoid process.

The **spinous process** is a shelf-like bony projection on the dorsal aspect of the body.

The **acromion process** projects forwards almost at right angle from the lateral end of the spine.

The **coracoid process** is like a bird's beak. It arises from the upper border of the head and bends sharply to project superoanteriorly.

ANATOMICAL POSITION AND SIDE DETERMINATION

The side of the scapula can be determined by holding the scapula in such a way that:

1. The **glenoid cavity** faces laterally, forwards, and slightly upwards (at an angle of 45° from the coronal plane).
2. The **coracoid process** is directed forwards.
3. The shelf-like **spinous process** is directed posteriorly.

FEATURES AND ATTACHMENTS (Fig. 2.7)

Surfaces

Costal surface (subscapular fossa)

1. It is concave and directed medially and forwards.
2. It presents three longitudinal ridges, which provide attachment to the intramuscular tendons of subscapularis muscle.
3. The **subscapularis muscle** (a multipennate muscle) arises from the medial two-third of subscapular fossa/costal surface except near the neck where a *subscapular bursa* intervenes between the neck and the subscapular tendon.
4. The **serratus anterior muscle** is inserted on this surface along the medial border and inferior angle.

Dorsal surface

1. The dorsal surface is convex and presents a shelf-like projection called **spinous process.**
2. The spinous process divides the dorsal surface into supraspinous and infraspinous fossae. The upper, supraspinous fossa is smaller (one-third) and lower, infraspinous fossa is larger (two-third).
3. The **spinoglenoid notch** lies between lateral border of the spinous process and the dorsal surface of the neck of scapula. Through this notch supraspinous fossa communicates with the infraspinous fossa and suprascapular nerve and vessels pass from supraspinous fossa to the infraspinous fossa.
4. The **supraspinatus muscle** arises from medial two-third of supraspinous fossa.
5. The **infraspinatus muscle** arises from medial two-third of infraspinous fossa.
6. The **teres minor muscle** arises from the upper two-third of the dorsal surface of lateral border. This origin is interrupted by the *circumflex scapular artery.*
7. The **teres major muscle** arises from the lower one-third of the dorsal surface of lateral border and inferior angle of scapula.
8. The **latissimus dorsi muscle** also arises from dorsal surface of the inferior angle by a small slip.

Borders

Superior border

1. The superior border is the shortest border and extends between superior and lateral angles.
2. The **suprascapular notch** is present on this border near the root of coracoid process.
3. The suprascapular notch is converted into **suprascapular foramen** by *superior transverse (suprascapular) ligament.*

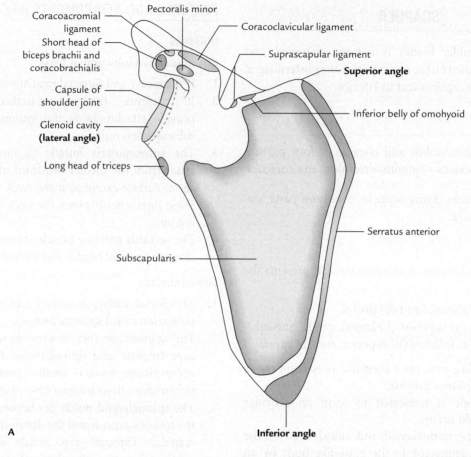

Coracoacromial ligament
Short head of biceps brachii and coracobrachialis
Capsule of shoulder joint
Glenoid cavity (lateral angle)
Long head of triceps
Subscapularis
Pectoralis minor
Coracoclavicular ligament
Suprascapular ligament
Superior angle
Inferior belly of omohyoid
Serratus anterior

A

Inferior angle

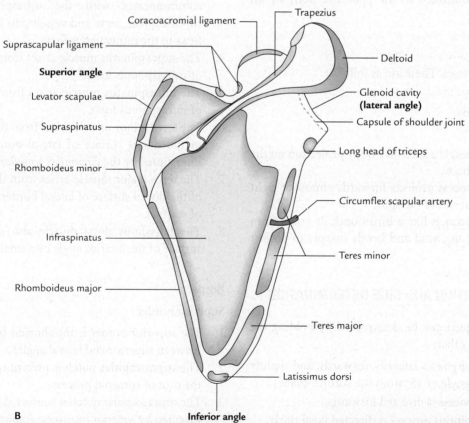

Coracoacromial ligament
Suprascapular ligament
Superior angle
Levator scapulae
Supraspinatus
Rhomboideus minor
Infraspinatus
Rhomboideus major
Trapezius
Deltoid
Glenoid cavity (lateral angle)
Capsule of shoulder joint
Long head of triceps
Circumflex scapular artery
Teres minor
Teres major
Latissimus dorsi

B

Inferior angle

Fig. 2.7 Right scapula showing attachments of the muscles and ligaments: A, costal surface; B, dorsal surface.

4. The suprascapular artery passes above the ligament and suprascapular nerve passes below the ligament, through suprascapular foramen. (*Mnemonic:* **Air force flies above the Navy**, i.e., **A:** artery is above and **N:** nerve is below the ligament.)

5. The **inferior belly of omohyoid** arises from the superior border near the suprascapular notch.

Lateral border

1. The lateral border is the thickest border and extends from inferior angle to the glenoid cavity.
2. The **infraglenoid tubercle** is present at its upper end, just below the glenoid cavity.
3. The **long head of triceps** muscle arises from the infraglenoid tubercle.

N.B. Lateral border of scapula is thick because it acts as fulcrum during rotation of the scapula.

Medial border (vertebral border)

1. It extends from superior angle to the inferior angle.
2. It is thin and angled at the root of spine of scapula.
3. The **serratus anterior muscle** is inserted on the costal surface of the medial border and the inferior angle.
4. The **levator scapulae muscle** is inserted on the dorsal aspect of the medial border from superior angle to the root of spine.
5. The **rhomboideus minor muscle** is inserted on the dorsal aspect of the medial border opposite the root of spine.
6. The **rhomboideus major muscle** is inserted on the dorsal aspect of the medial border from the root of spine to the inferior angle.

Angles

Inferior angle: It lies over the 7th rib or the 7th intercostal space.

Superior angle: It is at the junction of superior and medial borders, and lies over the 2nd rib.

Lateral angle (head of scapula)

1. It is truncated and bears a pear-shaped articular cavity called the **glenoid cavity,** which articulates with the head of humerus to form *glenohumeral (shoulder) joint.*
2. A fibrocartilaginous rim, the **glenoid labrum** is attached to the margins of glenoid cavity to deepen its concavity.
3. The **capsule of shoulder joint** is attached to the margins of glenoid cavity, proximal to the attachment of glenoid labrum.
4. The **long head of biceps brachii** arises from supraglenoid tubercle. This origin is intracapsular.

Processes

Spinous process (spine of scapula)

1. It is a triangular shelf-like bony projection, attached to the dorsal surface of scapula at the junction of its upper one-third and lower two-third.
2. It divides the dorsal surface of scapula into two parts—upper supraspinous fossa and lower infraspinous fossa.
3. The spine has two surfaces—(a) superior and (b) inferior, and three borders—(a) anterior, (b) posterior, and (c) lateral.

Surfaces

(a) The *superior surface of spine* forms the lower boundary of supraspinous fossa and gives origin to supraspinatus.
(b) The *inferior surface of spine* forms the upper limit of infraspinous fossa and gives origin to infraspinatus.

Borders

(a) The *anterior border of spine* is attached to the dorsal surface of scapula.
(b) The *lateral border of spine* bounds the **spinoglenoid notch** through which pass suprascapular nerve and vessels from supraspinous fossa to infraspinous fossa.
(c) The *posterior border of spine* is also called **crest of spine.** Trapezius is inserted to the upper lip of crest of spine, while posterior fibres of deltoid take origin from its lower lip.

Acromion process (acromion)

1. It projects forwards almost at right angle from the lateral end of spine and overhangs the glenoid cavity.
2. Its superior surface is subcutaneous.
3. It has a tip, two borders (medial and lateral), and two surfaces (superior and inferior).
4. The medial and lateral borders of acromion continue with the upper and lower lips of the crest of the spine of scapula, respectively.
5. Its superior surface is rough and subcutaneous.
6. Its inferior surface is smooth and related to **subacromial bursa.**
7. The medial border of acromion provides insertion to the trapezius muscle. Near the tip, medial border presents a circular facet, which articulates with the lateral end of clavicle to form the acromioclavicular joint.
8. The lateral border of acromion gives origin to intermediate fibres of the deltoid muscle.
9. The coracoacromial ligament is attached to the tip of acromion.
10. The acromial angle is at the junction of lateral border of acromion and lateral border of the crest of the spine of scapula.

Coracoid process

1. It arises from the upper part of the head of scapula and bent sharply so as to project forwards and slightly laterally.
2. The coracoid process provides attachment to **three muscles**—short head of biceps brachii, coracobrachialis, and pectoralis minor, and **three ligaments**—coracoacromial, coracoclavicular, and coracohumeral.
3. The *short head of biceps brachii* and *coracobrachialis* arise from its tip by a common tendon.
4. The *pectoralis minor* muscle is inserted on the medial border of the upper surface.
5. The *coracoacromial ligament* is attached to its lateral border.
6. The *conoid part of the coracoclavicular ligament* (**rhomboid ligament**) is attached to its knuckle.
7. The *trapezoid part of the coracoclavicular ligament* (**rhomboid ligament**) is attached to a ridge on its superior aspect between the pectoralis minor muscle and coracoacromial ligament.
8. The *coracohumeral ligament* is attached to its root adjacent to the glenoid cavity.

N.B.

- In living individual, the tip of coracoid process can be palpated 2.5 cm below the junction of lateral one-fourth and medial three-fourth of the clavicle.
- In reptiles, coracoid process is a separate bone, but in humans it is attached to scapula and thus it represents *atavistic epiphysis*.

OSSIFICATION

The ossification of scapula is cartilaginous. The cartilaginous scapula is ossified by **eight centres**—one primary and seven secondary.

The *primary centre* appears in the body.

The *secondary centres* appear as follows:

1. Two centres appear in the coracoid process.
2. Two centres appear in the acromion process.
3. One centre appears each in the (a) medial border, (b) inferior angle, and (c) in the lower part of the rim of glenoid cavity.

The primary centre in the body and first secondary centre in the coracoid process appears in eighth week of intrauterine life (IUL) and first year of postnatal life, respectively and they fuse at the age of 15 years.

All other secondary centres appear at about puberty and fuse by 20th year.

N.B. First coracoid centre represents *precoracoid element* and second coracoid (subcoracoid) centre represents *coracoid proper* of reptilian girdle.

Clinical correlation

Sprengel's deformity of the scapula (congenital high scapula): The scapula develops in the neck region during intrauterine life and then migrates downwards to its adult position (i.e., upper part of the back of the chest). Failure of descent leads to Sprengel's deformity of the scapula. In this condition the scapula is hypoplastic and situated in the neck region. It may be connected to the cervical part of vertebral column by a fibrous, cartilaginous, or bony bar called omovertebral body. An attempt to bring down scapula by a surgical procedure may cause injury to the brachial plexus.

HUMERUS

The humerus is the bone of arm. It is the longest and strongest bone of the upper limb.

PARTS (Fig. 2.8)

The humerus is a long bone and consists of three parts: upper end, lower end, and shaft.

Upper End

The upper end presents the following five features:

1. Head.
2. Neck.
3. Greater tubercle.
4. Lesser tubercle.
5. Intertubercular sulcus.

The head is smooth and rounded, and forms less than half of a sphere. It is directed medially backwards and upwards. It articulates with the glenoid cavity of scapula to form the glenohumeral (shoulder) joint.

Lower End

The lower end presents the following seven features:

1. **Capitulum**, a lateral rounded convex projection.
2. **Trochlea**, a medial pulley-shaped structure.
3. **Radial fossa**, a small fossa above the capitulum.
4. **Coronoid fossa**, a small fossa above the trochlea.
5. **Medial epicondyle**, a prominent projection on the medial side.
6. **Lateral epicondyle**, a prominent projection on the lateral side but less than the medial epicondyle.
7. **Olecranon fossa**, a large, deep hollow on the posterior aspect above the trochlea.

Shaft

The shaft is a long part of bone extending between its upper and lower ends. It is cylindrical in the upper half and flattened anteroposteriorly in the lower half.

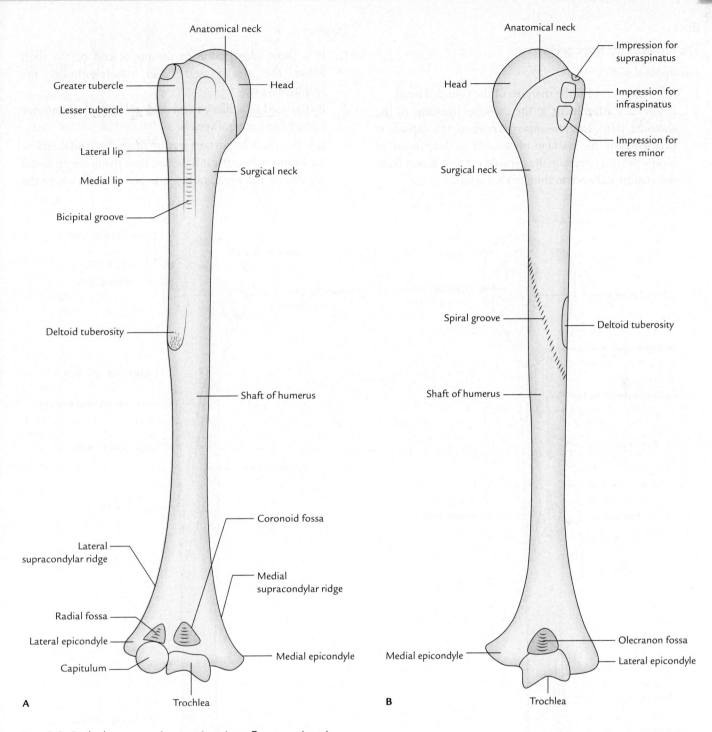

Fig. 2.8 Right humerus: **A**, anterior view; **B**, posterior view.

ANATOMICAL POSITION AND SIDE DETERMINATION

The side of humerus can be determined by holding it vertically in such a way that:

1. The **rounded head** at the upper end faces medially, backwards and upwards.
2. The **lesser tubercle**, **greater tubercle**, and **vertical groove** (**intertubercular groove**) at the upper end faces anteriorly.

3. The **olecranon fossa** on the lower flattened end faces posteriorly.

FEATURES AND ATTACHMENTS (Fig. 2.9)

Upper End Head

1. It is smooth, rounded and forms one-third of a sphere.
2. It is covered by an articular hyaline cartilage, which is thicker in the center and thinner at the periphery.

Neck

The humerus has three necks:

Anatomical neck

1. It is constriction at the margins of the rounded head.
2. It provides attachment to the capsular ligament of the shoulder joint, except—*superiorly* where the capsule is deficient, for the passage of tendon of long head of biceps brachii, *medially* the capsule extends down from the anatomical neck to the shaft for about 1–2 cm.

Surgical neck

1. It is short constriction in the upper end of the shaft below the greater and lesser tubercles/below the epiphyseal line.
2. It is related to axillary nerve and posterior and anterior circumflex humeral vessels.
3. It is the most important feature of the proximal end of the humerus because it is weaker than the more proximal regions of the bone, hence it is one of sites where the

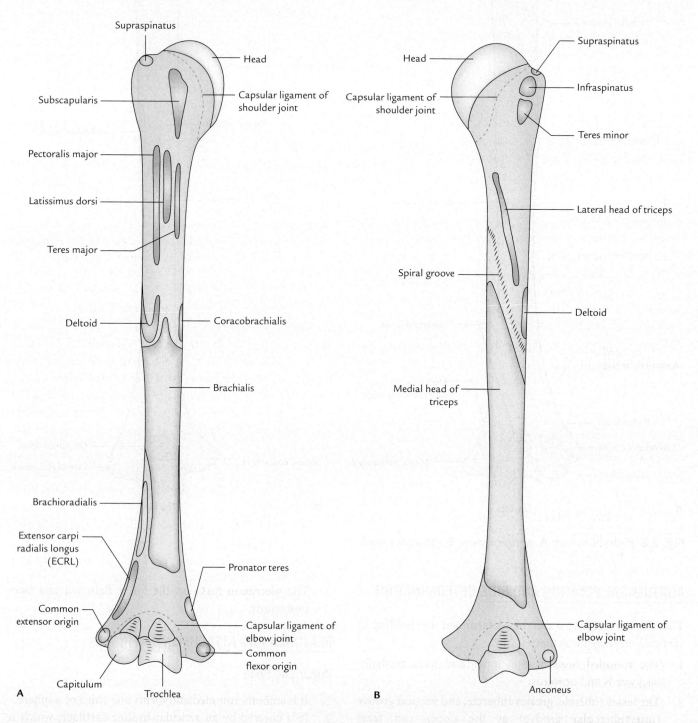

Fig. 2.9 Right humerus showing attachments of the muscles and ligaments: **A**, anterior aspect; **B**, posterior aspect.

humerus commonly fractures leading to damage of associated nerves and vessels.

Morphological neck

1. It is the junction between diaphysis and epiphysis.
2. It is represented by an epiphyseal line in the adult bone.
3. It is a true junction of head with the shaft.

Greater tubercle

1. It is the most lateral part of the proximal end of humerus.
2. Its posterosuperior aspect bears three flattened facet-like impressions: upper, middle, and lower, which provide attachment to *supraspinatus, infraspinatus,* and *teres minor muscles,* respectively.

Mnemonic: SIT, (supraspinatus, infraspinatus, teres minor).

Lesser tubercle

1. It is small elevation on the front of upper end of humerus, just above the surgical neck.
2. It provides attachment to *subscapularis muscle.*

Intertubercular Sulcus/Bicipital Groove

1. It is a vertical groove between lesser and greater tubercles.
2. It contains (a) long head of biceps, enclosed in the synovial sheath and (b) ascending branch of anterior circumflex humeral artery.
3. Three muscles are attached in the region of this groove:
   (a) Pectoralis major on the lateral lip of the groove.
   (b) Teres major on the medial lip of the groove.
   (c) Latissimus dorsi in the floor of the groove.

Mnemonic: Lady between 2 *Majors.* The 'L' of lady stands for latissimus dorsi and '2M' stands for pectoralis major and teres major.

Shaft

The upper part of the shaft is cylindrical and its lower part is triangular in cross section. It has three borders and three surfaces.

Borders

Anterior border: It starts from the lateral lip of the intertubercular sulcus, and extends down to the anterior margin of the deltoid tuberosity and become smooth and rounded in the lower half, where it ends in the radial fossa.

Medial border

1. It extends from the medial lip of the intertubercular sulcus down to the medial epicondyle. Its lower part is sharp and called medial **supracondylar ridge.** This ridge provides attachment to medial intermuscular septum.
2. A rough strip on the middle of this border provides insertion to the **coracobrachialis muscle.**
3. A narrow area above the medial epicondyle provides origin to the humeral head of the **pronator teres.**

Lateral border

1. Its upper part is indistinct while its lower part is prominent where it forms the **lateral supracondylar ridge.** Above the lateral supracondylar ridge, it is ill-defined but traceable to the posterior part of the greater tubercle.
2. About its middle, this border is crossed by the radial groove from behind.
3. The lower part of this border, lateral supracondylar ridge, provides attachment to the lateral intermuscular septum.

Surfaces

Anterolateral surface

1. It lies between the anterior and lateral borders.
2. A little above the middle, this surface presents a characteristic V-shaped tuberosity–the **deltoid tuberosity** which provides insertion to the deltoid muscle.

Anteromedial surface

1. It lies between the anterior and medial borders.
2. The upper part of this surface forms the floor of the intertubercular sulcus.
3. About its middle and close to the medial border it presents a nutrient foramen directed downwards.

Posterior surface

1. It lies between the medial and lateral borders.
2. In the upper one-third of this surface, there is an oblique ridge directed downwards and laterally. This ridge provides origin to the lateral head of the triceps brachii.
3. Below and medial to the ridge, is the radial/spiral groove, which lodges radial nerve and profunda brachii vessels.
4. The entire posterior surface below the spiral groove provides origin to the medial head of the triceps brachii.

Lower End

1. It is flattened from before backwards and expanded from side to side.
2. The capitulum (rounded convex projection laterally) articulates with the head of radius.
3. The trochlea (pulley-shaped projection medially) articulates with the trochlear notch of ulna.
4. The ulnar nerve is related to the posterior surface of the medial epicondyle.
5. The anterior surface of the medial epicondyle provides an area for common flexor origin of the superficial flexors of the forearm.
6. The anterolateral part of lateral epicondyle provides an area for common extensor origin.
7. The posterior surface of lateral epicondyle gives origin to anconeus muscle.

8. The coronoid process of ulna fits into *coronoid fossa* (above the trochlea) during full flexion of elbow.
9. The head of radius fits into *radial fossa* (above capitulum) during full flexion of elbow.
10. The olecranon process of ulna fits into *olecranon fossa* (on posterior aspect above the trochlea) during full extension of elbow.
11. The capsule of elbow joint is attached above the coronoid and radial fossae anteriorly and above the olecranon fossa posteriorly.

N.B.

• Sometimes a bony bar between the coronoid and olecranon fossae is perforated and forms 'supratrochlear foramen.'
• *Supratrochlear process* (Fig. 2.10): It is small hook-like bony process, which may sometimes arise from the anteromedial surface, about 5 cm above the lower end of the humerus. A fibrous band called *Struthers' ligament* stretches from it to the medial epicondyle. In such cases, the brachial artery along with median nerve deviates from their normal course and pass through the foramen thus formed.
• *The angle of humeral torsion*: It is an angle formed by the superimposition of the long axis of the upper and lower articular surfaces of the humerus.

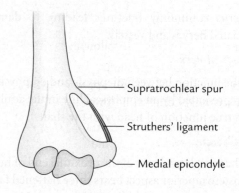

Fig. 2.10 Supratrochlear spur. (*Source: Fig. 17.1, Page 154, Anatomy for Excellence: Must Know Facts, 2e, Vishram Singh. Copyright Elsevier, 2013, All rights reserved.*)

Clinical correlation

• **Nerves directly related to the humerus:** The three nerves (axillary, radial, and ulnar) are closely related to the back of humerus as follows (Fig. 2.11):
  (a) *Axillary nerve* around the surgical neck.
  (b) *Radial nerve* in the radial/spiral groove.
  (c) *Ulnar nerve* behind the medial epicondyle.

Therefore, these nerves are often involved in the fracture of humerus at the above sites:

• **Common sites of fracture of the humerus:** These are (a) surgical neck, (b) shaft, and (c) supracondylar region.
• **Supracondylar fracture of the humerus** (Fig. 2.12): It is caused by a fall on the outstretched hand and commonly occurs in young age. Clinically it presents as backward displacement of the lower fragment with unduly prominent elbow, however the three bony points of elbow (viz. medial epicondyle, lateral epicondyle, and olecranon process) form the usual equilateral triangle because the olecranon process always moves with the lower fragment. This fracture may cause injury to median nerve and brachial artery. The injury to the brachial artery may cause Volkmann's ischemic contracture and myositis ossificans.
• Nonunion of fracture of the humerus is common, if fracture occurs at the junction of its upper one-third and middle one-third due to poor blood supply.
• Median nerve is most commonly involved in the supracondylar fracture of the humerus.

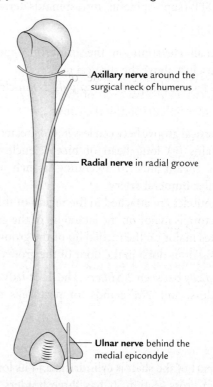

Fig. 2.11 Three nerves closely related to the back of the humerus.

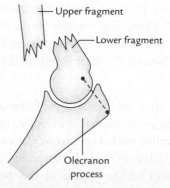

Fig. 2.12 Supracondylar fracture of the humerus. (*Source: Fig. 2.2(B): (C), Page 52, Clinical and Surgical Anatomy, 2e, Vishram Singh. Copyright Elsevier, 2007, All rights reserved.*)

OSSIFICATION

The humerus is ossified by the following ossification centres:

1. One primary centre for shaft.
2. Three secondary centres for upper end.
3. Four secondary centres for lower end.

The site of appearance, time of appearance, and time of fusion of these centres are given in the Table 2.3.

Clinical correlation

The separate centre for medial epicondyle and its late union with the shaft may be mistaken for the *fracture of medial epicondyle of humerus*.

RADIUS

The radius is the lateral bone of the forearm and is homologous to the medial bone of the leg, the tibia.

PARTS (Fig. 2.13)

The radius is a long bone and consists of three parts: upper end, shaft, and lower end.

Upper End

The **upper end** presents head, neck, and radial tuberosity. The head is disc shaped and articulates above with the capitulum of humerus. The neck is constricted part below the head. The radial tuberosity is just below the medial part of the neck.

Shaft

The **long shaft** extends between the upper and lower ends and presents a lateral convexity. It widens rapidly towards the distal end and is concave anteriorly in its distal part. Its sharpest interosseous border is located on the medial side.

Lower End

The **lower end** is the widest part and presents five surfaces. The lateral surface projects distally as the *styloid process*. The dorsal surface presents a palpable dorsal tubercle (*Lister's tubercle*), which is limited medially by an oblique groove.

ANATOMICAL POSITION AND SIDE DETERMINATION

The side of radius can be determined by keeping the bone vertically in such a way that:

1. The **narrow disc-shaped end** (head) is directed upwards.
2. The **sharpest border** (**interosseous border**) of the shaft is kept medially.
3. The **styloid process** at the lower end is directed laterally and prominent tubercle (*Lister's tubercle*) at lower end faces dorsally.
4. The **convexity of shaft** faces laterally, and concave anterior surface of shaft faces anteriorly.

FEATURES AND ATTACHMENTS (Fig. 2.14)

Upper End

Head

1. It is shaped like a disc and in living it is covered with an articular hyaline cartilage.
2. It articulates superiorly with capitulum to form *humero-radial articulation*.
3. The circumference of head is smooth and articulates medially with the radial notch of ulna, rest of it is encircled by the *annular ligament*.

Neck

1. It is the constricted part just below the head and is embraced by the lower part of annular ligament.
2. The **quadrate ligament** is attached to the medial side of the neck.

Table 2.3 Ossification centres of the humerus

Site of appearance	Time of appearance		Time of fusion
Shaft	8th week of IUL		
Upper end • Head • Greater tubercle • Lesser tubercle	1st year 3rd year 5th year	Fuse together at 7th year to form a conjoint upper epiphysis	Joins with shaft 20th year
Lower end • Capitulum and lateral flange of trochlea • Medial part of trochlea • Lateral epicondyle • Medial epicondyle	2nd year 10th year 12th year	Fuse together at 14th year to form most of the lower epiphysis	Joins with shaft 16–17th year
	6th year (form small part of the lower epiphysis)		18th year

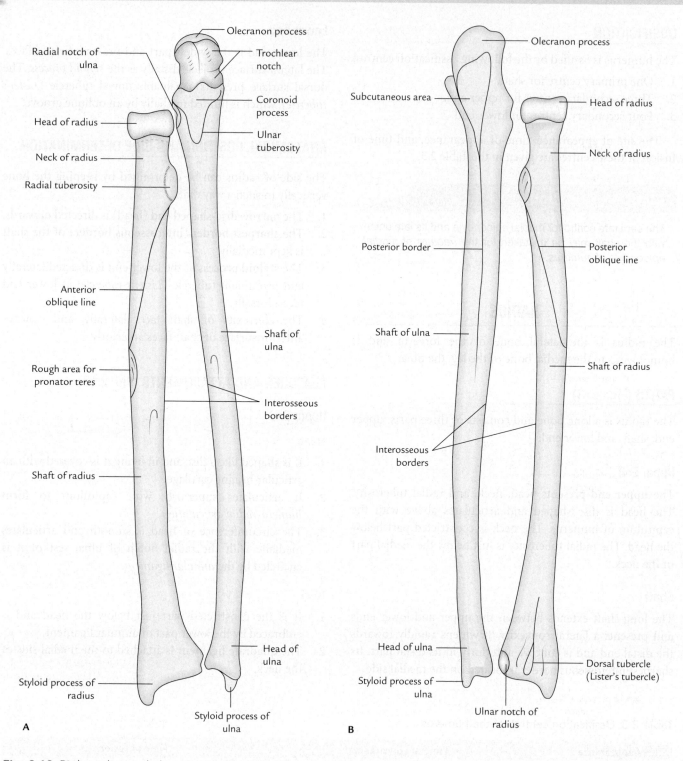

Fig. 2.13 Right radius and ulna: **A**, anterior view; **B**, posterior view.

Radial tuberosity

1. Biceps tendon is inserted to its rough, posterior part.
2. A small synovial bursa covers its smooth anterior part and separates it from the biceps tendon.

Shaft

The shaft has three borders and three surfaces.

Borders
Anterior border

1. It starts below the anterolateral part of radial tuberosity and runs downwards and laterally to the styloid process.
2. The upper part of this border is called **anterior oblique line** and lower part forms the sharp lateral border of the anterior surface.

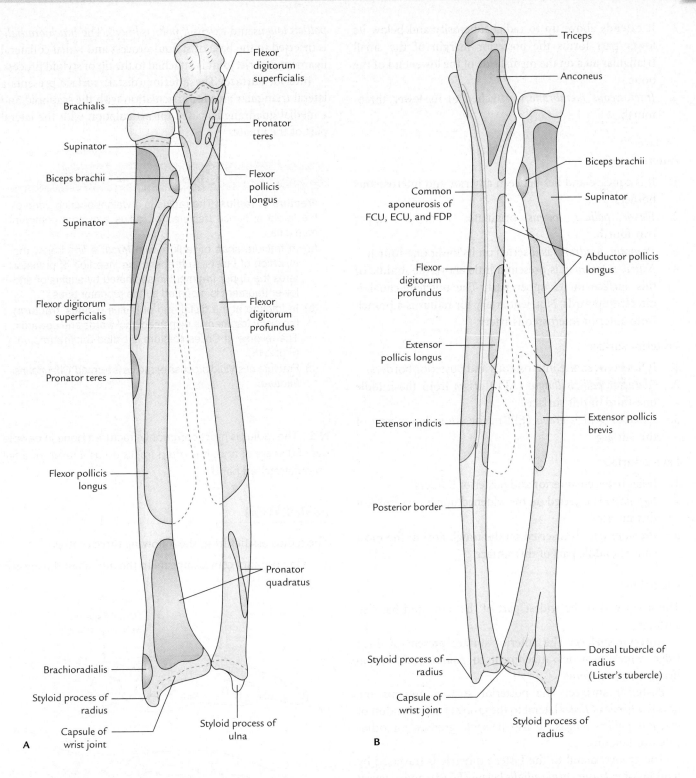

Fig. 2.14 Radius and ulna of right side showing attachments of the muscles and ligaments: **A**, anterior aspect; **B**, posterior aspect (FCU = flexor carpi ulnaris, ECU = extensor carpi ulnaris, FDP = flexor digitorum profundus).

3. Its anterior oblique line gives origin to radial head of flexor digitorum superficialis (FDS).

Posterior border

1. It is well-defined only in its middle third of the shaft.

2. Above it runs upwards and medially to the radial tuberosity and form the **posterior oblique line**.

Medial (interosseous) border

1. It is the sharpest border.

2. It extends above up to radial tuberosity and below its lower part forms the posterior margin of the small triangular area on the medial side of the lower end of the bone.
3. *Interosseous membrane* is attached to its lower three-fourth.

Surfaces

Anterior surface

1. It is concave and lies between anterior and interosseous borders.
2. *Flexor pollicis longus* originates from its upper two-fourth.
3. *Pronator quadratus* is inserted on its lower one-fourth.
4. *Nutrient foramen* is present a little above the middle of this surface in its upper part. The nutrient canal is directed upwards. Nutrient artery for radius is a branch from anterior interosseous artery.

Posterior surface

1. It lies between the interosseous and posterior borders.
2. *Abductor pollicis longus* (APL) arises from the middle one-third of this surface.
3. *Extensor pollicis brevis* (EPB) arises from lower part of this surface.

Lateral surface

1. It lies between anterior and posterior borders.
2. *Supinator* is inserted on the widened upper one-third of this surface.
3. *Pronator teres* is inserted on the rough area in the most convex middle part of this surface.

Lower End

The lower end is the widest part of the bone and has five surfaces.

Anterior surface: The anterior surface presents a thick ridge, which provides attachment to *palmar radio-carpal ligament of wrist joint.*

Posterior surface: The posterior surface presents the *dorsal tubercle of Lister* lateral to the groove for the tendon of *extensor pollicis longus*. It also presents grooves for other extensor tendons.

The groove lateral to the Lister's tubercle is traversed by tendons of *extensor carpi radialis longus* (ECRL) and *extensor carpi radialis brevis* (ECRB). Through the groove medial to groove for *extensor pollicis longus* passes tendons of extensor digitorum and extensor indicis.

Medial surface: The medial surface presents the ulnar notch for articulation with the head of ulna. *Articular disc of inferior radio-ulnar joint* is attached to the lower margin of ulnar notch.

Lateral surface: The lateral surface projects downward as the styloid process and is related to tendons of *adductor*

pollicis longus and *extensor pollicis brevis*. The *brachioradialis* is inserted to the base of styloid process and radial collateral ligament of wrist joint is attached to the tip of styloid process.

Inferior surface: The inferior (distal) surface presents a lateral triangular area for articulation with the scaphoid and a medial quadrangular area for articulation with the lateral part of the lunate.

Clinical correlation

Fracture of radius: The radius is a weight-bearing bone of the forearm; hence fractures of radius are more common than ulna.
(a) In fracture shaft of radius, with *fracture line* below the insertion of biceps and above the insertion of pronator teres the upper fragment is supinated by supinator and lower fragment is pronated by the pronator teres.
(b) In fracture at the distal end of radius **(Colles' fracture)** the distal fragment is displaced backwards and upwards. The reverse of Colles' fracture is called *Smith's fracture* (Fig. 2.15).
(c) Fracture of styloid process of radius is termed '*Chauffeur's fracture*'.

N.B. The radius is most commonly fractured bone in people over 50 years of age. It is often fractured as a result of a fall on outstretched hand.

OSSIFICATION

The radius ossifies from the following three centres:

1. One primary centre appears in the mid-shaft during 8th week of 1UL.

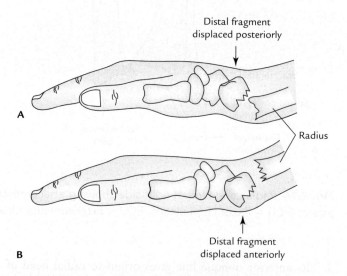

Fig. 2.15 Fracture at distal end of the radius: **A**, Colles' fracture; **B**, Smith's fracture. (*Source:* Fig. 2.3, Page 53, *Clinical and Surgical Anatomy*, 2e, Vishram Singh. Copyright 2007, All rights reserved.)

2. Two secondary centres, one for each end:
   (a) Centre for lower end appears at the age of first year.
   (b) Centre for upper end appears during fifth year.
3. The upper epiphysis fuses at the age of 12 years.
4. The lower epiphysis fuses at the age of 20th year.

Clinical correlation

Madelung deformity: It is a congenital anomaly of radius which presents the following clinical features:
- The anterior bowing of distal end of radius, due to an abnormal growth of distal epiphysis.
- It occurs between 10 and 14 years of age.
- There is premature disappearance of distal epiphyseal line.
- There may be subluxation or dislocation of distal end of ulna, due to defective development of distal radial epiphysis.

ULNA

The ulna is the medial bone of forearm and is homologous to the lateral bone of leg—the fibula.

PARTS (Fig. 2.13)

The ulna is a long bone and consists of three parts: upper end, lower end, and shaft.

Upper End

The **upper end** is expanded and hook-like with concavity of hook facing forwards. The concavity of upper end (**trochlear notch**) lies between large olecranon process above and the small coronoid process below.

Shaft

The **long shaft** extends between the upper and lower ends. Its thickness diminishes progressively from above downwards throughout its length. *The lateral border (interosseous border) is sharp crest-like.*

Lower End

The **lower end** is slightly expanded and has a *head* and *styloid process*. The styloid process is posteromedial to the head.

N.B. The ulna looks like a **pipe wrench** with olecranon process resembling the upper jaw, the coronoid fossa, the lower jaw, and the trochlear notch the mouth of the wrench.

ANATOMICAL POSITION AND SIDE DETERMINATION

The side of ulna can be determined by keeping the bone vertically in such a way that:

1. The **broad hook-like end** is directed upwards.
2. The **sharp crest-like interosseous border** of shaft is directed laterally.
3. The **concavity** of the hook-like upper end and the coronoid process are facing forwards.

FEATURES AND ATTACHMENTS (Fig. 2.14)

Upper End

The **upper end** has two processes: coronoid and olecranon, and two notches: trochlear and radial.

Processes

Olecranon process: It projects upwards from the upper end and bends forward at its summit like a beak. It has the following five surfaces:

1. **Upper surface**
   (a) Its rough posterior two-third provides insertion to the *triceps brachii.*
   (b) *Capsular ligament of elbow joint* is attached anteriorly near its margins.
   (c) A synovial bursa lies between the tendon of triceps and capsular ligament.
2. **Anterior surface:** It is smooth and forms upper part of the trochlear notch.
3. **Posterior surface**
   (a) It forms a subcutaneous triangular area.
   (b) A synovial bursa (**subcutaneous olecranon bursa**) lies between posterior surface and skin.
4. **Medial surface:** Its upper part provides attachments to three structures: (a) ulnar head of flexor carpi ulnaris (origin), (b) posterior, and (c) oblique bands of ulnar collateral ligament.

Coronoid process: It is bracket-like projection from the front of the upper end of the ulna below the olecranon process. It has four surfaces: superior, anterior, medial, and lateral.

1. **Superior surface:** It is smooth and forms the lower part of trochlear notch.
2. **Anterior surface:** It is triangular in shape.
   (a) Its lower corner presents an ulnar tuberosity.
   (b) Brachialis muscle is inserted to the whole of the anterior surface including ulnar tuberosity.
   (c) The medial margin of the anterior surface is sharp and has a tubercle at its upper end called **sublime tubercle**. The medial margin provides attachment to the following structures from proximal to distal:
       (i) Anterior band of ulnar collateral ligament.
       (ii) Oblique band of ulnar collateral ligament.
       (iii) Humero-ulnar head of flexor digitorum superficialis.

(iv)   Ulnar head of pronator teres.

(v)   Ulnar head of flexor pollicis longus.

3. **Medial surface:** It gives origin to flexor digitorum profundus.

4. **Lateral surface:** The upper part of this surface possesses a radial notch for articulation with the head of the radius.

   (a)   The *annular ligament* is attached to the anterior and posterior margins of the radial notch.

   (b)   The lower part of the lateral surface below radial notch has a depressed area called **supinator fossa**, which accommodates radial tuberosity during supination and pronation.

   (c)   **Supinator fossa** is bounded behind by supinator crest. Supinator crest and adjoining part of supinator fossa gives origin to the *supinator muscle*.

Notches (articular surfaces)

Trochlear notch

1. It is C-shaped (semilunar) and articulates with the trochlea of humerus.

2. It has a non-articular strip at the junction of its olecranon and coronoid parts.

3. Its superior, medial, and anterior margins provide attachment to capsule of the elbow joint.

Radial notch

It articulates with the head of radius to form the superior radio-ulnar joint.

Shaft

It has three borders—lateral, anterior, and posterior; and three surfaces—anterior, medial, and posterior.

Borders

Lateral (interosseous) border

1. It is sharpest and is continuous above with the supinator crest.

2. It is ill-defined below.

3. *Interosseous membrane* is attached to this border except for its upper part.

Anterior border

1. It extends from the medial side of the ulnar tuberosity to the base of styloid process.

2. It is thick and round.

3. It upper three-fourth gives origin to *flexor digitorum profundus*.

Posterior border

1. It starts from the apex of triangular subcutaneous area on the back of olecranon process and descends to the styloid process.

2. It is subcutaneous throughout, hence can be palpated along its entire length.

3. It provides attachment to three muscles by a common aponeurosis. The muscles are:

   (a)   Flexor digitorum profundus.

   (b)   Flexor carpi ulnaris.

   (c)   Extensor carpi ulnaris.

Surfaces

Anterior surface

1. It lies between anterior and interosseous borders.

2. The *flexor digitorum profundus* arises from its upper three-fourth.

3. The *pronator quadratus* arises from an oblique ridge on the lower one-fourth of this surface.

4. The *nutrient foramen* is located a little above the middle of this surface and is directed upwards.

Medial surface

1. It lies between the anterior and posterior borders.

2. The *flexor digitorum profundus* arises from the upper two-third of this surface.

Posterior surface

1. It lies between posterior and interosseous borders.

2. It is divided into smaller upper part and large lower part by an oblique line, which starts at the junction of upper and middle third of posterior border and runs towards the posterior edge of radial notch.

3. Area above the oblique line receives insertion of *anconeus muscle*.

4. Area below the oblique line is divided into larger medial and smaller lateral parts by a faint vertical line. The lateral part provides attachment to three muscles form proximal to distal as follows:

   (a)   Abductor pollicis longus in the upper one-fourth.

   (b)   Extensor pollicis longus in the middle one-fourth.

   (c)   Extensor indicis in the next one-fourth.

   (d)   The distal one-fourth is devoid of any attachments.

Lower End

The lower end consists of head and styloid process.

Head

1. It presents a convex articular surface on its lateral side for articulation with the ulnar notch of radius to form the **inferior radio-ulnar joint**.

2. Its inferior surface is smooth and separated from wrist joint by an articular disc of inferior radio-ulnar joint.

Styloid process

1. It projects downwards from the posteromedial aspect of the head of ulna.

2. Its tip provides attachment to medial collateral ligament of wrist joint.
3. The apex of triangular articular disc is attached to the depression between head and base of styloid process.
4. **Tendon of extensor carpi ulnaris** lies in the groove between the back of the head of ulna and styloid process.

N.B. The styloid process is subcutaneous, and may be felt in living individual slightly distal to the head when the forearm is pronated.

Clinical correlation

- When the elbow is fully extended, the tip of olecranon process and medial and lateral epicondyles of the humerus lie in a same horizontal line. When the elbow is fully flexed the three bony points form an equilateral triangle. In dislocation of elbow this relationship is disturbed.
- Ulna stabilizes the forearm by gripping the lower end of humerus by its trochlear notch and provides foundation for radius to produce supination and pronation at superior and inferior radio-ulnar joints.
- The fracture of upper third of shaft of ulna with dislocation of radial head at superior radio-ulnar joint is called *Monteggia fracture dislocations.*
- The fracture of lower third of the shaft of radius associated with dislocation of inferior radio-ulnar joint is called *Galeazzi fracture dislocation.*
- A fracture of the shaft of ulna due to direct injury when a night watchman reflexly raises his forearm to ward off the blow of the stick is termed *night-stick fracture.*

OSSIFICATION

The ulna ossifies from the three main centres: one primary centre for the shaft and two secondary centres, one each for the lower end and the upper end.

Primary centre

It appears in the mid-shaft during eighth week of IUL.

Secondary centres

Upper end

Appearance: 9 years (upper part of trochlear surface and top of olecranon process).
Fusion: 18 years.

Lower end (middle of head)

Appearance: 6 years.
Fusion: 20 years.

N.B. Distal part of olecranon process is formed as an upward extension of the shaft.

CARPAL BONES (Fig. 2.16)

The carpus (G. Corpus = wrist) consists of eight carpal bones, which are arranged in two rows: proximal and distal. Each row consists of four bones.

The **proximal row** of carpal bones consists of the following bones from lateral to medial side:

1. Scaphoid.
2. Lunate.
3. Triquetral.
4. Pisiform.

The **distal row** of carpal bones consists of the following bones from lateral to medial side:

1. Trapezium.
2. Trapezoid.
3. Capitate.
4. Hamate.

Mnemonic: She Looks Too Pretty. Try To Catch Her.

IDENTIFICATION OF INDIVIDUAL CARPAL BONES

The individual carpal bones can be identified by looking at their shape and few other features. These are given in the Table 2.4.

N.B. *Morphology:* Carpus of primitive tetrapods consists of three bones in the proximal row, five bones in the distal row and an 'Os centrale' between the two rows.

The pisiform bone is usually regarded as a sesamoid bone developed in the tendon of flexor carpi ulnaris, but some authorities regard it as a displaced 'Os centrale'.

Clinical correlation

Scaphoid fracture (Fig. 2.17): Fracture of scaphoid is the most common fracture of carpus and usually occurs due to fall on the outstretched hand. Fracture occurs at the narrow waist of the scaphoid. Clinically it presents as tenderness in the anatomical box. Blood vessels mostly enter the scaphoid through its both ends. But in 10–15% cases, all the blood vessels supplying proximal segment enter it through its distal pole. In this condition when waist of scaphoid is fractured, the proximal segment is deprived of blood supply and may undergo avascular necrosis.

OSSIFICATION

The carpal bones are cartilaginous at birth. Each carpal bone ossifies by one centre and all these centres appear after birth.

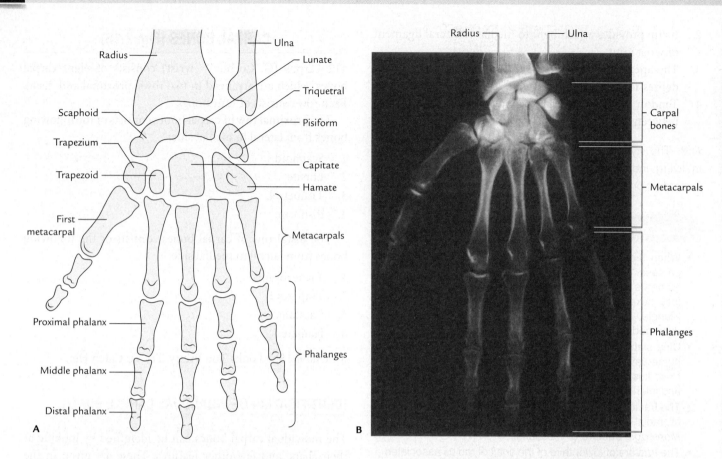

Fig. 2.16 Bones of the hand: **A**, schematic diagram; **B**, as seen in radiographs. (*Source:* Fig. 7.91B, Page 710, *Gray's Anatomy for Students*, Richard L Drake, Wayne Vogl, Adam WM Mitchell. Copyright Elsevier Inc. 2005, All rights reserved.)

Table 2.4 Identification of the carpal bones

Carpal bone	Identifying features
1. Scaphoid	– Boat-shaped – Has constriction (neck) – Has tubercle on distal part of its palmar surface
2. Lunate	Moon-shaped/crescentic
3. Triquetral	– Pyramidal in shape – Oval facet on the distal part of its palmar surface for articulation with pisiform
4. Pisiform	– Pea-shaped/pea-like – Oval facet on the proximal part of its dorsal surface
5. Trapezium	– Quadrilateral in shape – Has groove and crest (tubercle) on its palmar surface
6. Trapezoid	– Shoe-shaped
7. Capitate	– Largest carpal bone – Has rounded head on its proximal surface
8. Hamate	– Wedge-shaped – Hook-like process projects from distal part of its palmar surface

The centres appear as follows:

Capitate	Second month
Hamate	End of third month
Triquetral	Third year
Lunate Scaphoid Trapezium Trapezoid	}Fourth year, in females and fifth year in males
Pisiform	Twelfth year in males, 9th to 10th year in females

N.B. The capitate is the first bone to ossify and pisiform is the last bone to ossify.

The spiral sequence of ossification of the carpal bones and approximate ages in years is given in Figure 2.18.

Clinical correlation

The knowledge of ossification of carpal bones is important in determining the bone age of the child.

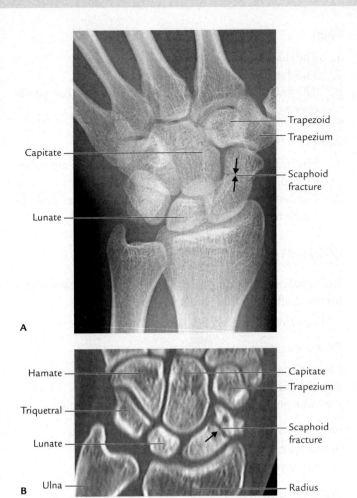

A

B

Fig. 2.17 Fracture of scaphoid bone (arrow): **A**, in radiograph of the hand (AP view); **B**, CT scan of the wrist. (*Source*: Fig. 5.6, Page 131, *Integrated Anatomy*, David JA Heylings, Roy AJ Spence, Barry E Kelly. Copyright Elsevier Limited 2007, All rights reserved.)

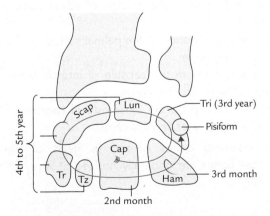

Fig. 2.18 Ossification of the carpal bones (Scap = scaphoid, Lun = lunate, Tri = triquetral, Tr = trapezium, Tz = trapezoid, Cap = capitate, Ham = hamate).

METACARPAL BONES

The metacarpus consists of five metacarpal bones. They are conventionally numbered one to five from lateral (radial) to medial (ulnar) side.

PARTS

Each metacarpal is a small long bone and consists of three parts: (a) head, (b) shaft, and (c) base.

Head

The **head** is at distal end and rounded.

Shaft

The **shaft** extends between head and base. It is concave on palmar aspect and on sides. The dorsal surface of shaft presents a triangular area in its distal part.

Base

The **base** is proximal end and expanded.

PECULIARITIES OF FIRST METACARPAL

1. The first metacarpal is the shortest and stoutest bone.
2. It is rotated medially through 90° so that its dorsal surface faces laterally.
3. Its base possesses concavo-convex (saddle-shaped) articular surface for articulation with trapezium.
4. The head is less convex and broader than other metacarpals.
5. The sesamoid bones glide on radial and ulnar corners of head and produces impressions of gliding.
6. Its base dose not articulate with any other metacarpal.
7. It has epiphysis at its proximal end unlike other metacarpals, which have epiphysis at their distal end.

OSSIFICATION

Each metacarpal ossifies by two centres: one primary centre for the shaft and the one secondary centre for the head.

N.B. The secondary centre of first metacarpal appears in its base.

The time of appearance of centres and their fusion is given in the box below:

Center	Time of appearance	Fusion
Primary centre for shaft	9th week of IUL	
Secondary centre for head of second, third, fourth, and fifth metacarpal	2 years	16 years
Secondary centre for base for first metacarpal	2 years	18 years

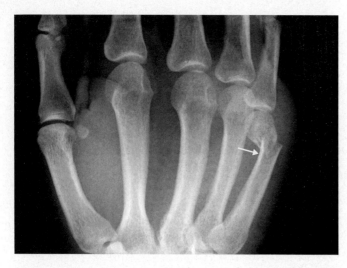

Fig. 2.19 An X-ray of hand showing boxer's fracture—neck of 5th metacarpal (arrow). (*Source:* Fig. 5.8, Page 131, *Integrated Anatomy*, David JA Heylings, Roy AJ Spence, Barry E Kelly. Copyright Elsevier Limited 2007, All rights reserved.)

Clinical correlation

- **Bennet's fracture:** It is an oblique fracture of the base of 1st metacarpal. It is intra-articular and may be associated with subluxation or dislocation of metacarpal.
- **Boxer's fracture** (Fig. 2.19): It is fracture of neck of metacarpal, and most commonly involves neck of 5th metacarpal.

PHALANGES

There are 14 phalanges in each hand: two in thumb and three in each finger.

PARTS AND FEATURES

Each phalanx is a short long bone and has three parts: (a) base (proximal end), (b) head (distal end), and (c) shaft (extending between the two ends).

Base

1. The bases of proximal phalanges have concave oval facet for articulation with the heads of metacarpals.
2. The bases of middle and distal phalanges possess pulley-shaped articular surfaces.

Shaft

1. The shaft tapers towards the head.
2. The dorsal surface is convex from side to side.
3. The palmar surface is flat from side to side but gently concave in the long axis.

Head

1. The heads of proximal and middle phalanges are pulley shaped.
2. The heads of distal phalanges is non-articular and has rough horseshoe-shaped tuberosity.

OSSIFICATION

Each phalanx ossifies by the two centres: one primary centre for the shaft and one secondary centre for the base.

Their time of appearance is as follows:

Primary centres

For proximal phalanx: 10th week of IUL.
For middle phalanx: 12th week of IUL.
For distal phalanx: 8th week of IUL.

Secondary centres

Appearance: 2 years.
Fusion: 16 years.

Clinical correlation

An *undisplaced fracture of phalanx* can be treated satisfactorily by strapping the fractured finger with the neighboring finger.

N.B. The *sesamoid bones in region of hand* are found on the following sites:

(a) Sesamoid bone in the tendon of flexor carpi ulnaris (pisiform).
(b) Two sesamoid bones on the palmar surface of the head of first metacarpal.
(c) Sesamoid bone in the capsule of interphalangeal (IP) joint of thumb (in 75% cases).
(d) Sesamoid bone on the ulnar side of capsule of MCP joint of little finger (in 75% cases).

The sesamoid bones related to head of the first metacarpal bones are generally noticed in X-ray of hand (Fig. 2.15).

Golden Facts to Remember

▶ Most commonly fractured bone in the body	Clavicle
▶ Most important feature of the proximal end of humerus	Surgical neck
▶ Commonest site of fracture clavicle	Junction of its lateral one-third and medial two-third
▶ Strongest ligament of the upper limb	Coracoclavicular ligament
▶ Thickest border of the scapula	Lateral border
▶ Commonest fracture of the humerus	Supracondylar/supraepicondylar fracture
▶ Most commonly injured nerve in supracondylar	Median nerve fracture of humerus
▶ Most common site of the fracture of radius	Fracture of distal end of radius 2.5 cm proximal to the wrist (Colles' fracture)
▶ Most commonly fractured carpal bone	Scaphoid
▶ Most commonly dislocated carpal bone	Lunate
▶ Largest carpal bone	Capitate
▶ First carpal bone to ossify	Capitate
▶ Shortest and stoutest metacarpal	First metacarpal
▶ All metacarpals have epiphysis at their distal end (i.e., head) *except*	First metacarpal, which has epiphysis at its proximal end (i.e., base)

Clinical Case Study

A 55-year-old individual sustained a severe blow on his right flexed elbow. He developed pain and swelling in the elbow region. He was taken to an orthopedic surgeon, who on examination found that the three bony points (olecranon, medial epicondyle, and lateral epicondyle) in the elbow region were forming an equilateral triangle. He suspected a fracture and advised X-ray of elbow region. The X-ray revealed **supraepicondylar/supracondylar fracture of the humerus.**

Questions
1. What are the three common sites of fracture of the shaft of humerus? Name the nerves related to these sites.
2. Why the triangular relation of three bony points is not disturbed in the supracondylar fracture of humerus?
3. Which is the most commonly injured nerve in the supracondylar fracture of humerus?
4. On clinical examination, how will you differentiate the supracondylar fracture of humerus from the posterior dislocation of elbow?

Answers
1. Sites: (a) surgical neck, (b) midshaft, and (c) supracondylar.
   Nerves: (a) axillary nerve, (b) radial nerve, and (c) median nerve.
2. In flexed elbow, the three bony points of elbow (olecranon, medial, and lateral epicondyles) form an equilateral triangle. It is not disturbed in supracondylar fracture because the line of fracture lies above these points.
3. Median nerve.
4. In supracondylar fracture of the humerus, the triangular relationship of three bony points in elbow region is not disturbed (*vide supra*) but in posterior dislocation of elbow, it is disturbed because the olecranon shifts posterosuperiorly.

Pectoral Region

The pectoral region is the anterior aspect of the thorax (chest). The important structures are present in this region are:

1. Muscles that connect the upper limb with the anterolateral chest wall.
2. Breasts (mammary glands) which secrete milk (in female).

SURFACE LANDMARKS

The following landmarks can be felt on the surface of the body in this region (Fig. 3.1):

1. **Clavicle:** Being subcutaneous in location, it is palpable along its whole length at the junction of root of the neck and front of the chest.
2. **Suprasternal notch (jugular notch):** It is a palpable notch at the upper border of manubrium sterni between the medial ends of two clavicles.
3. **Sternal angle (angle of Louis):** It is felt as a transverse ridge about 5 cm below the suprasternal notch. It marks the junction of manubrium and the body of the sternum. On either side, the costal cartilage of 2nd rib articulates with the sternum at this level. *The sternal angle thus serves as a useful landmark to identify the 2nd rib and subsequently helps in counting down the other ribs.*
4. **Infraclavicular fossa:** It is a triangular depression below the junction of middle and lateral third of the clavicle.
5. **Coracoid process:** The tip of coracoid process is felt in the infraclavicular fossa, 2.5 cm below the clavicle.
6. **Nipple:** It is the most important surface feature of the pectoral region. Its position varies considerably in the female but in the male, it usually lies in the 4th intercostal space just medial to the midclavicular line.

LINES OF ORIENTATION

The following lines are often used to describe the surface features on the anterior chest wall:

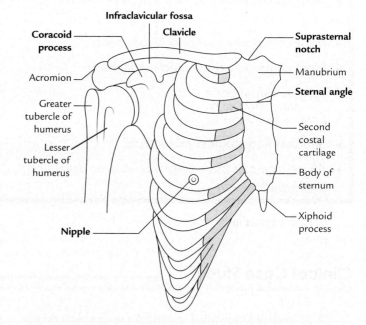

Fig. 3.1 Skeletal framework and surface landmarks of the pectoral region.

1. **Midsternal line:** It runs vertically downwards in the median plane on the front of the sternum.
2. **Midclavicular line:** It runs vertically downwards from the midpoint of the clavicle to the midinguinal point.
3. **Anterior axillary line:** It runs vertically downwards from the anterior axillary fold.
4. **Midaxillary line:** It runs vertically downwards from a point located midway between the anterior and posterior axillary folds.
5. **Posterior axillary line:** It runs vertically downwards from the posterior axillary fold.

CUTANEOUS INNERVATION

The skin of the pectoral region is supplied by the following cutaneous nerves (Fig. 3.2):

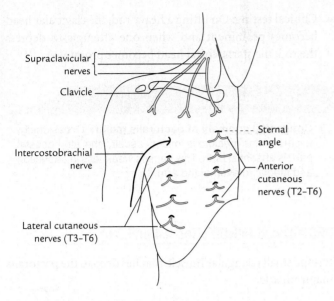

Fig. 3.2 Cutaneous nerves of the pectoral region.

1. The skin above the horizontal line drawn at the level of sternal angle is supplied by supraclavicular nerves (C3 and C4).
2. The skin below this horizontal line is supplied by anterior and lateral cutaneous branches of the 2nd–6th intercostal nerves (T2–T6).

N.B. The area supplied by C4 spinal segment directly meets the area supplied by T2 spinal segment. This is because the nerves derived from C5–T1 spinal segments form *brachial plexus* to supply the upper limb (Fig. 3.3).

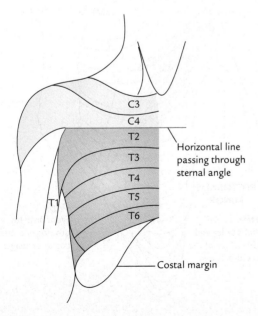

Fig. 3.3 Dermatomes in the pectoral region.

MUSCLES

The muscles of the pectoral region are:

1. Pectoralis major.
2. Pectoralis minor.
3. Subclavius.
4. Serratus anterior.*

PECTORALIS MAJOR (Figs 3.4 and 3.5)

It is the largest muscle of the pectoral region.

Origin

Pectoralis major muscle is thin fan shaped and arises by two heads, viz.

1. Small clavicular head.
2. Large sternocostal head.

Clavicular head—arises from the medial half of the anterior aspect of the clavicle.

Sternocostal head—arises from the (a) lateral half of the anterior surface of the sternum, up to 6th costal cartilage, (b) medial parts of 2nd–6th costal cartilages, and (c) aponeurosis of the external oblique muscle of the abdomen.

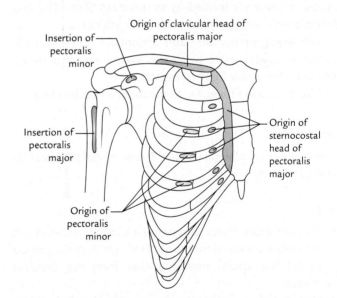

Fig. 3.4 Bony attachments of the pectoralis major and minor muscles.

*The serratus anterior is a thin muscular sheet overlying the lateral aspect of chest wall, hence, it is not a muscle of pectoral region but grouped with pectoral muscles for convenience of study and surgical significance.

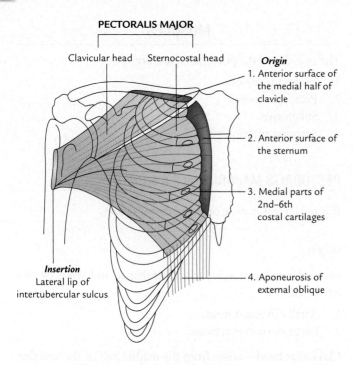

Fig. 3.5 Origin and insertion of the pectoralis major muscle.

Insertion

Pectoralis major is inserted by a U-shaped (bilaminar) tendon on to the lateral lip of the bicipital groove. The anterior lamina of the tendon is formed by the clavicular fibres, while posterior lamina is formed by sternocostal fibres. The two laminae are continuous with each other inferiorly.

The lower sternocostal and abdominal fibres in their course to insertion are twisted in such a way that fibres, which are lowest are inserted highest.

This twisting of fibres forms the rounded axillary fold.

Nerve Supply

Nerve supply is by lateral (C5 to C7) and medial pectoral (C8 and T1) nerves.

N.B.

- The pectoralis major and pectoralis minor muscles are the only muscles of the upper limb, which are supplied by all five spinal segments that form the *brachial plexus*.
- Occasionally a vertical sheet of muscle fibres extending from root of the neck to the upper part of the abdomen passes superficial to the medial part of pectoralis major. It is termed **rectus sternalis/sternalis muscle**.

Actions

The clavicular head flexes the arm, whereas sternocostal head adducts and medially rotates the arm.

- **Clinical testing:** On lifting a heavy rod, the clavicular head becomes prominent and when one attempts to depress the rod, the sternocostal head becomes prominent.

Clinical correlation

- **Congenital anomaly of pectoralis major:** Occasionally, a part of the pectoralis major, usually the sternocostal part, is absent at birth. This causes weakness in adduction and medial rotation of the arm.

PECTORALIS MINOR (Figs 3.4 and 3.6)

It is the small triangular muscle that lies deep to the pectoralis major muscle.

Origin

It arises from 3rd, 4th, and 5th ribs, near their costal cartilages.

Insertion

It is inserted by a short thick tendon into the medial border and upper surface of the coracoid process of the scapula.

Nerve Supply

Nerve supply is by medial and lateral pectoral nerves.

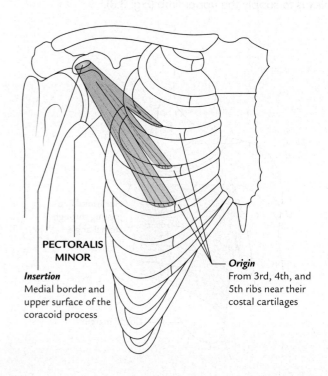

Fig. 3.6 Origin and insertion of the pectoralis minor muscle.

Actions

1. Assists the serratus anterior in drawing the scapula forward (*protraction*) for punching action.
2. Depresses the point of shoulder.
3. Acts as an accessory muscle of respiration, during forced inspiration.

N.B.

- The pectoralis minor is considered as the 'key muscle' of axilla because it crosses in front of the axillary artery and thus used to divide this artery into three parts.
- The origin of pectoralis minor is variable. It may be prefixed (i.e., arises from 2nd to 5th ribs) or postfixed (i.e., arises from 4th to 6th ribs).
- Rarely some fibres of the pectoralis minor separate and pass from first rib to the coracoid process to constitute what is called *pectoralis minimus muscle*.

SUBCLAVIUS (Fig. 3.7)

It is the small rounded muscle that lies horizontally inferior to the clavicle.

Origin

It arises from the first rib at the costochondral junction.

Insertion

Subclavius is inserted into the subclavian groove on the inferior surface (middle-third) of the clavicle.

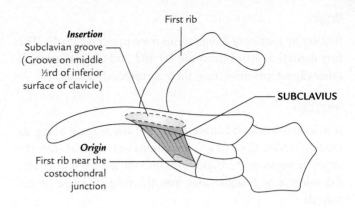

Fig. 3.7 Origin and insertion of the subclavius muscle.

Nerve Supply

It is by nerve to subclavius, which arises from the upper trunk of the brachial plexus.

Actions

The subclavius stabilizes the clavicle by pulling it inferiorly and medially, during movement at the shoulder joint.

SERRATUS ANTERIOR (Fig. 3.8)

The serratus anterior is a broad sheet of muscle that clothes the side wall of the thorax. Thus strictly speaking, it is not a muscle of the pectoral region. But for convenience, it is described with the muscles of pectoral region.

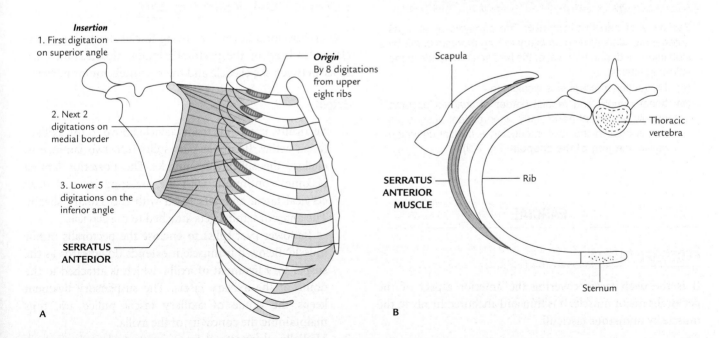

Fig. 3.8 Serratus anterior muscle: A, origin and insertion; B, horizontal section through axilla showing relationship to the thoracic wall.

Origin

It arises by a series of 8 digitations from upper eight ribs. The first digitation arises from the 1st and 2nd ribs, whereas all other digitations arise from their corresponding ribs.

Insertion

It is inserted into the costal surface of the scapula along its medial border. (The first 2 digitations are inserted into the superior angle, next 2 digitations into the medial border and the lower 4 or 5 digitations into the inferior angle of the scapula.)

Nerve Supply

It is by long thoracic nerve/nerve to serratus anterior (C5, C6, and C7).

Actions

1. It is a powerful protractor of the scapula, i.e., it pulls the scapula forward around the chest wall for pushing and punching movements as required during boxing. Hence, serratus anterior is also called **boxer's muscle.**
2. It keeps the medial/vertebral border of scapula in firm contact with the chest wall.
3. Its lower 4 or 5 digitations along with lower part of the trapezius rotate the scapula laterally and upwards during overhead abduction of the arm.

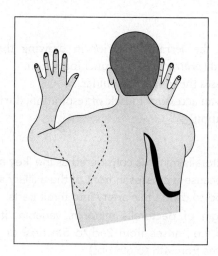

Fig. 3.9 The winging of right scapula. The vertebral border and inferior angle of scapula protrude posteriorly, when the patient is asked to press his hands against the wall.

> ### Clinical correlation
>
> **Paralysis of serratus anterior:** The paralysis of serratus anterior muscle following an injury to *long thoracic nerve* by stab injury or during removal of the breast tumor leads to the following effects:
> (a) Protraction of scapula is weakened.
> (b) Inferior angle and medial border of scapula become unduly prominent particularly when patient pushes his hands against the wall, producing a clinical condition called **winging of the scapula** (Fig. 3.9).

FASCIAE

PECTORAL FASCIA

It is the deep fascia covering the anterior aspect of the pectoralis major muscle. It is thin and anchored firmly to the muscle by numerous fasciculi.

Extent

1. **Superiorly**, it is attached to the clavicle.
2. **Inferiorly**, it is continuous with the fascia of anterior abdominal wall.
3. **Superolaterally**, it passes over the deltopectoral groove to become continuous with the fascia covering the deltoid muscle.
4. **Inferolaterally**, it curves round the inferolateral border of the pectoralis major to become continuous with the axillary fascia. The axillary fascia is a dense fibrous sheet that extends across the base of the axilla.

CLAVIPECTORAL FASCIA (Fig. 3.10)

The clavipectoral fascia is a strong fascial sheet deep to the clavicular head of the pectoralis major muscle, filling the space between the clavicle and the pectoralis minor muscle.

Extent

1. **Vertically**, it extends from clavicle above to the axillary fascia below. Its upper part splits into two laminae to enclose the subclavius muscle. The posterior lamina becomes continuous with the investing layer of deep cervical fascia and gets fused with the axillary sheath. The anterior lamina gets attached to the clavicle.

    Its lower part splits to enclose the pectoralis minor muscle. Below this muscle it extends downwards as the **suspensory ligament of axilla**, which is attached to the dome of the axillary fascia. The suspensory ligament keeps the dome of axillary fascia pulled up, thus maintaining the concavity of the axilla.
2. **Medially**, clavipectoral fascia is attached to the first rib and costoclavicular ligament and blends with external intercostal membrane of the upper two intercostal spaces.

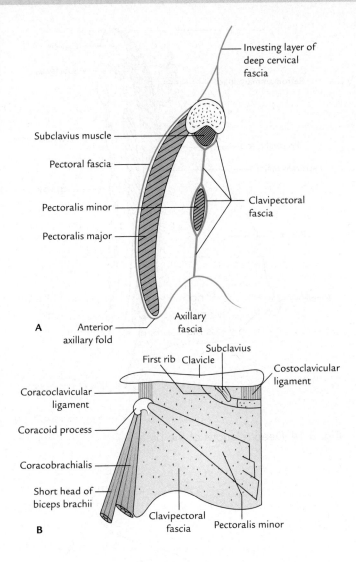

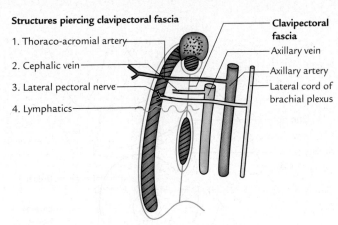

Fig. 3.11 Structures piercing the clavipectoral fascia. (*Source:* Fig. 1.9, Page 11, *Selective Anatomy Prep Manual for Undergraduates*, Vol. I, Vishram Singh. Copyright Elsevier 2014, All rights reserved.)

Fig. 3.10 Clavipectoral fascia: **A**, as seen in sagittal section of anterior axillary wall; **B**, as seen from front.

3. **Laterally**, it is attached to the coracoid process and blends with the coracoclavicular ligament. The thick upper part of the fascia extending from first rib near costochondral junction to the coracoid process is called **costocoracoid ligament.**

N.B. The clavipectoral fascia encloses two muscles—subclavius and pectoralis minor.

Structures Piercing the Clavipectoral Fascia

These are as follows (Fig. 3.11):
1. Lateral pectoral nerve.
2. Thoraco-acromial artery.
3. Lymphatics from the breast to the apical group of axillary group of lymph nodes.
4. Cephalic vein. The first two structures pass outwards, whereas the lower two structures pass inwards.

BREAST (MAMMARY GLAND)

The mammary gland is a modified sweat gland present in the superficial fascia of the pectoral region. The mammary gland is found in both sexes. However, it remains rudimentary in male but becomes well-developed in female at puberty. On rare occasions the breasts of male become enlarged, this condition is called **gynecomastia.** In female, it forms an accessory sex organ of female reproductive system and provides milk to the newborn baby. The anatomy of breast is of great surgical importance, and therefore, needs to be studied in detail.

LOCATION (Figs 3.12 and 3.13)

The breast is located in the superficial fascia of the pectoral region. A small extension from its superolateral part (**axillary tail of Spence**) however pierces the deep fascia and extends into the axilla. The aperture in the deep fascia through which axillary tail passes into the axilla is called **foramen of Langer.** The *axillary tail is the site of high percentage of breast tumor.*

SHAPE AND EXTENT (Figs 3.12 and 3.13)

Shape
Hemispherical bulge.

Extent

1. **Vertically,** it extends from 2nd rib to 6th rib.
2. **Horizontally,** it extends from lateral border of the sternum to the midaxillary line.

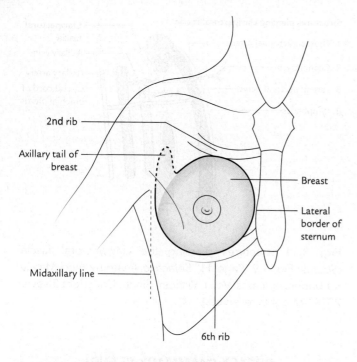

Fig. 3.12 Location and extent of the breast.

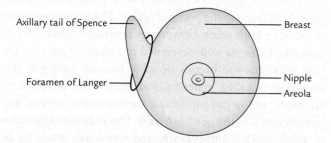

Fig. 3.13 Axillary tail of the breast (of Spence) passing through the foramen of Langer.

RELATIONS (Figs 3.14 and 3.15)

The deep aspect of breast is related to the following structures from superficial to deep:

1. **Pectoral fascia**, the deep fascia covering the anterior aspect of the pectoralis major.
2. **Three muscles**—pectoralis major, serratus anterior, and external oblique (Fig. 3.15).

N.B. The breast is separated from *pectoral fascia* by a space (retromammary space), which is filled with loose areolar tissue. Due to the presence of loose areolar tissue, deep to the breast, the breast can be moved freely up and down and from side to side over the pectoral fascia.

STRUCTURE (Fig. 3.16)

The breast consists of the following three structures:

1. Skin.

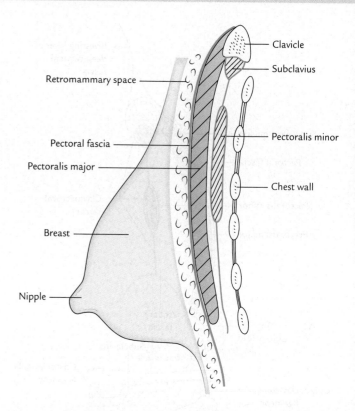

Fig. 3.14 Deep relations of the breast.

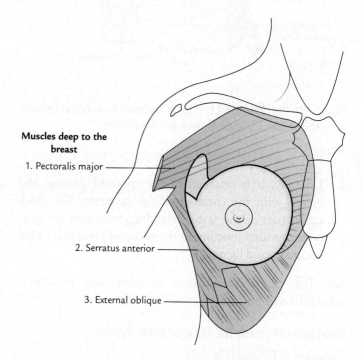

Fig. 3.15 Muscles lying deep to the breast.

2. Stroma.
3. Parenchyma/glandular tissue/mammary gland proper.

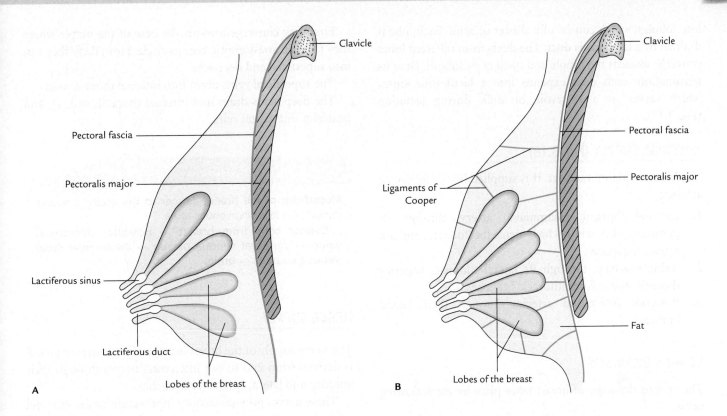

Fig. 3.16 Structure of the breast: A, parenchyma (lobes of the breast); B, stroma of the breast (suspensory ligaments of Cooper and fat).

Skin: It is the covering for the breast and presents the following features:

1. **Nipple:** It is a conical projection below the center of the breast, usually at the level of the 4th intercostal space. It contains smooth muscle fibres, which can make the nipple stiff and erect or flatten it. Being richly innervated by sensory nerve endings, the nipple is the most sensitive part of the breast to tactile stimulation and become erect during sexual arousal.

2. **Areola:** It is the circular area of pigmented skin surrounding the base of the nipple. It contains large number of modified sebaceous glands, particularly at its outer margin. They produce oily secretion, which lubricates the nipple and areola, and thus prevents them from drying and cracking. The color of the areola and nipple varies with the complexion of the woman. During pregnancy the areola becomes darker and enlarged.

N.B. The sebaceous glands in the areola are enlarged during pregnancy and appear as small nodular elevations called **Montgomery's tubercles.**

Stroma: The stroma of breast consists of connective tissue and fat. It forms the supporting framework of the breast.

The connective tissue condenses to form fibrous strands/septa, called **suspensory ligaments of Cooper.**

The suspensory ligaments of Cooper are arranged in a radial fashion. They connect the dermis of the overlying skin to the ducts of the breast and pectoral fascia. The ligaments of the Cooper maintain the protuberance of the breast. Their atrophy due to ageing makes the breast pendulous in old age.

The fat forms the most of the bulk of the breast. It is distributed all over the breast except beneath the areola and the nipple.

Parenchyma: The parenchyma/glandular tissue of the breast secrete milk to feed the newborn baby. It consists of about **15–20 lobes** arranged in a radial fashion like the spokes of a wheel and converge towards the nipple. Each lobe is divided

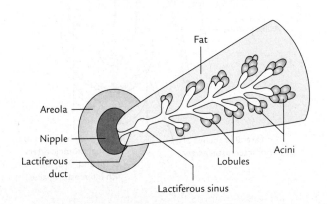

Fig. 3.17 Structure of the lobe of the mammary gland.

into lobules, which consist of a cluster of acini. Each lobe is drained by a **lactiferous duct**. The ducts from different lobes converge towards the nipple and open at its submit. Near its termination, each duct expands into a **lactiferous sinus,** which serves as a reservoir of milk during lactation (Fig. 3.17).

ARTERIAL SUPPLY (Fig. 3.18)

The breast is highly vascular. It is supplied by the following arteries:

1. **Internal thoracic (mammary) artery**, through its perforating branches, which pierce the 2nd, 3rd, and 4th intercostal spaces.
2. **Axillary artery**, through its lateral thoracic, superior thoracic, and acromiothoracic branches.
3. **Posterior intercostal arteries** through their lateral branches.

VENOUS DRAINAGE

The venous drainage of breast takes place by the following veins:

1. Axillary vein.
2. Internal thoracic vein.
3. Posterior intercostal veins.

The veins follow the arteries.

First they converge towards the base of the nipple where they form an anastomotic venous circle. From there they run into superficial and deep sets.

The **superficial veins** drain into internal thoracic vein.

The **deep veins** drain into internal thoracic, axillary, and posterior intercostal veins.

Clinical correlation

Metastasis of the breast cancer to the brain: It occurs through the following venous route:

Cancer cells from breast → posterior intercostal veins → vertebral venous plexus → intracranial dural venous sinuses → brain.

NERVE SUPPLY

The nerve supply of the breast is primarily somatosensory. It is derived from 2nd to 6th intercostal nerves through their anterior and lateral cutaneous branches.

These nerves provide sensory innervation to the skin and carry autonomic fibres to the smooth muscle and blood vessels of the breast.

The sensory nerve endings in nipple and areola play an important role in stimulating the release of milk from mammary gland in response to suckling by the infant.

N.B. The secretion of milk from breast is not under neural control but by **prolactin hormone** secreted by the pituitary gland.

LYMPHATIC DRAINAGE

Lymph Nodes Draining the Breast (Fig. 3.19)

The lymph from the breast is drained into the following group of lymph nodes:

1. **Axillary lymph nodes** lying in the axilla and divided into four groups: (a) anterior/pectoral, (b) posterior, (c) central and lateral (for details see page 53).
2. **Internal mammary nodes** lying along the internal thoracic vessels.
3. **Supraclavicular nodes** lying above the clavicle.
4. **Posterior intercostal nodes** lying in the posterior parts of intercostal spaces in front of the head of the ribs.
5. **Cephalic (deltopectoral) nodes** lying in the deltopectoral groove.

N.B. In addition to the above-mentioned nodes, the lymph from breast also drains into subdiaphragmatic and subperitoneal lymph plexuses.

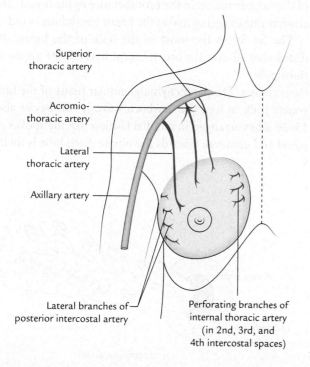

Superior thoracic artery
Acromio-thoracic artery
Lateral thoracic artery
Axillary artery
Lateral branches of posterior intercostal artery
Perforating branches of internal thoracic artery (in 2nd, 3rd, and 4th intercostal spaces)

Fig. 3.18 Arterial supply of the breast.

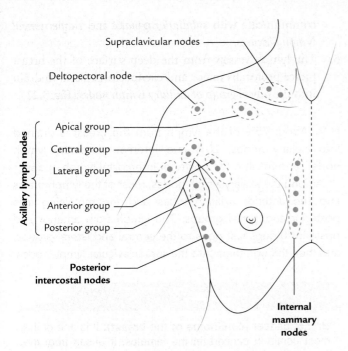

Supraclavicular nodes

Deltopectoral node

Axillary lymph nodes
- Apical group
- Central group
- Lateral group
- Anterior group
- Posterior group

Posterior intercostal nodes

Internal mammary nodes

Fig. 3.19 Lymph nodes draining the breast.

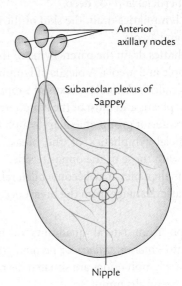

Anterior axillary nodes

Subareolar plexus of Sappey

Nipple

Fig. 3.20 Subareolar plexus of Sappey.

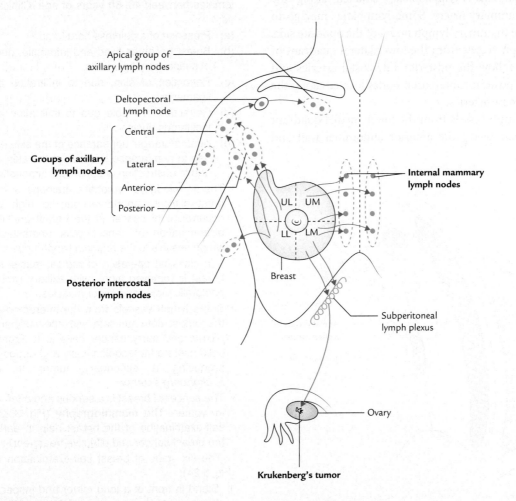

Apical group of axillary lymph nodes

Deltopectoral lymph node

Groups of axillary lymph nodes
- Central
- Lateral
- Anterior
- Posterior

Internal mammary lymph nodes

UL   UM

LL   LM

Breast

Posterior intercostal lymph nodes

Subperitoneal lymph plexus

Ovary

Krukenberg's tumor

Fig. 3.21 Mode of lymphatic drainage of the breast (UL = upper lateral quadrant, LL = lower lateral quadrant, UM = upper medial quadrant, LM = lower medial quadrant).

Lymphatics Draining the Breast

The lymphatics draining the breast are divided into two groups: (a) superficial and (b) deep.

Superficial lymphatics drain the skin of the breast except that of nipple and areola.

Deep lymphatics drain the parenchyma of the breast, and skin of the nipple and areola. A plexus of lymph vessels deep to the areola is called **subareolar plexus of Sappey** (Fig. 3.20). The subareolar plexus and most of the lymph from the breast drain into the anterior group of axillary lymph nodes.

The superficial lymphatics of the breast of one side communicate with those of the opposite side. Consequently the unilateral malignancy may become bilateral.

The **lymphatic drainage from the breast** occurs as follows (Fig. 3.21):

1. The lymph from lateral quadrants of the breast is drained into *anterior axillary* or *pectoral group of lymph nodes.* These lymph nodes are situated deep to the lower border of pectoralis minor.
2. The lymph from medial quadrants is drained into *internal mammary lymph nodes* situated along the internal mammary artery. Some lymphatics may go to the internal mammary lymph nodes of the opposite side.
3. A few lymph vessels from the lower lateral quadrant of the breast follow the posterior intercostal arteries and drain into posterior intercostal nodes located along the course of these arteries.
4. The few lymph vessels from the lower medial quadrant of the breast pierce the anterior abdominal wall and communicate with *subdiaphragmatic* and *subperitoneal lymph plexuses.*
5. The lymph vessels from the deep surface of the breast pierce pectoralis major and clavipectoral fascia to drain into the *apical group of axillary lymph nodes* (Fig. 3.22).

N.B. About 75% of the lymph from the breast is drained into axillary nodes, 20% into internal mammary lymph nodes, and 5% into the posterior intercostal lymph nodes.

Among the axillary lymph nodes, most of the lymph drains into the anterior axillary nodes and the remaining into posterior and apical groups. The lymph from anterior and posterior groups first goes to the central and lateral groups, and then through them into the supraclavicular lymph nodes.

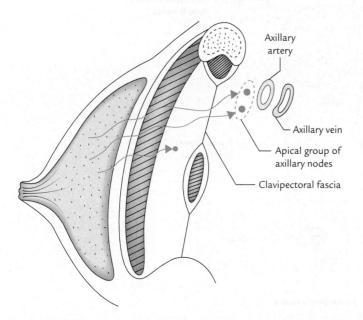

Fig. 3.22 Direct pathway of deep lymphatics of the breast through pectoralis major and clavipectoral fascia to the apical group of axillary nodes.

Labels: Axillary artery; Axillary vein; Apical group of axillary nodes; Clavipectoral fascia

---

Clinical correlation

Breast cancer (carcinoma of the breast): It is one of the most common cancers in the females. It arises from the epithelial cells of the **lactiferous** ducts. In about 60% cases, it occurs in the upper lateral quadrant and commonly affects females between 40–60 years of age. Clinically it presents as:

(a) Presence of a painless hard lump.
(b) Breast becomes fixed and immobile, due to infiltration of suspensory ligaments.
(c) Retraction of skin, due to infiltration of suspensory ligaments.
(d) Retraction of nipple due to infiltration and fibrosis of lactiferous ducts.
(e) *peau d'orange'* appearance of the skin (i.e., skin giving rise to appearance like that of the skin of the orange) due to obstruction of superficial lymphatics.

- The knowledge of lymphatic drainage of the breast is of great clinical importance due to high percentage of occurrence of cancer in the breast and its subsequent dissemination of cancer cells (metastasis) along the lymph vessels to the regional lymph nodes.

  In classical operation of *radical mastectomy,* whole of breast is removed along with axillary lymph nodes, and pectoralis major and minor muscles.

- Some lymph vessels from the inferomedial quadrant of the breast communicate with the *subperitoneal lymph plexus* and carry cancer cells to it. From here cancer cells migrate transcoelomically and deposit on the ovary producing a secondary tumor in ovary called *Krukenberg's tumor.*

- The cancer of breast is a serious and often a fatal disease in women. The **mammography** (Fig. 3.23) and regular self-examination of the breast help in early detection of the breast cancer and effective treatment.

  The six steps of breast self-examination are as follows (Fig. 3.24):

1. Stand in front of a long mirror and inspect both breasts for any discharge from the nipples, puckering, or dimpling of the skin. Now look for any change in shape or contour of the breasts.

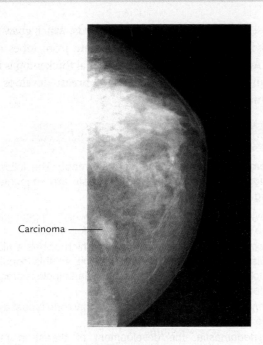

Carcinoma —

Fig. 3.23 Mammogram depicting carcinoma.

2. Clasp hands behind your head and press hands forward.
3. Press hands firmly on the hips and bow slightly forward.
4. During shower raise your one arm and use the fingers of the other hand to palpate the breast in a circular fashion from periphery to the nipple for unusual lump or mass under the skin.
5. Gently squeeze the nipple and look for any discharge. Do similar examination on the other side.
6. The steps 4 and 5 should be repeated in lying down position. In this position the breasts are flattened and make it easier to palpate them (Fig. 3.24).

DEVELOPMENT OF THE BREAST (Fig. 3.25)

The breast develops from an ectodermal thickening called **milk line/ridge (of Schultz)**. This line appears in young embryo and extends from axilla to the groin. In lower animals several mammary glands develop along this line but in human beings this ridge disappears except for its small part in the pectoral region. Here it thickens, becomes

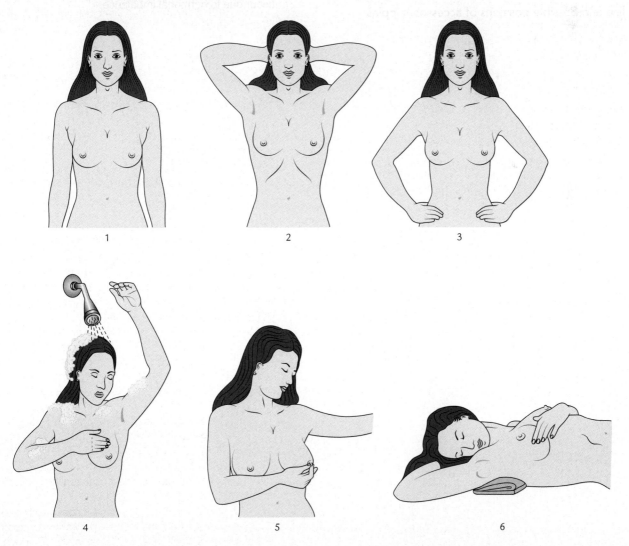

Fig. 3.24 Steps of self-examination of the breast.

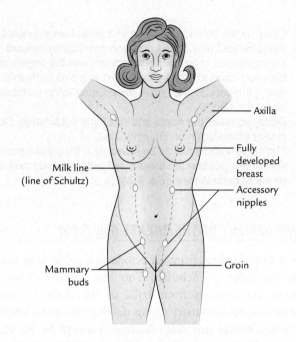

Fig. 3.25 Development of the breast. Note the extent of milk line and possible positions of accessory nipples.

Labels: Axilla; Fully developed breast; Accessory nipples; Groin; Mammary buds; Milk line (line of Schultz)

depressed, and gives off 15–20 solid cords, which grow in the underlying mesenchyme and proliferate from lobes of the gland. At birth, the depressed ectodermal thickening is raised to form the nipple. The stroma of breast develops from surrounding mesoderm.

Clinical correlation

Developmental anomalies of the breast: The following developmental anomalies of the breasts are encountered during clinical practice:

- *Polythelia/supernumerary nipples*, which appear along the milk ridge and is often mistaken for moles.
- *Retracted nipple/inserted nipple*, which occurs if nipple fails to develop from ectodermal pit. In this condition suckling of infant cannot take place and nipple is prone to infection.
- *Polymastia*, the development more than one breast along the milk line.
- *Gynecomastia*, the development of breast in male, mainly at puberty. Usually it is bilateral and thought to occur due to hormonal imbalance.

Golden Facts to Remember

▶ Most important structure of the pectoral region in female	Breast
▶ Largest muscle of the pectoral region	Pectoralis major
▶ Key muscle of the pectoral region	Pectoralis minor
▶ Most of the lymph from breast is drained into	Anterior axillary lymph nodes
▶ Subareolar plexus of Sappey	Plexus of lymph vessels deep to the areola which drain into anterior axillary lymph nodes
▶ Rotter's lymph nodes	Interpectoral lymph nodes
▶ Most common site of the cancer breast	Upper and outer quadrant of the breast

Clinical Case Study

A 55-year-old female complained to her family physician of hard painless lump in the upper and outer portion of her right breast. The examination of breast revealed peau d'orange appearance of the skin, loss of mobility of breast, and retraction of nipple. The examination of axilla revealed the enlargement of axillary lymph nodes. The X-ray of vertebral column revealed irregular shadow in the vertebral bodies of T6 and T7 vertebrae. She was diagnosed as a case of the *breast cancer*.

Questions

1. What do you understand of **lump in the breast**? What are its common causes?
2. Mention the anatomical basis of peau d'orange appearance of skin, retraction of nipple and loss of mobility of the breast.
3. Name the three muscles lying deep to the base of the breast.
4. What is the venous route of the spread of breast cancer?
5. What is the commonest site of the breast cancer?

Answers

1. Any abnormal mass or thickening of the breast tissue is called **lump in the breast**. Lump in the breast may occur due to **fibroadenoma** (a benign tumor of the breast, which is usually a firm solitary mass that is mobile beneath the skin) or **breast cancer** (a malignant tumor of the breast, which is adherent to underlying tissue and immobile).
2. The peau d'orange **appearance of skin** (i.e., skin like orange peel) is due to retraction of pits of hair follicles beneath the edematous skin following retraction of ligaments of Cooper. The condition is due to blockage of lymphatics draining the skin, leading to a stagnation of lymph and edema of skin.

   Retraction of nipple occurs due to infiltration of lactiferous ducts by the cancer cells and their subsequent fibrosis.
3. Pectoralis major, serratus anterior, and aponeurosis of external oblique muscle of the abdomen.
4. Cancer cells of the breast → posterior intercostal veins → vertebral venous plexus → vertebral bodies (also see page 42).
5. Upper and outer quadrant of the breast.

Axilla (Armpit)

The **axilla** or **armpit** is a fat-filled pyramid-shaped space, between the upper part of the arm and the side of the chest wall (Fig. 4.1). It contains the brachial plexus, axillary vessels, and lymph nodes. It also acts as a funnel shaped tunnel for neurovascular structures to pass from the root of the neck to the upper limb and vice versa. Groups of lymph nodes within it drain the upper limb and the breast. The study of axilla is clinically important because axillary lymph nodes are often enlarged and hence routinely palpated during physical examination of the patient. Abscess in this region is also common.

BOUNDARIES (Figs 4.2–4.4)

The axilla resembles a truncated four-sided pyramid and presents an apex, a base and four walls (anterior, posterior, medial, and lateral) (Fig. 4.2).

- **Apex/cervico-axillary canal**: It is a passageway between the neck and axilla. It is directed upwards and medially into the root of the neck and corresponds to the triangular space bounded in front by the clavicle, behind by the upper border of the scapula and medially by the outer border of the first rib (Fig. 4.3). The axillary artery and brachial plexus enter the axilla from neck through this gap, hence it is also termed **cervico-axillary canal**. The

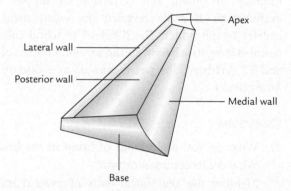

Fig. 4.2 Boundaries of the axilla (Note anterior wall is not seen).

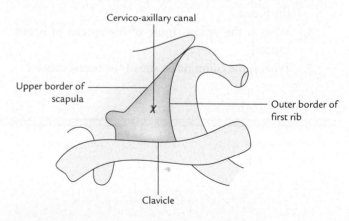

Fig. 4.3 Boundaries of the cervico-axillary canal (apex of the axilla).

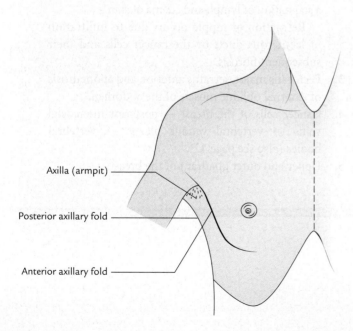

Fig. 4.1 Location of the axilla.

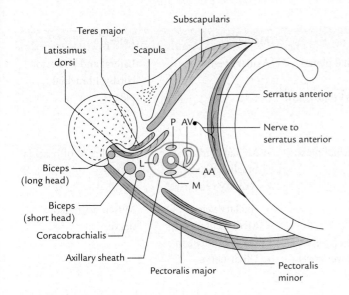

Fig. 4.4 Boundaries and contents of the axilla as seen in a horizontal section (AV = axillary vein, AA = axillary artery, P = posterior cord, L = lateral cord, M = medial cord).

axillary vein enters the neck from axilla into the neck through this canal.

- **Base/floor:** It is at the *lower end of the axilla* and directed downwards. It is formed by the axillary fascia. The base corresponds to the hollow bounded in front by the *anterior axillary fold*, formed by the lower border of the pectoralis major muscle, behind by the *posterior axillary fold* formed by the tendon of latissimus dorsi and teres major muscles, and medially by the lateral aspect of the chest wall.

N.B. The perpendicular line dropped from a point midway between the anterior and posterior axillary folds is called *midaxillary line*—an important surface landmark.

- **Anterior wall:** It is formed by the pectoralis major, subclavius, and pectoralis minor muscles.
- **Posterior wall:** It is formed by the subscapularis muscle above and latissimus dorsi and teres major muscles below.
- **Medial wall:** It is formed by the upper four or five ribs, and corresponding intercostal spaces covered by the serratus anterior muscle.
- **Lateral wall:** It is formed by tendon of biceps brachii in the bicipital groove of humerus coracobrachialis and short head of biceps brachii. The lateral wall is extremely narrow because anterior and posterior walls of the axilla converge at this site.

CONTENTS OF THE AXILLA

The contents of axilla are:

1. Axillary artery and its branches.
2. Axillary vein and its tributaries.
3. Cords of brachial plexus.
4. Axillary lymph nodes.
5. Fibrofatty tissue.
6. Axillary tail of breast.
7. Long thoracic and intercostobrachial nerves.

N.B. The neurovascular structures in the axilla are normally protected by the arm on the side of the body and the cushioning matrix—the axillary fat, but they are vulnerable to injury when the arm is abducted.

AXILLARY ARTERY (Fig. 4.5)

The axillary artery is the main artery of the upper limb. It begins at the outer border of the first rib as the continuation of subclavian artery and ends by becoming brachial artery at the lower border of teres major. In axilla, it runs from its apex to the base along the lateral wall nearer to the anterior wall than the posterior wall. During its course through axilla, it is crossed on its superficial aspect by the pectoralis minor muscle, which divides it into three parts. The axillary vein is medial to the artery and the cords of brachial plexus are arranged around the second part of the artery (i.e., part deep to the pectoralis minor); the lateral cord being lateral, the medial cord medial, and posterior cord behind.

Parts

The axillary artery is divided into the following three parts by the pectoralis minor:

1. **First part,** superior (or proximal) to the muscle.
2. **Second part,** posterior (or deep) to the muscle.
3. **Third part,** inferior (or distal) to the muscle.

Relations (Fig. 4.6)

The axillary vein lies medial to the axillary artery throughout its course, but the relationship of cords of brachial plexus and their branches are different for each of the three parts of the artery. The relations of the three parts of the axillary artery are given in the Table 4.1.

Branches of the Axillary Artery (Fig. 4.5)

The axillary artery gives six branches: one branch from first part, two branches from the second part, and three branches from the third part. Most of these branches go to and supply walls of the axilla.

A. From first part
Superior thoracic artery, a very small branch, arises near the subclavius, passes between the pectoralis major and minor muscles, and supplies these muscles and medial wall of the axilla.

Table 4.1 Relations of the axillary artery

Part	Anterior	Posterior	Medial	Lateral
First part	• Pectoralis major (clavicular part) • Loop of communication between lateral and medial pectoral nerves	• Medial cord of brachial plexus • Long thoracic nerve • Serratus anterior (first digitation)	Axillary vein	Lateral and posterior cords of brachial plexus
Second part	Pectoralis minor	• Posterior cord of brachial plexus • Subscapularis	• Medial cord of brachial plexus • Axillary vein	Lateral cord of brachial plexus
Third part	Medial root of median nerve	• Radial nerve • Axillary nerve • Subscapularis (in the upper part) • Teres major (in the lower part)	• Axillary vein • Medial cutaneous nerve of forearm • Ulnar nerve	Musculocutaneous nerve

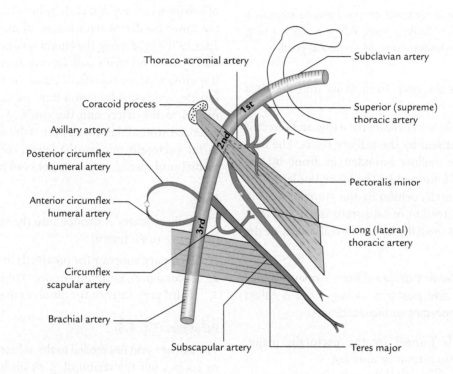

Fig. 4.5 Course and branches of the axillary artery.

B. From second part

1. **Thoraco-acromial artery (acromiothoracic artery)**, emerges at the upper border of pectoralis minor, pierces clavipectoral fascia and soon breaks up into four branches: (a) *pectoral branch*, (b) *deltoid branch*, (c) *acromial branch*, and (d) *clavicular branch*. These branches radiate at right angle to each other. The pectoral branch supplies pectoral muscles, deltoid branch, ends by joining anastomosis over the acromion, clavicular branch supplied sternoclavicular joint.

2. **Lateral thoracic artery**, emerges at and runs along the inferior border of pectoralis minor, supplying the branches to pectoralis major and minor and serratus anterior muscles. In the females, the lateral thoracic artery is large and provides important supply to the breast through its lateral mammary branches.

C. From third part

1. **Subscapular artery**, the *largest branch of axillary artery*, runs along the lower border of the subscapularis and ends near the inferior angle of the scapula. It gives a

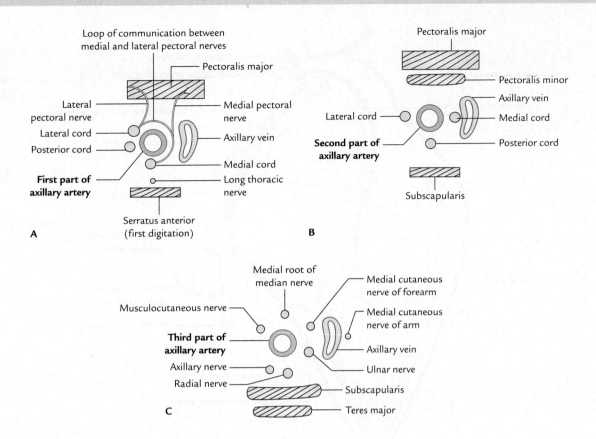

Fig. 4.6 Relations of the axillary artery: **A**, first part; **B**, second part; **C**, third part.

large branch, the *circumflex scapular artery,* which passes through upper triangular intermuscular space, winds round the lateral border of scapula to enter infraspinous fossa. In addition, it gives numerous small branches.

2. **Anterior circumflex humeral artery,** a small branch, passes in front of surgical neck of humerus and anastomoses with the posterior circumflex humeral artery to form an arterial circle around the surgical neck of humerus. It gives an *ascending branch*, which runs upwards into the intertubercular sulcus of humerus to supply the head of humerus and shoulder joint.

3. **Posterior circumflex humeral artery,** larger than the anterior circumflex humeral artery, passes backwards, along with axillary nerve through the quadrangular intermuscular space, crosses the posterior aspect of surgical neck of humerus to anastomose with the anterior circumflex humeral artery. It supplies the deltoid muscle and shoulder joint.

Arterial Anastomosis Around Scapula (Scapular Anastomosis; Fig. 4.7)

The arterial anastomosis around scapula is principally formed between the branches of the first part of the subclavian and the third part of the axillary arteries.

The scapular anastomosis takes place at two sites: around the body of scapula and over the acromion process of the scapula.

1. **Around the body of scapula:** It occurs between the
   (a) *suprascapular artery,* a branch of the thyrocervical trunk from the first part of the subclavian artery,
   (b) *circumflex scapular artery,* a branch of the subscapular artery from the third part of the axillary artery, and
   (c) *deep branch of the transverse cervical artery, a branch of the thyrocervical trunk.*

2. **Over the acromion process:** It occurs between the
   (a) *acromial branch of the thoraco-acromial artery,*
   (b) *acromial branch of the suprascapular artery, and*
   (c) *acromial branch of the posterior circumflex humeral artery.*

Clinical correlation

Collateral circulation through scapular anastomosis: If the subclavian and axillary arteries are blocked anywhere between 1st part of subclavian artery and 3rd part of axillary artery, the scapular anastomosis serves as a potential pathway (collateral circulation) between the first part of the subclavian artery and the third part of the axillary artery, to ensure the adequate circulation to the upper limb.

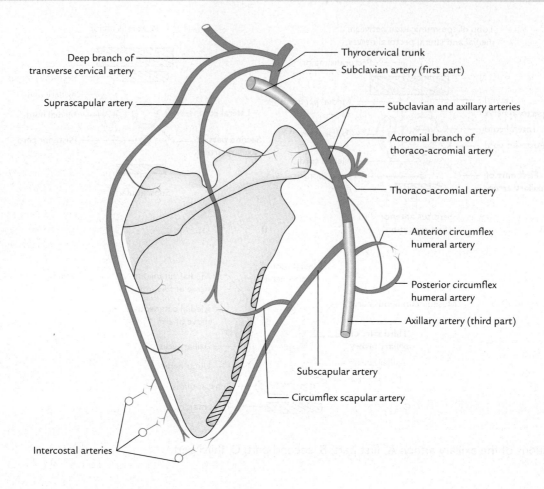

Fig. 4.7 Anastomosis around the scapula (scapular anastomosis).

AXILLARY VEIN (Fig. 4.8)

The axillary vein is formed at the lower border of teres major muscle by the union of *basilic vein* and *venae comitantes of*

the brachial artery. It runs upwards along the medial side of the axillary artery and ends at the outer border of the first rib by becoming the subclavian vein.

Tributaries

The tributaries of axillary vein are as follows:

1. Veins, which correspond to the branches of axillary artery, namely, lateral thoracic vein and subscapular vein.
2. Cephalic vein, which joins it after piercing the clavipectoral fascia.

N.B. There is no or very thin axillary sheath around the axillary vein, hence it can freely expand during increased venous return.

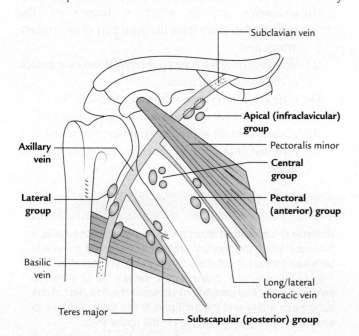

Fig. 4.8 Axillary lymph nodes.

Clinical correlation

- **Spontaneous thrombosis of the axillary vein:** Occasionally, a muscular band—the *axillary arch*, overlies the vein. It may compress the vein, following excessive and unaccustomed movements of the arm at the shoulder joint and cause spontaneous thrombosis of the axillary vein.

AXILLARY LYMPH NODES (Fig. 4.8)

The axillary lymph nodes are scattered in the fibrofatty tissue of the axilla. Their number varies between 20 and 30. They are divided into the following five groups:

1. **Anterior or pectoral group:** They lie along the lateral thoracic vein at the lower border of the pectoralis minor. They receive the lymph from the upper half of the trunk anteriorly and from the major part of the breast. The axillary tail of Spence is in actual contact with these lymph nodes. Therefore, cancer involving axillary tail of the breast may be misdiagnosed as an enlarged lymph node.
2. **Posterior or subscapular group:** They lie on the posterior axillary fold along the subscapular vein. They receive the lymph from the upper half of the trunk posteriorly, and from the axillary tail of the breast.
3. **Lateral group:** They lie along the upper part of the humerus in relation to the axillary vein. They drain the lymph from the upper limb.
4. **Central group:** They are situated in the upper part of the axilla. They receive the lymph from the other groups and drain into the apical group (vide infra). The intercostobrachial nerve passes amongst these nodes. Therefore, enlargement of these nodes such as in cancer may compress this nerve, causing pain in the area of distribution of this nerve, i.e., along the inner border of the arm.
5. **Apical or infraclavicular group:** They are situated deep to the clavipectoral fascia at the apex of the axilla along the axillary vein. They are of great clinical importance, because they receive lymph directly from the upper part of the breast and indirectly from the rest of the breast through central group of nodes. They drain into *subclavian lymph trunk on the right side* and *into the thoracic duct* on the left side. A few efferents from this group drain into the supraclavicular lymph nodes. Although these lymph nodes are located very deeply but can be palpated by pushing the fingers of one hand into the apex of axilla from below and fingers of the other hand behind the clavicle from above.

N.B. The axillary lymph nodes are also described in terms of levels at which they are situated, viz.

- **Level I nodes:** They lie lateral to the lower border of pectoralis minor muscle.
- **Level II nodes:** They lie deep to the pectoralis minor muscle.
- **Level III nodes:** They lie medial to the upper border of pectoralis minor muscle.

The lymph nodes first receive the lymph from the area of breast involved in cancer are termed *sentinel lymph nodes.* These are usually the level I lymph nodes. The **sentinel nodes** are confirmed by injecting a radioactive substance into the affected area of the breast.

Clinical correlation

- **Palpation of axillary lymph nodes:** The palpation of axillary lymph nodes is part of clinical examination of the breast due to their involvement in cancer breast.
- **Axillary abscess:** An abscess in the axilla arises from infection and suppuration of the axillary lymph nodes. The abscess may grow to a considerable size before the patient feels pain. The pus of axillary abscess may track into the neck or into the arm if it enters the axillary sheath, or between the pectoral muscles if it breaks through the clavipectoral fascia. The axillary abscess is drained by giving an incision in the floor of axilla, for it being the most dependant part, midway between the anterior and posterior axillary folds nearer to the medial wall to avoid injury to the main vessels running along the anterior, posterior, and lateral walls of the axilla.

BRACHIAL PLEXUS

The brachial plexus is the plexus of nerves formed by the anterior (ventral) **rami** of lower four cervical and the first thoracic (i.e., C5, C6, C7, C8, and T1) spinal nerves with little contribution from C4 to T2 spinal nerves.

N.B. If the contribution from C4 is large and that from T2 is absent, it is called *prefixed brachial plexus.* On the other hand, if contribution from T2 is large and that from C4 is absent, it is termed *postfixed brachial plexus.*

Components (Fig. 4.9)

The brachial plexus consists of four components: (a) roots, (b) trunks, (c) divisions, and (d) cords. The roots and trunks are located in the neck, divisions behind the clavicle and the cords in the axilla.

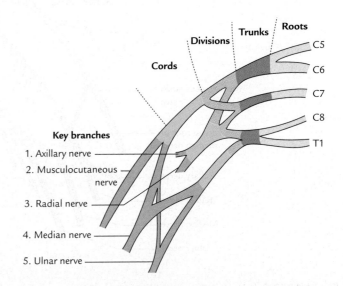

Fig. 4.9 Components and key branches of the brachial plexus.

Roots

The roots (five) are constituted of anterior primary rami of C5 to T1 spinal nerves. They are located in neck, deep to scalenus anterior muscle.

Trunks

The trunks (three) are formed as follows:

The C5 and C6 roots join to form the upper trunk; the C7 root alone forms the middle trunk and, C8 and T1 roots join to form the lower trunk. They lie in the neck occupying the cleft between scalenus medius behind and the scalenus anterior in front.

Divisions

Each trunk divides into anterior and posterior divisions. They lie behind the clavicle.

Cords

The cords (three) are formed as follows: the anterior divisions of the upper and middle trunks unite to form the lateral cord and the anterior division of the lower trunk continues as the medial cord. The posterior divisions of the three trunks unite to form the posterior cord.

Branches (Fig. 4.10)

A. From roots

1. Long thoracic nerve/nerve to serratus anterior (C5, C6, and C7).
2. Dorsal scapular nerve/nerve to rhomboids (C5).

In addition to the long thoracic nerve and dorsal scapular nerve, branches are given by the roots to supply scalene muscles and longus colli (C5, C6, C7, and C8) and there is contribution to phrenic nerve (C5).

B. From trunks

1. Suprascapular nerve (C5 and C6)
2. Nerve to subclavius (C5 and C6)

N.B. The branches arising from roots and trunks are supraclavicular branches of brachial plexus.

C. From cords

1. **From lateral cord**
   (a) Lateral pectoral nerve (C5, C6, and C7).
   (b) Lateral root of median nerve (C5, C6, and C7).
   (c) Musculocutaneous nerve (C5, C6, and C7).

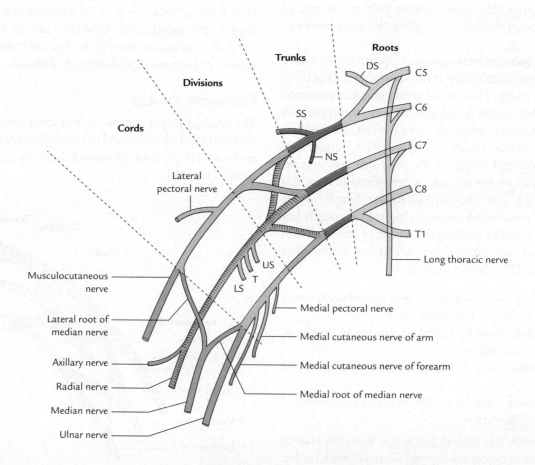

Fig. 4.10 Brachial plexus and its branches (SS = suprascapular nerve, NS = nerve to subclavius, US = upper subscapular nerve, LS = lower subscapular nerve, T = thoraco-dorsal nerve, DS = dorsal scapular nerve).

2. **From medial cord**
   (a) Medial pectoral nerve (C8 and T1).
   (b) Medial cutaneous nerve of arm (T1).
   (c) Medial cutaneous nerve of forearm (C8 and T1).
   (d) Medial root of median nerve (C8 and T1).
   (e) Ulnar nerve (C7, C8, and T1).

3. **From posterior cord**
   (a) Radial nerve (C5, C6, C7, C8, and T1).
   (b) Axillary nerve (C5 and C6).
   (c) Thoraco-dorsal nerve/nerve to latissimus dorsi (C6, C7, and C8).
   (d) Upper subscapular nerve (C5 and C6).
   (e) Lower subscapular nerve (C5 and C6).

N.B. *Erb's point (Fig. 4.11):* It is the region of upper trunk of brachial plexus where six nerves meet as follows: 5th and 6th cervical roots join to form the upper trunk, which gives off two nerves—suprascapular and nerve to subclavius, and then divides into anterior and posterior divisions.

Clinical correlation

- **Lesions of the Brachial plexus:** For understanding the effects of the lesions of the brachial plexus, the student will find it helpful to know the spinal segments, which control the various movements of the upper limb:
  - Adduction of the shoulder is controlled by C5 segment.
  - Abduction of the shoulder is controlled by C6 and C7 segments.
  - Flexion of the elbow is controlled by C5 and C6 segments.
  - Extension of the elbow is controlled by C6 and C7 segments.
  - Flexion of the wrist and fingers is controlled by C8 and T1 segments.

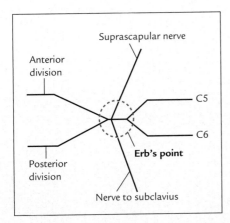

Fig. 4.11 Erb's point.

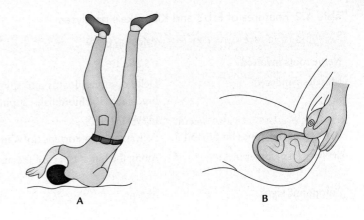

Fig. 4.12 Injury of the upper brachial plexus leading to excessive increase in the angle between the head and shoulder: A, fall from the height and landing on a shoulder; B, Traction of the arm and hyperextension of the neck.

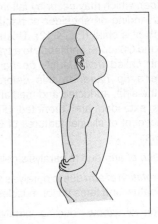

Fig. 4.13 Policeman receiving a tip position of the upper limb in Erb's paralysis.

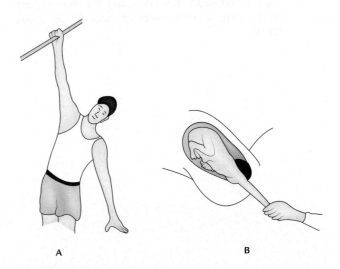

Fig. 4.14 Injury of the lower brachial plexus leading to excessive increase in the angle between the trunk and shoulder: A, sudden upward pull of the arm; B, arm pulled during delivery.

Table 4.2 Features of Erb's and Klumpke's paralyses

	Erb's paralysis	Klumpke's paralysis
Nerve roots involved	C5 and C6	C8 and T1
Muscles paralyzed	Deltoid, supraspinatus infraspinatus, biceps brachii, brachialis, brachioradialis, supinator and extensor carpi radialis longus	All intrinsic muscles of the hand
Position of the upper limb/hand	Policeman's tip/Porter's tip/Waiter's tip position	Claw hand
Sensory loss (sometimes)	Along the outer aspect of the arm	Along the medial border of forearm and hand
Autonomic signs	Absent	Present (Horner's syndrome)

The important lesions of the brachial plexus are as follows:

(a) *Erb's paralysis (upper plexus injury):* It is caused by the excessive increase in the angle between the head and shoulder, which may occur by fall from the back of horse and landing on shoulder or traction of the arm during birth of a child (Fig. 4.12). This involves upper trunk (C5 and C6 roots) and leads to a typical deformity of the limb called *policeman's tip hand/porter's tip hand/waiter's tip hand.* In this deformity, the arm hangs by the side, adducted and medially rotated, and forearm is extended and pronated (Fig. 4.13). The detailed account of clinical features of Erb's paralysis is as follows:

– *Adduction of arm* due to paralysis deltoid muscle.

– *Medial rotation of arm* due to paralysis supraspinatus, infraspinatus, and teres minor muscles.

– *Extension of elbow,* due to paralysis of biceps brachii.

– *Pronation of forearm* due to paralysis of biceps brachii.

– *Loss of sensation (minimal) along the outer aspect of arm* due to involvement of roots of C6 spinal nerve.

(b) *Klumpke's paralysis (lower plexus injury):* It is caused by the hyperabduction of the arm, which may occur when one falls on an outstretched hand or an arm is pulled into machinery or during delivery (extended arm in a breech presentation (Fig. 4.14). The nerve roots involved in this injury are C8 and T1 and sometimes C7. The clinical features of Klumpke's paralysis are as follows:

– *Claw hand,* due to paralysis of the flexors of the wrist and fingers (C6, C7, and C8), and all intrinsic muscles of the hand (C8 and T1).

– *Loss of sensations along the medial border of the forearm and hand (T1).*

– *Horner's syndrome,* (characterized by partial ptosis, miosis, anhydrosis, and enophthalmos) due to involvement of sympathetic fibres supplying head and neck, which leave the spinal cord through T1.

The important features of Erb's and Klumpke's paralysis are enumerated in Table 4.2.

• **Surgical approach to axilla:** The axilla is approached surgically through the skin of the floor of axilla for the excision of axillary lymph nodes to treat the cancer of the breast. The structures at risk during this procedure are (a) intercostobrachial nerve, (b) long thoracic nerve, (c) thoraco-dorsal nerve, and (d) thoraco-dorsal artery. Effort should be made to safeguard the above structures.

Golden Facts to Remember

► Most dependant part of the axilla	Floor of the axilla
► Axillary lymph node group receiving most of the lymph from the breast	Anterior or pectoral group
► Largest branch of the brachial plexus	Radial nerve
► Kuntz's nerve	Communicating branch between T1 and T2 nerves, which carry sympathetic fibres from 3rd thoracic ganglion to the upper limb via T2 nerve
► Cervico-axillary canal	Truncated apex of the axilla through which the axillary artery and brachial plexus enter the axilla from neck

Clinical Case Study

A baby boy was delivered in the hospital by an obstetrician by pulling baby's head using forceps (*forceps delivery*). Two weeks later the parents took the baby to the pediatrician for check-up. While examining the baby, the pediatrician found that baby's right arm was medially rotated and adducted while his forearm was extended and pronated. He also noticed sensory loss on the lateral aspect of the right upper limb.

Questions

1. Name the position of upper limb of baby observed by the pediatrician.
2. Which position of the limb is characteristic of this clinical condition?
3. Name the site of lesion and the cause that produced this condition.
4. What is the cause of sensory loss in the upper limb?

Answers

1. Policeman's tip hand/Porter's tip hand.
2. Erb's paralysis.
3. Erb's point due to excessive separation of neck and shoulder caused by pulling the baby's head during delivery.
4. Involvement of ventral root of C5 and C6 spinal nerves.

Back of the Body and Scapular Region

The superficial structures on the back of the body are studied with the upper limb because the shoulder girdle is attached posteriorly with the axial skeleton by a number of muscles. These muscles are called **posterior axio-appendicular muscles.** They play an important role in the movements of the scapula. Further removal of the scapula in malignant disease (e.g., fibrosarcoma) requires detailed knowledge of the muscles, nerves, and vessels on the back.

SURFACE LANDMARKS (Fig. 5.1)

1. **Scapula (shoulder blade)** is the most important surface landmark on the back. It is placed at a tangent on the posterolateral aspect of the rib cage. Vertically, it extends from 2nd to 7th rib. Although it is thickly covered by the muscles, still most of its outline can be felt in the living individual:

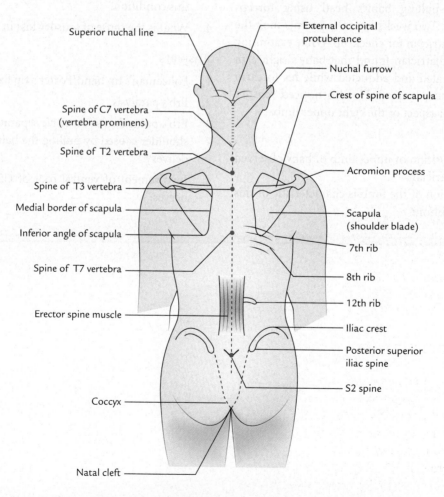

Fig. 5.1 Surface landmarks on the back of the body.

(a) *Acromion process* can be easily felt at the top of the shoulder.

(b) *Crest of the spine of the scapula*, runs medially and slightly downwards from the acromion to the medial border of the scapula, hence it can be easily palpated by finger drawn along it.

(c) *Medial border* can be traced upwards to the superior angle and downwards to the inferior angle. The superior angle of the scapula lies opposite the spine of T2 vertebra, the root of the spine lies at the level of T3 vertebra and the inferior angle of the scapula lies at the level of T7 vertebra.

N.B. The scapula is freely mobile as about 15 muscles are attached to its processes and fossae. The two scapulae are drawn apart when the arms are folded across the chest. The medial borders of the two scapulae are close to the midline when shoulders are drawn back.

2. **Eighth rib** is palpable, immediately inferior to the inferior angle of the scapula. The lower ribs can be counted from it.

3. **Twelfth rib** can be palpated if it projects beyond the lateral margin of the erector spinae muscle, about 3 cm above the iliac crest.

4. **Iliac crest** is felt as a curved bony ridge below the waist. When traced forwards and backwards, it ends as *anterior* and *posterior superior iliac spines,* respectively. The posterior superior iliac spine may be felt in shallow dimple of skin above the buttock, about 5 cm from the median line.

5. **Sacrum**—the back of sacrum lies between the right and left dimples (vide supra) and its spines can be palpated in the median plane.

6. **Coccyx** is a slightly movable bone and may be felt deep between the buttocks in the *natal cleft.*

7. **Spines of vertebrae** lie in the median furrow of the back and may be felt. The spine of 7th cervical vertebra (*vertebra prominens*) is readily felt at the root of the neck at the lower end of nuchal furrow.

    The approximate levels of other spines are given in Table 5.1.

8. **External occipital protuberance and superior nuchal lines**—the *external occipital protuberance* is a bony projection felt in the midline on the back of the head. The curved bony ridge extending laterally on each side from external occipital protuberance is the *superior nuchal line.* These bony features demarcate the junction between the head and neck posteriorly.

9. **Nuchal groove furrow** is the median furrow, which extends from external occipital protuberance to the spine of C7 vertebra.

Table 5.1 Approximate levels of some spines on the back of the body

Vertebral spine	Level
T2	Superior angle of the scapula
T3	Where crest of spine of the scapula meets its medial border
T7	Inferior angle of the scapula
L4	Highest point of iliac crest
S2	Posterior-superior iliac spine

10. **Ligamentum nuchae** is the median fibrous partition on the back of neck, which extends from external occipital protuberance to the spine of C7 vertebra and separates the short cervical spines from the skin.

CUTANEOUS NERVES (Fig. 5.2)

The cutaneous nerves on the back are derived from the posterior rami of the spinal nerves. Each primary ramus divides into medial and lateral branches:

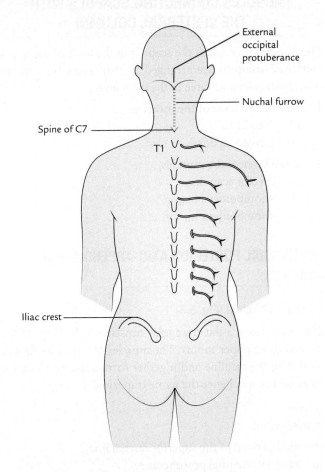

Fig. 5.2 Cutaneous nerves of the back.

1. Up to T6, the cutaneous innervation is provided by medial branches, which emerge close to the median plane.
2. Below T6, the cutaneous innervation is provided by lateral branches, which emerge in line with the lateral edge of the erector spinae muscle.

The cutaneous branches of upper three lumbar nerves emerge a short distance above the iliac crest and turn down over it to supply the skin of the gluteal region.

N.B. The posterior rami of C1, C7, C8, L4, and L5 do not give any cutaneous branches.

CUTANEOUS ARTERIES

The arteries which accompany the cutaneous nerves on the back of body in the thoracic and lumbar regions are the dorsal branches of the posterior intercostal and lumbar arteries, respectively.

POSTERIOR AXIO-APPENDICULAR MUSCLES (MUSCLES CONNECTING SCAPULA WITH THE VERTEBRAL COLUMN)

The muscles that attach the scapula to the back of the trunk (vertebral column) are arranged in two layers (two in the superficial layer and three in the deep layer).

1. **Superficial layer of the muscles**
   (a) Trapezius.
   (b) Latissimus dorsi.

2. **Deep layer of the muscles**
   (a) Levator scapulae.
   (b) Rhomboideus major.
   (c) Rhomboideus minor.

SUPERFICIAL POSTERIOR AXIO-APPENDICULAR MUSCLES

Trapezius Muscle (Fig. 5.3)

The trapezius is a flat triangular muscle on the back of the neck and the upper thorax. The muscles of two sides lie side by side in the midline and together form a diamond shape/trapezoid shape, hence the name trapezius.

Origin

It arises from:

(a) medial third of the superior nuchal line,
(b) external occipital protuberance,
(c) ligamentum nuchae,
(d) spine of 7th cervical vertebra, and
(e) spines of all thoracic vertebrae.

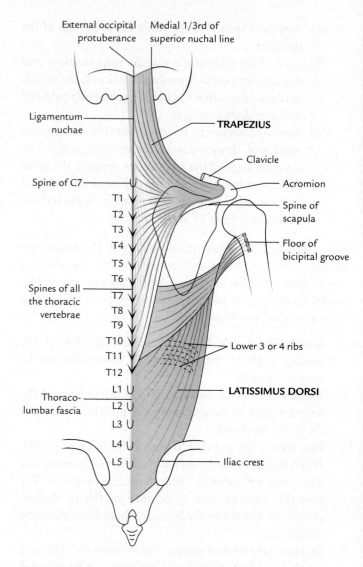

Fig. 5.3 Origin and insertion of the trapezius and latissimus dorsi muscles.

Insertion

The insertion occurs as follows:

1. The **superior fibres** runs downwards and laterally to be inserted on to the posterior border of the lateral third of the clavicle.
2. The **middle fibres** proceed horizontally to be inserted on to the medial margin of the acromion and upper lip of the crest of the spine of the scapula.
3. The **lower fibres** pass upward and laterally to be inserted on to the deltoid tubercle at the junction of medial and middle third of the spine of the scapula.

Nerve supply

It is by:

(a) spinal part of the accessory nerve (provides motor supply), and
(b) ventral rami of C3 and C4 (carry proprioceptive sensations).

Actions

1. The upper fibres of trapezius along with levator scapulae elevate the scapula as in *shrugging the shoulder.*
2. The middle fibres of trapezius along with rhomboids retract the scapula as in *bracing back the shoulder.*
3. The lower fibres of trapezius depress the medial part of the spine of the scapula.
4. Acting with serratus anterior, the trapezius rotates the scapula forward so that the arm can be abducted beyond 90°.

Clinical testing

Palpate the trapezius while the shoulder is shrugged against the resistance. Inability to shrug (to raise) the shoulder is suggestive of muscle weakness.

Latissimus Dorsi (L. *Latissimus* = widest, *Dorsi* = back)

The latissimus dorsi is a wide, flat, triangular muscle on the back (lumbar region and lower thorax). It is mostly superficial except a small portion, covered posteriorly by the lower part of trapezius.

Origin

It arises from:

(a) spines of lower six thoracic vertebrae anterior to the trapezius, by tendinous fibres,
(b) posterior lamina of thoraco-lumbar fascia (by which it is attached to the spines of lumbar and sacral vertebrae) by tendinous fibres,
(c) outer lip of the posterior part of the iliac crest by muscular slips,
(d) lower three or four ribs by fleshy slips,
(e) inferior angle of the scapula.

Insertion

From its extensive origin the fibres pass laterally with different degrees of obliquity (the upper fibres are nearly horizontal, the middle are oblique, and lower are almost vertical) to form a sheet that overlaps the inferior angle of the scapula. This sheet curves around the inferolateral border of the teres major to gain its anterior surface. Here it ends as flattened tendon, which is inserted into the floor of intertubercular sulcus (bicipital groove) of the humerus.

The latissimus dorsi and teres major together form the **posterior axillary fold.**

Nerve supply

The latissimus dorsi is supplied by *thoraco-dorsal nerve* from the posterior cord of the brachial plexus.

Actions

1. Latissimus dorsi is active in adduction, extension, and rotation, especially medial rotation of the humerus.

2. It pulls up the trunk upwards and forwards during climbing. This action is in conjunction with the pectoralis major muscle.
3. It assists backward swinging of the arm during walking.
4. It takes part in all violent expiratory efforts.

N.B. Because of its attachment on the ilium and sacrum, the latissimus dorsi is able to elevate the pelvis if the arms are stabilized. This action occurs when the arms are stabilized on crutch-handles. This is a very good example of 'reversal of muscle action' where proximal attachment (i.e., *origin*) pulls the distal attachment (i.e., *insertion*).

Clinical testing

The posterior axillary fold becomes accentuated when a 90° abducted arm is adducted against the resistance or when patient coughs violently.

Clinical correlation

- **Musculocutaneous flap of latissimus dorsi:** The latissimus dorsi is supplied by a *single dominant vascular pedicle* formed by the thoraco-*dorsal artery,* a continuation of the subscapular artery. This artery and its accompanying venae comitantes and *thoraco-dorsal nerve* descend in the posterior wall of axilla and enter the costal surface of the muscle at a single neuro-vascular hilum about 1–4 cm medial to the lateral border of the muscle. The presence of single dominant vascular pedicle provides the anatomical basis for raising the muscle above, or along with the overlying skin in the form of *musculocutaneous flap.* The musculocutaneous flap of latissimus dorsi is often used in reconstructing a breast following mastectomy.
- **Conditioning of latissimus dorsi to act as a cardiac muscle:** The latissimus dorsi if conditioned with pulsated electrical impulses, starts functioning like a cardiac muscle, i.e., it will be non-fatigable and use oxygen at a steady pace. Thus following conditioning, the latissimus dorsi can be used as an autotransplant to repair a surgically removed portion of heart. The procedure involves detaching the latissimus dorsi from its vertebral origin keeping the neurovascular pedicle intact and slipping it into the pericardial cavity, where it is wrapped around the heart like a towel. A pacemaker is required to provide the continuous rhythmic contractions.

DEEP POSTERIOR AXIO-APPENDICULAR MUSCLES (Fig. 5.4)

Levator Scapulae

Origin

The levator scapula is a slender muscle. It arises by tendinous slips from

(a) transverse processes of atlas and axis vertebrae, and
(b) posterior tubercles of the transverse processes of the 3rd and 4th cervical vertebrae.

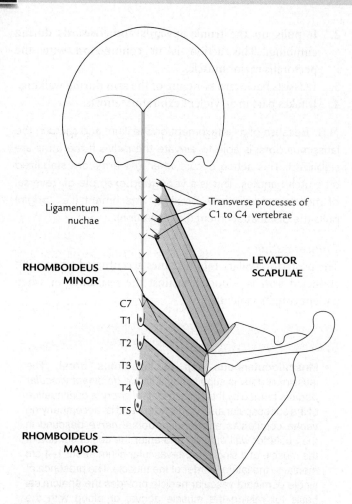

Fig. 5.4 Origin and insertion of the levator scapulae rhomboideus major and rhomboideus minor muscles.

Insertion

The four discrete slips of the muscles fibres descend diagonally towards the scapula to be inserted on to the upper part of its medial border between superior angle and the triangular smooth surface at the medial end of the scapular spine.

Nerve supply

The levator scapulae is innervated by:

(a) direct branches of C3 and C4 spinal nerves, and
(b) C5 spinal nerve through the dorsal scapulae nerve.

Action

The levator scapulae elevate and steady the scapula during movements of the arm.

Rhomboideus Minor

Origin

The rhomboideus minor is a thick cylindrical muscle, which arises from:

(a) lower part of the ligamentum nuchae, and
(b) spines of the 7th cervical and 1st thoracic vertebrae.

Insertion

It is inserted on to the base of triangular area at the root of the spine of the scapula.

Rhomboideus Major

Origin

The thin flat rhomboideus major muscle is about two times wider than the rhomboideus minor. It arises from spine of T2, T3, T4, and T5 vertebrae and intervening supraspinous ligaments.

Insertion

The fibres run downwards and laterally to be inserted on the medial border of the scapula between the root of the spine and inferior angle of the scapula.

Nerve supply of rhomboids

Both the rhomboideus major and minor are supplied by the dorsal scapular nerve (C5).

Actions of the rhomboids

Both the rhomboideus major and minor retract the scapula as in squaring the shoulders.

Clinical testing of the rhomboids

The rhomboids can be palpated along the medial borders of the scapulae deep to trapezius on bracing the shoulder back against the resistance.

Dorsal scapular nerve (nerve to rhomboids)

The dorsal scapular nerve arises from C5 spinal nerve root in the neck. The nerve pierces the scalenus medius and comes to lie on the anterior surface of the levator scapulae in the posterior triangle of the neck. Here it is accompanied by deep branch of the transverse cervical artery (or dorsal scapular artery). Then the dorsal scapular nerve and artery descend to the back along the anterior surface of the levator scapulae. [Note: The spinal accessory nerve and superficial branch of the transverse cervical artery runs on the posterior surface of the levator scapulae (Fig. 5.5)].

Clinical correlation

Triangle of auscultation (Fig. 5.6): It is small triangular gap in the musculature on the back of the thorax near the inferior angle of the scapula. Its boundaries are:
• Superior horizontal border of the latissimus dorsi.
• Medial border of the scapula.
• Inferolateral border of the trapezius.
   The floor *of this triangle* is formed by, 6th and 7th ribs and the 6th intercostal space.
   The upper part of the lower lobe of the lung lies deep to this triangle. When the scapulae are drawn anteriorly by folding the arm across the chest and the trunk is flexed, this triangle enlarges and becomes more subcutaneous. Now the lower lobe of the lung can be auscultated by putting the stethoscope in this region.
   The sounds are not muffled by the muscles of back in this area.

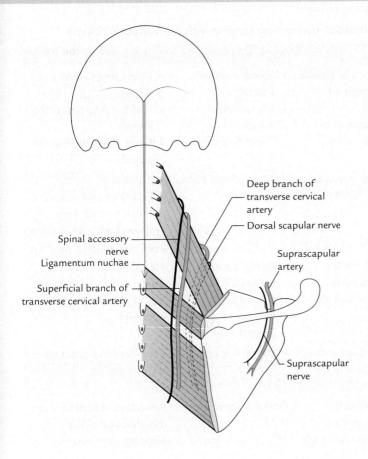

Fig. 5.5 Nerves and vessels related to deep posterior axio-appendicular muscles.

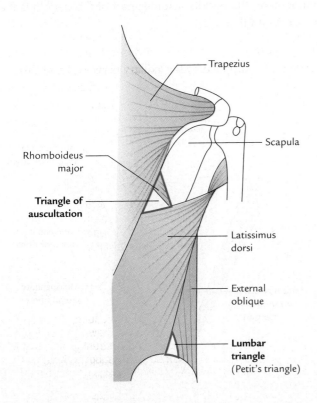

Fig. 5.6 Triangle of auscultation.

The origin, insertion, nerve supply, and actions of the muscles, which connect scapula with the vertebral column are summarized in Table 5.2.

SCAPULAR REGION

The scapular region includes parts/structures around the scapula. The following text deals with the scapulohumeral muscles, intermuscular spaces in the subscapular region, nerve and vessels and anastomosis around the scapula.

SCAPULOHUMERAL MUSCLES

The **scapulohumeral muscles** are relatively short muscles, which pass from scapula to the humerus and act on the glenohumeral joint (shoulder joint proper). They are also called **intrinsic shoulder muscles**. There are six in number as follows:

1. Deltoid.
2. Supraspinatus.
3. Infraspinatus.
4. Teres minor.
5. Teres major.
6. Subscapularis.

Deltoid (Fig. 5.7)

The deltoid is a 'three-in-one muscle'. It is thick, powerful, and curved triangular muscle covering the shoulder and forming its rounded contour. The deltoid is shaped like the inverted Greek letter Delta (D), hence its name deltoid. The deltoid muscle is divided into three parts: (a) anterior unipennate part, (b) posterior unipennate part, and (c) middle multipennate part.

Origin

The deltoid has a V-shaped origin from the subcutaneous bony arch formed by (a) lateral 1/3rd of clavicle, (b) acromion process, and (c) crest of spine of the scapula. The details are as under:

1. The *anterior unipennate part*—arises from the upper surface and anterior border of the lateral third of the clavicle.
2. The *middle multipennate part*—arises from the lateral margin and upper surface of the acromion.
3. The *posterior unipennate part*—arises from the lower lip of the crest of the spine of the scapula.

Insertion

The fibres converge inferiorly to form a short thick tendon, which is inserted onto the V-shaped deltoid tuberosity/tubercle on the lateral aspect of the midshaft of the humerus.

N.B. The fibres of multipennate middle part arise from four septa that are attached above to the acromion. These fibres

Table 5.2 Origin, insertion, nerve supply, and actions of the muscles connecting scapula with the vertebral column

Muscle	Origin	Insertion	Nerve supply	Actions
Trapezius	• Medial 1/3rd of superior nuchal line • Ligamentum nuchae • External occipital protuberance • Spines of C7–T12 vertebrae	• Lateral 1/3rd of clavicle • Medial margin of acromion • Superior margin of spine of the scapula	• Spinal accessory (motor) • C3, C4 spinal nerves (proprioceptive)	• Upper fibres elevates the scapula • Middle fibres retract the scapula • Lower fibres depress the scapula
Latissimus dorsi	• Spines of T7–T12 vertebrae • Thoraco-lumbar fascia • Iliac crest • Lower 3 or 4 ribs • Inferior angle of the scapula	Floor of intertubercular sulcus of the humerus	Thoraco-dorsal nerve (C6, C7, C8)	• Adduction, • Extension and medial rotation of the arm • Raises body towards arm as in climbing
Levator scapulae	Transverse processes of C1–C4 vertebrae	Medial border of the scapula between the superior angle and root of spine	• Dorsal scapular nerve (C5) • C3 and C4 spinal nerves (proprioceptive)	Elevation and medial rotation of the scapula and tilts its glenoid cavity inferiorly
Rhomboideus minor	• Lower part of the ligamentum nuchae • Spines of C7 and T1 vertebrae	Base of triangular area at the root of spine of the scapula	• Dorsal scapular nerve (C5)	Retraction and elevation of the scapula
Rhomboideus major	Spines of T2–T5 vertebrae	Medial border of the scapula from root of spine to the inferior angle	Dorsal scapular nerve (C5)	Retraction, medial rotation, and elevation of the scapula

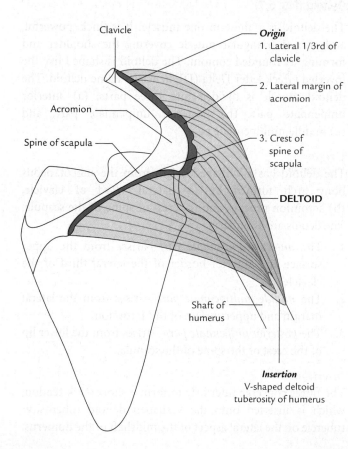

Fig. 5.7 Origin and insertion of the deltoid muscle.

converge onto the three septa of insertion, which are attached to the deltoid tuberosity. Due to multipennate arrangement, the middle acromial part of the deltoid is the strongest part (Fig. 5.8).

Nerve supply
The deltoid is supplied by the axillary nerve (C5 and C6).

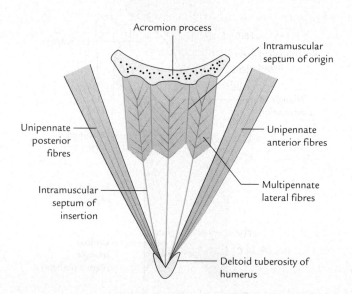

Fig. 5.8 Architecture of the deltoid muscle.

Actions

1. The anterior (clavicular) fibres are flexors and medial rotators of the arm.
2. The posterior (spinous) fibres are the extensors and lateral rotators of the arm.
3. The middle (acromial) fibres are the strong abductor of the arm from 15° to 90°.

Middle (acromial) fibres cannot abduct the arm from 0° to 15° when the arm is by the side of body because its vertical pull corresponds to the long axis of the arm.

N.B. The deltoid muscle is like three muscles in one: the anterior fibres flex the arm, lateral fibres abduct the arm and posterior fibres extend the arm.

Clinical testing

The deltoid can be easily seen and felt to contract when the arm is abducted against resistance.

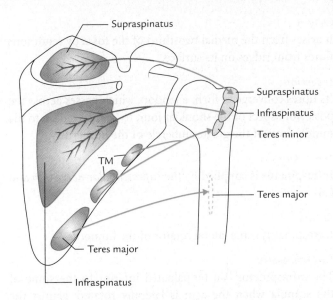

Fig. 5.9 Origin and insertion of the supraspinatus, infraspinatus, teres minor, and teres major muscles (TM = teres minor).

Clinical correlation

Site of the intramuscular injection in deltoid: The intramuscular injections are commonly given in the lower half of the deltoid to avoid injury to the axillary nerve, which winds around the surgical neck of the humerus.

N.B. In actual clinical practice, the intramuscular injection is given in the upper and outer quadrant of the deltoid region.

Structures under cover of deltoid

- **Bones:** Upper end of the humerus and coracoid process.
- **Joints and ligaments:** Shoulder (glenohumeral) joint and coracoacromial ligament.
- **Bursae around the shoulder joint:** Subscapular, subacromial/subdeltoid, and infraspinatus.
- **Muscles:**
  (a) Insertions of pectoralis minor, pectoralis major, teres major, latissimus dorsi, subscapularis, supraspinatus, infraspinatus, and teres minor.
  (b) Origins of long head of biceps, short head of biceps, coracobrachialis, long and lateral heads of triceps.
- **Vessels:** Anterior and posterior circumflex humeral.
- **Nerves:** Axillary nerve.
- **Spaces:** Quadrangular and triangular subscapular intermuscular spaces.

Supraspinatus (Fig. 5.9)

Origin

Supraspinatus arises from medial two-third of the supraspinous fossa of the scapula.

Insertion

The fibres pass forward and converge under the acromion, into a tendon, which crosses above the shoulder joint and is inserted on to the superior facet on the greater tubercle of the humerus.

Nerve supply

Supraspinatus is supplied by the *suprascapular nerve* (C5 and C6).

Actions

Supraspinatus initiates the abduction of shoulder. It is responsible for first 15° of abduction of the shoulder and thus assists the deltoid in carrying abduction thereafter, i.e., from 15° to 90°.

Clinical testing

The supraspinatus can be palpated deep to the trapezius and above the spine of the scapula when the arm is abducted against the resistance.

Clinical correlation

Rupture of supraspinatus tendon: It is a common soft tissue injury in the shoulder region. The patient with ruptured supraspinatus tendon when asked to raise his hand above the head on the affected side, he will first tilt his body on the affected side so that arm swings away from the body leading to an initial abduction of 15° or he will slightly (about 15°) raise the affected arm by the hand of the healthy side—a common 'trick-device' learned by the patients with ruptured supraspinatus tendon.

Infraspinatus (Fig. 5.9)

It is a thick triangular muscle, which occupies most of the infraspinous fossa.

Origin

It arises from the medial two-third of the fossa by tendinous fibres from ridges on its surface.

Insertion

Its fibres converge to form a tendon, which passes across the posterior aspect of the shoulder joint to be inserted on to the middle facet of the greater tubercle of the humerus.

Nerve supply

Infraspinatus is supplied by the *suprascapular nerve* (C5 and C6).

Action

Infraspinatus is the lateral rotator of the humerus.

Clinical testing

The infraspinatus can be palpated inferior to the spine of the scapula when the arm is laterally rotated against the resistance.

Teres Minor (Fig. 5.9)

Origin

This narrow elongated muscle arises from posterior aspect of the lateral border of the scapula.

Insertion

The fibres run upwards and laterally across the shoulder joint to be inserted on to the lower facet of the greater tubercle of the humerus.

Nerve supply

Teres minor is supplied by a branch of the axillary nerve (C5 and C6). The *nerve to teres minor possesses a pseudoganglion.*

Actions

Teres minor acts as a lateral rotator and weak adductor of the humerus.

Teres Major (Fig. 5.9)

Origin

This thick flat muscle arises from the oval area on the dorsal surface of the inferior angle and adjoining lateral border of the scapula.

Insertion

The fibres run upwards and laterally, and end in a flat tendon, which is inserted on to the medial lip of the intertubercular sulcus of the humerus.

Nerve supply

Teres major is supplied by the *lower subscapular nerve* (C5, C6, and C7).

Action

Teres major acts as a medial rotator of the arm.

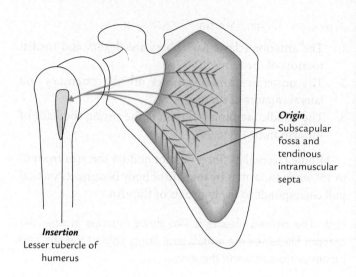

Origin
Subscapular fossa and tendinous intramuscular septa

Insertion
Lesser tubercle of humerus

Fig. 5.10 Origin and insertion of the subscapularis muscle.

Subscapularis (Fig. 5.10)

It is a bulky triangular muscle, which fills the subscapular fossa.

Origin

Subscapularis arises from (a) medial two-third of the costal surface of the scapula and (b) tendinous intermuscular septa attached to the ridges on the bone.

Insertion

The fibres converge laterally into a broad tendon, which passes in front of the capsule of glenohumeral joint to be inserted on to the lesser tubercle of the humerus. The tendon is separated from the neck of the scapula by a large **subscapular bursa,** which generally communicates with the synovial cavity of the shoulder joint.

Nerve supply

The subscapularis is supplied by the *upper and lower subscapular nerves* (C5, C6).

Actions

Subscapularis is the medial rotator of the humerus. Together with supraspinatus, infraspinatus, and teres minor it stabilizes the head of the humerus in glenoid fossa during shoulder movements.

The origin, insertion, nerve supply, and actions of the scapulohumeral muscles are described in Table 5.3.

ROTATOR CUFF MUSCLES

The four of scapulohumeral muscles, viz. supraspinatus infraspinatus, teres minor, and subscapularis (often referred to as *SITS muscles*) are called **rotator cuff muscles** for they form musculotendinous/rotator cuff around the glenohumeral joint.

Table 5.3 Origin, insertion, nerve supply, and actions of the scapulohumeral muscles

Muscle	Origin	Insertion	Nerve supply	Actions
Deltoid (a) Clavicular part – unipennate (b) Acromial part – multipennate (c) Spinous part – unipennate	• Anterior aspect of lateral 1/3rd of clavicle • Lateral border of acromion • Lower lip of the spine of scapula	Deltoid tuberosity of humerus	Axillary nerve (C5, C6)	• Flexion and medial rotation by the anterior fibres • Abduction (15°–90°) of the arm by middle fibres • Extension and medial rotation of the arm by posterior fibres
Supraspinatus (multipennate)	• Medial 2/3rd of the supraspinous fossa of scapula	Superior facet of greater tubercle of the humerus	Suprascapular nerve (C5, C6)	Initiates abduction of the arm and carries it up to 15°
Infraspinatus (multipennate)	• Medial 2/3rd of the infraspinous fossa of scapula	Middle facet of greater tubercle of the humerus	Suprascapular nerve (C5, C6)	Lateral rotation of the arm
Teres minor	Upper 2/3rd of the dorsal aspect of the lateral border of scapula	Inferior facet of greater tubercle of the humerus	Axillary nerve (C5, C6)	Lateral rotation of the arm
Teres major	Inferior 1/3rd of the dorsal aspect of the lateral border and inferior angle of scapula	Medial lip of the intertubercular sulcus of the humerus	Lower subscapular nerve (C5, C6)	Abduction and medial rotation of the arm
Subscapularis (multipennate)	• Medial 2/3rd of the subscapular fossa • Tendinous intermuscular septa	Lesser tubercle of the humerus	Upper and lower subscapular nerves (C5, C6, C7)	• Adduction and medial rotation of the arm • Helps to hold the humeral head in glenoid cavity

ROTATOR CUFF (MUSCULOTENDINOUS CUFF)

The rotator cuff (Fig. 5.11) is the name given to the tendons of supraspinatus, infraspinatus, teres minor, and subscapularis which are fused with the underlying capsule of the glenohumeral joint. Tendon of supraspinatus fuse superiorly, tendons of infraspinatus and teres minor fuse posteriorly, and that of subscapularis fuse anteriorly. This cuff plays an important role in stabilizing the shoulder joint. *The primary function of rotator cuff muscles is to grasp the relatively large head of humerus and hold it against the smaller, shallow glenoid cavity* (Fig. 6.8A).

MOVEMENTS OF THE SCAPULA (Fig. 5.12)

The scapula is able to glide freely on the posterior chest wall because of the loose connective tissue between the serratus anterior and the chest wall.

The movements of scapula are produced by the muscles that attach it to the trunk and indirectly by the muscles passing from trunk to the humerus when the glenohumeral joint is fixed.

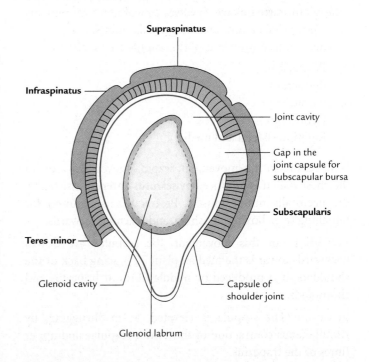

Fig. 5.11 Musculotendinous (rotator) cuff.

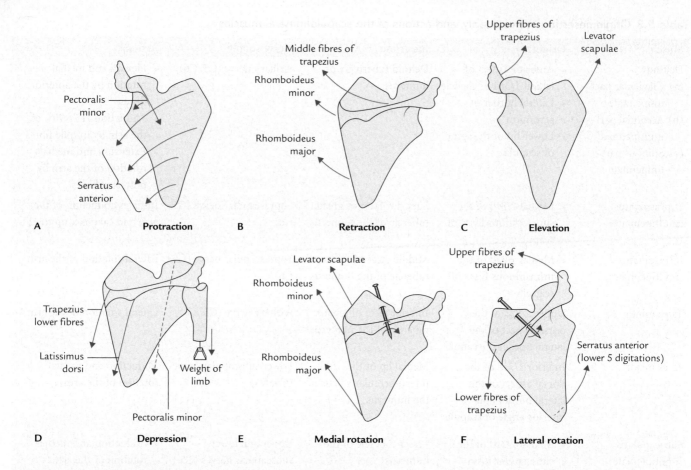

Fig. 5.12 Movements of the scapula (A–F).

All the movements of scapula occurring on the chest wall (**scapulothoracic linkage**) involves concomitant movements at sternoclavicular and acromioclavicular joints.

The various movements of the scapula are as follows:

1. Protraction.
2. Retraction.
3. Elevation.
4. Depression.
5. Rotation (lateral and medial).

Protraction: In this movement, scapula moves forwards on the chest wall. It is produced by **serratus anterior** assisted by the pectoralis minor muscle. Protraction is required for punching (e.g., boxing), pushing, and reaching forwards.

Retraction: In this movement, the scapulae are drawn backwards towards the median plane in bracing back of the shoulders. It is produced by middle fibres of trapezius and rhomboids.

Elevation: The scapula is elevated, as in shrugging, by simultaneous contraction of the levator scapulae and upper fibres of the trapezius.

Depression: The scapula is depressed by simultaneous contraction of the pectoralis minor, lower fibres of trapezius, and latissimus dorsi.

Rotation: The rotation of scapula takes place around the horizontal axis passing through the middle of the spine of scapula and sternoclavicular joint.

1. **Medial rotation** is brought about by simultaneous contraction of levator scapulae, rhomboids, and latissimus dorsi. The gravity (e.g., weight of the upper limb) plays a key role in this movement.

2. **Lateral rotation** is brought about by the *trapezius* (its upper fibres raise the acromion process and its lower fibres depress the medial end of the spine of the scapula) and *serratus anterior* (its lower 5 digitations pull the inferior angle of the scapula forwards and laterally). The lateral rotation of the scapula tilts its glenoid cavity upwards—which is essential for abduction of the upper limb above 90°.

The movements of scapula and the muscles, which produce them are summarized in Table 5.4 and Figure 5.12.

Table 5.4 Movements of the scapula and the muscles producing them

Movement of scapula	Muscles producing the movements
Protraction	• Serratus anterior • Pectoralis minor (assists)
Retraction	• Trapezius (middle fibres) • Rhomboideus minor • Rhomboideus major
Elevation	• Trapezius (upper fibres) • Levator Scapulae
Depression	• Pectoralis minor • Trapezius (lower fibres) • Latissimus dorsi • Weight of the upper limb
Medial rotation*	• Levator scapulae • Rhomboideus minor • Rhomboideus major
Lateral rotation	• Trapezius (upper and lower fibres) • Serratus anterior (lower 5 digitations)

*The gravity (e.g., weight of the upper limb) plays a major part in medial rotation of the scapula.

SUBSCAPULAR SPACES (INTERMUSCULAR SPACES IN THE SCAPULAR REGION; Fig. 5.13)

These are quadrangular (one) and triangular (two) intermuscular spaces in the scapular region, which are clearly seen from behind after reflecting the posterior part of the deltoid. The knowledge of these spaces is essential during surgery in the shoulder region.

QUADRANGULAR SPACE

Boundaries

Superior: – Teres minor (posteriorly)
 – Subscapularis (anteriorly)
 – Capsule of shoulder joint between the above two muscles
Inferior: Teres major
Medial: Long head of the triceps
Lateral: Surgical neck of the humerus

Structures passing through this space (Fig. 5.14)
• Axillary nerve
• Posterior circumflex humeral artery and vein

UPPER TRIANGULAR SPACE

Boundaries

Superior: Teres minor
Lateral: Long head of triceps
Inferior: Teres major

Structure passing through this space (Fig. 5.14): Circumflex scapular artery (this artery interrupts the origin of teres minor to reach the infraspinous fossa).

LOWER TRIANGULAR SPACE

Boundaries

Medial: Long head of triceps
Lateral: Shaft of humerus
Superior: Teres major

Structures passing through this space (Fig. 5.14)
• Radial nerve
• Profunda brachii artery and vein

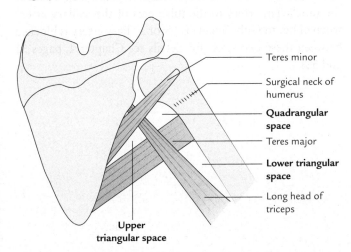

Fig. 5.13 Intermuscular spaces of the subscapular region (subscapular spaces).

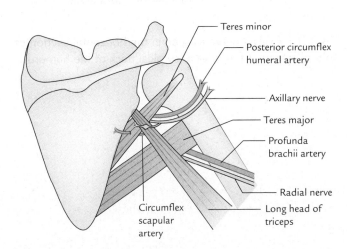

Fig. 5.14 Intermuscular spaces of the scapular region (subscapular spaces) and structures passing through them.

NERVES AND VESSELS

AXILLARY NERVE (Fig. 5.15)

The axillary nerve (C5, C6) arises from the posterior cord of the brachial plexus near the lower border of the subscapularis. It runs backwards on subscapularis to pass through the quadrangular space along with the posterior circumflex humeral artery. Here it is intimately related to the medial aspect of the surgical neck of the humerus immediately inferior to the capsule of the shoulder joint. The nerve gives a branch to the shoulder joint, and then runs laterally to divide into the anterior and posterior divisions/branches, deep to deltoid.

The *posterior branch* supplies teres minor and posterior part of the deltoid. It then continues over the posterior border of the deltoid as *upper lateral cutaneous nerve of the arm* and supplies the skin over the lower half of the deltoid. The nerve to teres minor possesses a *'pseudoganglion'*.

The *anterior branch* continues horizontally between the deltoid and surgical neck of the humerus with posterior circumflex humeral vessels. It supplies deltoid and sends a few branches through it to innervate the overlying skin.

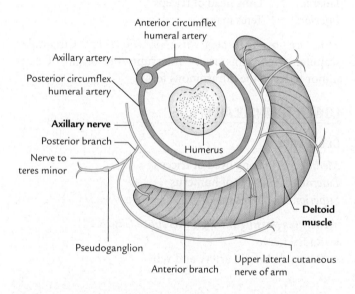

Fig. 5.15 Axillary nerve as seen in the horizontal section of deltoid region at the level of surgical neck of the humerus.

Clinical correlation

Injury of the axillary nerve: The axillary nerve is at risk of damage in inferior dislocation of the head of humerus from shoulder joint and in fractures of the surgical neck of the humerus because of its close relation to these structures (Fig. 6.2B). The damage of axillary nerve presents the following clinical features:

- *Impaired abduction of the shoulder*—due to paralysis of the deltoid and teres minor muscles.
- *Loss of sensations over the lower half of the deltoid ('regimental badge' area of the sensory loss)*—due to involvement of the upper lateral cutaneous nerve of the arm.
- *Loss of shoulder contour with prominence of greater tubercle of the humerus*—due to wasting of the deltoid muscle.

CIRCUMFLEX HUMERAL ARTERIES

These arteries arise from the third part of the axillary artery and together form a **circular anastomosis** around the surgical neck of the humerus.

ARTERIAL ANASTOMOSIS AROUND THE SCAPULA

This anastomosis is clinically important because it ensures adequate arterial supply to scapula and provides a subsidiary route through which the blood can pass from the first part of the subclavian artery to the third part of the axillary artery when either the subclavian artery or axillary artery is blocked between these two sites (for details see Chapter 4, pages 51 and 52).

Golden Facts to Remember

▶ Only muscle that suspends the pectoral girdle from the cranium	Trapezius
▶ Widest muscle on the back of the body	Latissimus dorsi
▶ Climbing muscles	Latissimus dorsi and pectoralis major
▶ Largest cutaneous nerve on the back of shoulder region	T2 which lies across the spine of the scapula
▶ All the rotator cuff muscles are the rotators of the humerus *except*	Supraspinatus
▶ Tendon most commonly torn in rotator cuff injury	Tendon of supraspinatus
▶ Best site for hearing lung sounds on the back of chest	Triangle of auscultation

Clinical Case Study

A 45-year-old man, a chronic user of crutch went to his family physician and complained that he had noticed loss of shoulder contour on the right side during the last 2 months. He also told that he feels no sensations in this region and could see the bony projection at the upper end. On examination, the physician found that patient could not abduct his arm up to the 90° and there was a loss of skin sensation over the lower half of the deltoid muscle. He could also notice the prominence of greater tubercle of the humerus. He was diagnosed as a case of **axillary nerve injury**.

Questions

1. Mention the origin and root value of axillary nerve.
2. What are the three common causes of axillary nerve injury?
3. Mention the cause of loss of skin sensation over the lower half of the deltoid.
4. What is the cause of loss of shoulder contour and prominence of greater tubercle of humerus?
5. Name the muscles supplied by the axillary nerve.

Answers

1. The axillary nerve arises from the posterior cord of the brachial plexus (C5 and C6).
2. Axillary nerve can be injured: (a) by the pressure of a badly adjusted crutch, pressuring upwards, into the armpit, (b) by inferior dislocation of the shoulder joint, and (c) by the intramuscular injection.
3. Due to involvement of the upper lateral cutaneous nerve of the arm.
4. Due to wasting of the deltoid muscle.
5. Deltoid and teres minor.

Shoulder Joint Complex (Joints of Shoulder Girdle)

The 'shoulder joint complex' consists of four basic articulations, namely (Fig. 6.1),

1. Glenohumeral joint.
2. Acromioclavicular joint.
3. Sternoclavicular joint.
4. Scapulothoracic articulation/scapulothoracic linkage (functional linkage between the scapula and thorax).

Normal function of the shoulder girdle requires smooth coordination of movements on all these joints. The impairment of any one of these joints leads to functional defect of the whole complex.

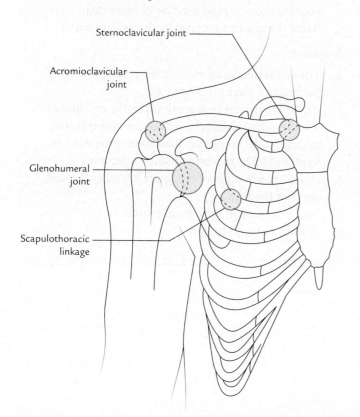

Fig. 6.1 Articulations of the shoulder complex (joints of the shoulder girdle).

The main function of the shoulder in man is to enable him to place his hand where he wishes to in a coordinated and controlled manner.

From weight-bearing forelimb of a quadruped to a freely mobile upper limb in human beings, substantial phylogenetic changes have occurred in the shoulder girdle. In human beings, shoulder girdle has sacrificed stability for mobility, which is responsible for most of the pathological changes that take place in it.

The **glenohumeral joint** is the primary articulation of the shoulder girdle and generally termed shoulder joint by the clinicians. It is quite commonly affected by disease hence it needs to be described in detail.

SHOULDER JOINT (GLENOHUMERAL JOINT)

It is a joint between the head of humerus and glenoid cavity of the scapula.

The shoulder joint is the most movable joint of the body and consequently one of the least stable. It is most common joint to dislocate and to undergo recurrent dislocations. Therefore, the students must study it very thoroughly.

Type

The shoulder joint is a ball-and-socket type of synovial joint (Fig. 6.2).

ARTICULAR SURFACES (Fig. 6.2)

The shoulder joint is formed by articulation of large round **head of humerus** with the relatively shallow **glenoid cavity of the scapula**. The glenoid cavity is deepened slightly but effectively by the fibrocartilaginous ring called **glenoid labrum**.

LIGAMENTS (Figs 6.3–6.5)

The ligaments of the shoulder joint are as follows:

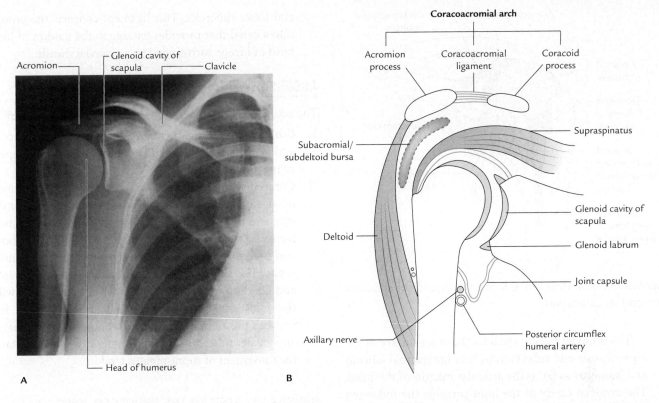

Coracoacromial arch

Acromion process

Coracoacromial ligament

Coracoid process

Supraspinatus

Subacromial/ subdeltoid bursa

Glenoid cavity of scapula

Glenoid labrum

Joint capsule

Deltoid

Acromion

Glenoid cavity of scapula

Clavicle

Head of humerus

A

B

Axillary nerve

Posterior circumflex humeral artery

Fig. 6.2 Shoulder joint: **A**, a radiograph showing articular surfaces; **B**, coronal section. (*Source:* Fig. 7.25, Page 628, *Gray's Anatomy for Students*, Richard L Drake, Wayne Vogl, Adam WM Mitchell. Copyright Elsevier Inc. 2005, All rights reserved.)

1. **Capsular ligament (joint capsule):** The thin fibrous layer of the joint capsule surrounds the glenohumeral joint. It is attached medially to the margins of the glenoid cavity beyond the glenoid labrum and laterally to the anatomical neck of the humerus, except inferiorly where it extends downwards 1.5 cm or more on the surgical neck of the humerus. Medially the attachment extends beyond the supraglenoid tubercle thus enclosing the long head of biceps brachii within the joint cavity.

Clinical correlation

A portion of epiphyseal line of proximal humerus is intracapsular, therefore, septic arthritis of the shoulder joint may occur following *metaphyseal osteomyelitis*.

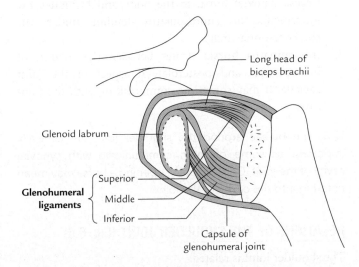

Long head of biceps brachii

Glenoid labrum

Glenohumeral ligaments { Superior Middle Inferior

Capsule of glenohumeral joint

Fig. 6.3 Interior of the shoulder joint exposed from behind to show the glenohumeral ligaments.

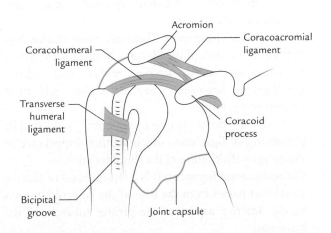

Acromion

Coracoacromial ligament

Coracohumeral ligament

Transverse humeral ligament

Coracoid process

Bicipital groove

Joint capsule

Fig. 6.4 Coracoacromial, coracohumeral, and transverse humeral ligaments as seen from the anterior aspect.

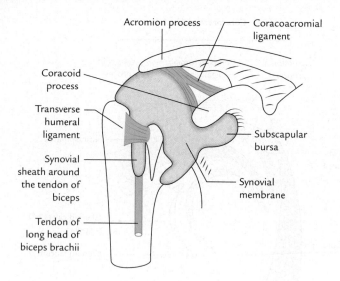

Fig. 6.5 Synovial membrane lining the interior of shoulder joint and its extensions.

The **synovial membrane** lines the inner surface of the joint capsule and reflects from it to the glenoid labrum and humerus as far as the articular margin of the head. The synovial cavity of the joint presents the following features:

(a) It forms tubular sheath around the tendon of biceps brachii where it lies in the bicipital groove of the humerus.

(b) It communicates with subscapular and infraspinatus bursae, around the joint.

Thus there are three apertures in the joint capsule:

(a) An opening between the tubercles of the humerus for the passage of tendon of long head of biceps brachii.

(b) An opening situated anteriorly inferior to the coracoid process to allow communication between the synovial cavity and subscapular bursa.

(c) An opening situated posteriorly to allow communication between synovial cavity and infraspinatus bursa.

2. **Glenohumeral ligaments:** There are three thickenings in the anterior part of the fibrous capsule; to strengthen it. These are called *superior, middle,* and *inferior glenohumeral ligaments.* They are visible only from interior of the joint.

A defect exists between superior and middle glenohumeral ligaments, which acquire importance in the anterior dislocation of the shoulder joint.

3. **Coracohumeral ligament:** It is a strong band of fibrous tissue that passes from the base of the coracoid process to the anterior aspect of the greater tubercle of the humerus.

4. **Transverse humeral ligament:** It is a broad fibrous band, which bridges the bicipital groove between the greater

and lesser tubercles. This ligament converts the groove into a canal that provides passage to the tendon of long head of biceps surrounded by a synovial sheath.

ACCESSORY LIGAMENTS

The accessory ligaments of the shoulder joint are as follows:

1. **Coracoacromial ligament:** It extends between coracoid and acromion processes. It protects the superior aspect of the joint.

2. **Coracoacromial arch:** The coracoacromial arch is formed by coracoid process, acromion process, and coracoacromial ligament between them. This osseoligamentous structure forms a protective arch for the head of humerus above and prevents its superior displacement above the glenoid cavity. The **supraspinatus muscle** passes under this arch and lies deep to the deltoid where its tendon blends with the joint capsule. The large **subacromial bursa** lies between the arch superiorly and tendon of supraspinatus and greater tubercle of humerus inferiorly. This facilitates the movement of supraspinatus tendon.

BURSAE RELATED TO THE SHOULDER JOINT

Several bursae are related to the shoulder joint but the important ones are as follows (Fig. 6.6):

1. **Subscapular bursa:** It lies between the tendon of subscapularis and the neck of the scapula; and protects the tendon from friction against the neck. This bursa usually communicates with the joint cavity.

2. **Subacromial bursa (Fig. 6.7):** It lies between the coracoacromial ligament and acromion process above, and supraspinatus tendon and joint capsule below. It continues downwards beneath the deltoid, hence it is sometimes also referred to as *subdeltoid bursa.* It is the largest synovial bursa in the body and facilitates the movements of supraspinatus tendon under the coracoacromial arch.

3. **Infraspinatus bursa:** It lies between the tendon of infraspinatus and posterolateral aspect of the joint capsule. It may sometime communicate with the joint cavity.

N.B. The bursae around the shoulder joint are clinically important as some of them communicate with synovial cavity of the joint. Consequently, opening a bursa may mean entering into the cavity of the joint.

RELATIONS OF THE SHOULDER JOINT (Fig. 6.6)

The shoulder joint is related:

Superiorly: to coracoacromial arch, subacromial bursa, supraspinatus muscle, and deltoid muscle.

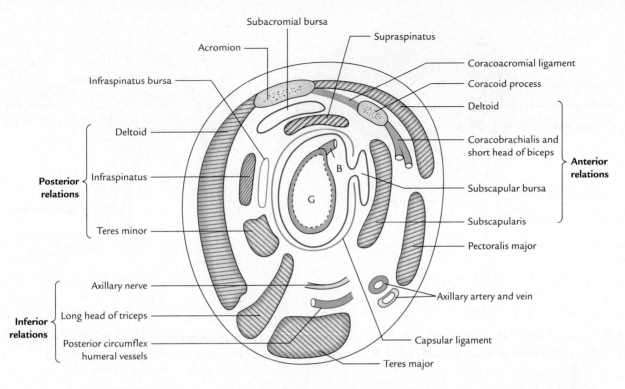

Fig. 6.6 Relations of the shoulder joint as seen in sagittal section (G = glenoid fossa, B = long head of biceps).

Inferiorly: to long head of triceps, axillary nerve and posterior circumflex humeral vessels.

Anteriorly: to subscapularis, subscapular bursa, coraco-brachialis, short head of biceps brachii, and deltoid.

Posteriorly: to infraspinatus, teres minor, and deltoid.

ARTERIAL SUPPLY

The glenohumeral joint is supplied by the following arteries:

1. Anterior and posterior circumflex humeral arteries.
2. Suprascapular artery.
3. Subscapular artery.

NERVE SUPPLY

The glenohumeral joint is supplied by the following nerves:

1. Axillary nerve.
2. Suprascapular nerve.
3. Musculocutaneous nerve.

FACTORS PROVIDING STABILITY TO THE SHOULDER JOINT

The factors providing stability to the joint are as follows:

1. Rotator cuff (musculotendinous cuff).
2. Coracoacromial arch.

3. Long head of biceps tendon.
4. Glenoid labrum.

The **rotator cuff/musculotendinous cuff** is formed by the blending together of the tendons of subscapularis, supraspinatus, infraspinatus, and teres minor around the joint capsule (for details see Chapter 5, page 67).

The *tone of rotator cuff muscles* grasp the head of humerus and pull it medially to hold it against the smaller and shallow glenoid cavity. It also helps the head of humerus rotating against the glenoid fossa during joint motion, which is what the term *rotator* refers to (Fig. 6.8).

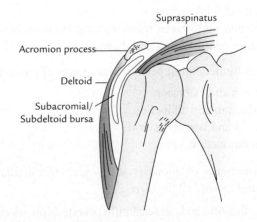

Fig. 6.7 Subacromial/subdeltoid bursa. (*Source*: Fig. 2.6, Page 57, *Clinical and Surgical Anatomy*, 2e, Vishram Singh. Copyright Elsevier 2007, All rights reserved.)

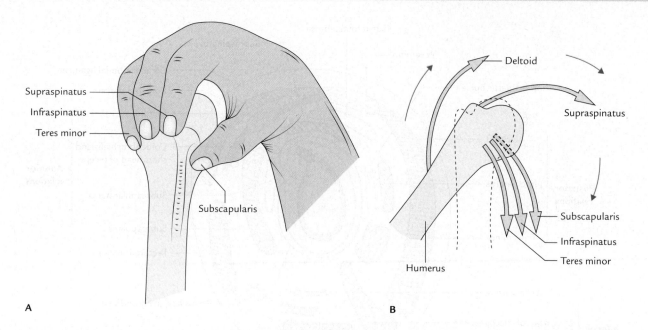

Fig. 6.8 Action of the rotator cuff muscles: **A**, they grasp and pull the relatively large head of the humerus medially to hold it against the smaller and shallow glenoid cavity; **B**, combined function of the rotator cuff muscles and deltoid.

The **coracoacromial arch** forms, the **secondary socket of the glenohumeral joint** and protects the joint from the above and prevents the upward dislocation of the head of humerus.

The **long head of biceps brachii**, passes above the head of humerus intracapsular, hence prevents its upward displacement.

The **glenoid labrum** provides protection by deepening the shallow glenoid cavity.

MOVEMENTS OF THE SHOULDER JOINT
(Figs 6.9 and 6.10)

The shoulder joint has more freedom of mobility than any other joint in the body, due to the following factors:

1. Laxity of joint capsule.
2. Articulation between relatively large humeral head and smaller and shallow glenoid cavity.

The glenohumeral joint permits four groups of movements:

1. Flexion and extension.
2. Abduction and adduction.
3. Medial and lateral rotation.
4. Circumduction.

The movements of shoulder joint occur in all the three planes and around all the three axes:

- The **flexion** and **extension**/hyperextension occur in sagittal plane around the frontal axis.
- The **abduction** and **adduction** occur in frontal plane around the sagittal axis.

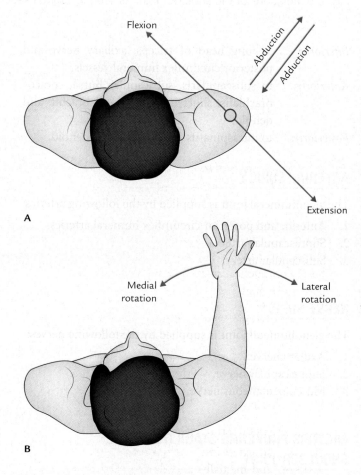

Fig. 6.9 Planes of movements of the shoulder joint: **A**, planes of flexion and extension, and abduction and adduction; **B**, plane of medial and lateral rotation.

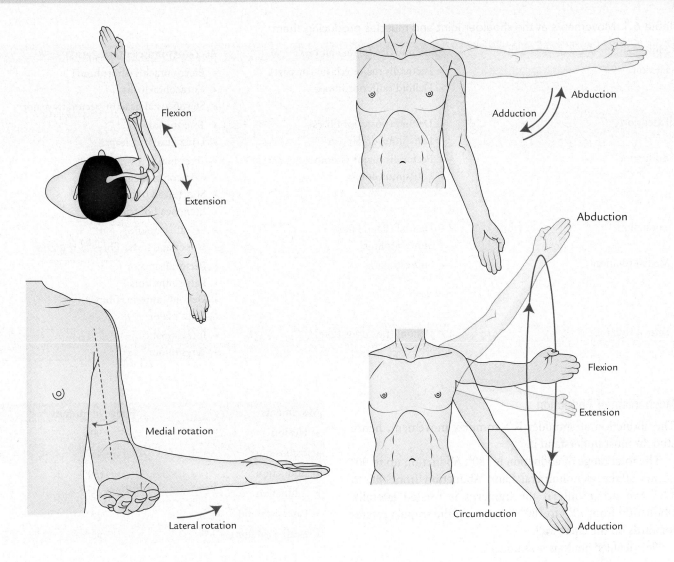

Fig. 6.10 Movements of the shoulder joint. (*Source:* Fig. 7.4, Page 611, *Gray's Anatomy for Students*, Richard L Drake, Wayne Vogl, Adam WM Mitchell. Copyright Elsevier Inc. 2005, All rights reserved.)

- The **medial** and **lateral rotation** occur in transverse plane around the vertical axis.
- The circumduction is really only a combination of all above movements.

N.B. *Plane of the glenohumeral joint:* The scapula does not lie in the coronal plane but is so oriented that its glenoid cavity faces forwards and laterally, therefore the plane of this joint lies obliquely at about 45° to the sagittal plane. The movements of shoulder joint are, therefore, described in relation to this plane.

The details are as under:

1. **Flexion and extension:** During flexion, the arm moves forwards and medially, and during extension it moves backwards and laterally. These movements take place parallel to the plane of glenoid cavity (i.e., midway between the coronal and sagittal plane).

2. **Abduction and adduction:** During abduction, the arm moves anterolaterally away from the trunk and during adduction the arm moves posteromedially towards the trunk. These movements occur at right angle to the plane of flexion and extension (i.e., in the plane of the body of the scapula).

3. **Medial and lateral rotation:** These movements are best demonstrated in midflexed elbow. In this position, the hand moves medially in medial rotation and laterally in lateral rotation.

4. **Circumduction:** The circumduction at glenohumeral joint is an orderly sequence of flexion, abduction, extension and adduction or the reverse. During this movement the upper limb moves along a circle.

The muscles producing the various movements at the shoulder joint are listed in Table 6.1.

Table 6.1 Movements at the shoulder joint and muscles producing them

Movements	Main muscles (prime movers)	Accessory muscles (synergists)
Flexion	• Pectoralis major (clavicular part) • Deltoid (anterior fibres)	• Biceps brachii (short head) • Coracobrachialis • Sternocostal head of pectoralis major
Extension	• Deltoid (posterior fibres) • Latissimus dorsi	• Teres major • Long head of triceps
Adduction	• Pectoralis major (sternocostal part) • Latissimus dorsi	• Teres major • Coracobrachialis • Short head of biceps • Long head of triceps
Abduction	• Deltoid (lateral fibres) • Supraspinatus	• Serratus anterior • Upper and lower fibres of trapezius
Medial rotation	• Subscapularis	• Pectoralis major • Latissimus dorsi • Deltoid (anterior fibres) • Teres major
Lateral rotation	• Deltoid (posterior fibres)	• Infraspinatus • Teres minor

Mechanism of Abduction

The abduction at shoulder is a complex movement, hence student must understand it.

The total range of abduction is 180°. Abduction up to 90° occurs at the glenohumeral joint. Abduction from 90° to 120° can occur only if the humerus is rotated laterally. Abduction from 120° to 180° can occur if the scapula rotates forwards on the chest wall.

The detailed analysis is as under:

1. The articular surface of the head of humerus permits elevation of arm only up to 90°, because when the upper end of humerus is elevated, to 90° its greater tubercle impinges upon the under surface of the acromion and can only be released by lateral rotation of the arm.
2. Therefore, the arm rotates laterally and carries abduction up to 120°.
3. Abduction above 120° can occur only if scapula rotates. So that the scapula rotates forwards on the chest wall.

N.B.

• The humerus and scapula move in the ratio of 2:1 during abduction, i.e., for every 15° elevation, the humerus moves 10° and scapula moves 5°.
• During early and terminal stages of elevation, the sternoclavicular and acromioclavicular joints move maximum, respectively.

Range of motion (ROM) of various movements

During clinical examination, the knowledge of range of motion of various movements is very important. It is given in the box below:

Movements	Range of motion
• Flexion	90°
• Extension	45°
• Abduction	180°
• Adduction	45°
• Lateral rotation	45°
• Medial rotation	55°

Clinical correlation

• **Dislocation of the shoulder joint:** Dislocation of shoulder joint mostly occurs inferiorly because the joint is least supported on this aspect. It often injures the axillary nerve because of its close relation to the inferior part of the joint capsule. However, clinically, it is described as anterior or posterior dislocation indicating whether the humeral head has descended anterior or posterior or to the infraglenoid tubercle of the scapula and long head of the triceps.

  The dislocation is usually caused by excessive extension and lateral rotation of the humerus.

  Clinically, it presents as (Fig. 6.11):
  (a) Hollow in rounded contour of the shoulder
  (b) Prominence of shoulder tip

• **Frozen shoulder (adhesive capsulitis):** It is a clinical condition characterized by pain and uniform limitation of all movements of the shoulder joint, though there are no radiological changes in the joint. It occurs due to shrinkage of the joint capsule, hence the name *adhesive capsulitis*. This condition is generally seen in individuals with 40–60 years of age.

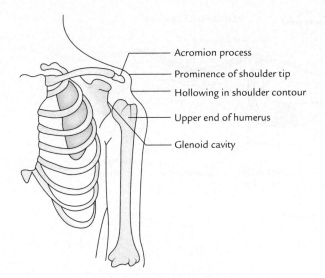

- Acromion process
- Prominence of shoulder tip
- Hollowing in shoulder contour
- Upper end of humerus
- Glenoid cavity

Fig. 6.11 Dislocation of the shoulder joint. Note the changes in the contour of shoulder.

- **Rotator cuff disorders:** The rotator cuff disorders include calcific supraspinatus tendinitis, subacromial the rotator cuff represent overall the most common cause of shoulder pain. The rotator cuff is commonly injured during repetitive use of the upper limb above the horizontal level (e.g., in throwing sports, swimming, and weight lifting). The deposition of calcium in the supraspinatus tendon is common. The calcium deposition irritates the overlying subacromial bursa causing *subacromial bursitis*. Consequently, when the arm is abducted the inflamed bursa is caught between tendon and acromion impingement, which causes severe pain. In most people, pain occurs during 60°–120° of abduction (*painful arc syndrome*). The rotator cuff disorders usually occur in males after 50 years of age.

  The pain due to *subacromial bursitis* is elicited when the deltoid is pressed just below the acromion, when the arm is adducted. The pain cannot be elicited by the pressure on the same point when the arm is abducted because the bursa slips/disappears under the acromion process (**Dawbarn's sign**).

ACROMIOCLAVICULAR JOINT (Fig. 6.12)

Type

It is a plane type of the synovial joint between the lateral end of the clavicle and acromion process of the scapula. The acromioclavicular joint is located about 2.5 cm medial to the point of the shoulder.

Articular Surfaces

These are small facets present on the lateral end of clavicle and the medial margin of the acromion process of the scapula. The articular surfaces are covered with fibrocartilage. The joint cavity is subdivided by an incomplete wedge-shaped articular disc.

Joint Capsule

It is thin, lax fibrous sac attached to the margins of articular surfaces.

Ligaments

These are acromioclavicular and coracoclavicular ligaments.

1. **Acromioclavicular ligament:** It is a fibrous band that extends from acromion to the clavicle. It strengthens the acromioclavicular joint superiorly.
2. **Coracoclavicular ligament:** It lies a little away from the joint itself but play an important role in maintaining the integrity of the joint.

   The coracoclavicular ligament consists of two parts: (a) conoid and (b) trapezoid, which are united posteriorly and often separated by a bursa.
   - *The conoid ligament* is an inverted cone-shaped fibrous band. The apex is attached to the root of the coracoid process just lateral to the scapular notch and base is attached to the conoid tubercle on the inferior surface of the clavicle.
   - *The trapezoid ligament* is a horizontal fibrous band that stretches from upper surface of the coracoid process to the trapezoid line on the inferior surface of lateral end of the clavicle.

N.B. The *coracoclavicular ligament* is largely responsible for suspending the weight of the scapula and upper limb from clavicle.

The coracoclavicular ligament is the strongest ligament of the upper limb.

Movements

The acromioclavicular joint permits the rotation of acromion of scapula at the acromial end of the clavicle. These movements are associated with movements of scapula at the scapulothoracic joint/linkage.

STERNOCLAVICULAR JOINT (Fig. 6.12)

Type

The sternoclavicular joint is a saddle type of the synovial joint.

Articular Surfaces

The rounded sternal end of clavicle articulates with the shallow socket at the superolateral angle of the manubrium sterni and adjacent part of the 1st costal cartilage. The medial

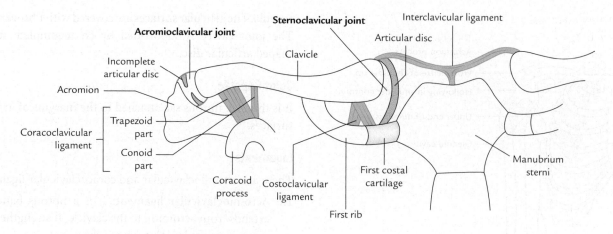

Fig. 6.12 Sternoclavicular and acromioclavicular joints.

end of clavicle rises higher than the manubrium, hence it poorly fits into its shallow socket. But a strong thick articular disc of fibrocartilage attached superiorly to the clavicle and 1st costal cartilage inferiorly prevents the displacement of the medial end of the clavicle.

The articular surface of clavicle is convex from above downwards and slightly concave from front to back. The articular surface of sternum is reciprocally curved. The articular surfaces are covered with fibrocartilage.

Articular Capsule

The joint capsule is attached to the margins of the articular surfaces including the periphery of the articular disc. The synovial membrane lines the internal surface of the fibrous joint capsule, extending to the edges of the articular disc.

Ligaments

1. **Anterior and posterior sternoclavicular ligaments:** They reinforce the joint capsule anteriorly and posteriorly. The posterior ligament is weaker than the anterior ligament.
2. **Interclavicular ligament:** It is T-shaped and connects the sternal ends of two clavicles and strengthens the joint capsule superiorly. In between, it is attached to the superior border of the suprasternal notch.
3. **Costoclavicular ligament:** It anchors the inferior surface of the sternal end of clavicle to the first rib and adjoining part of its cartilage.

Movements

The sternoclavicular joint allows the movements of pectoral girdle. This joint is critical to the movement of the clavicle.

Clinical correlation

- **Dislocation of the sternoclavicular joint:** It is rare because the sternoclavicular (SC) joint is extremely strong. However, dislocation of this joint in people below 25 years of age may result from fractures through the epiphyseal plate because epiphysis at the sternal end of clavicle does not unite until 23–25 years of age. The medial end is usually dislocated anteriorly. Backward dislocation is prevented by the costoclavicular ligament.

- **Transmission of weight of the upper limb:** The weight of the upper limb is transmitted from scapula to the clavicle through *coracoclavicular ligament*, and then from clavicle to sternum through *sternoclavicular joint*. Some of the weight is transmitted to the first rib through *costoclavicular ligament* (Fig. 1.4). When a person falls on the outstretched hand the force of blow is usually transmitted along the length of the clavicle, i.e., along its long axis. The clavicle may fracture at the junction of its middle and lateral third but it is rare for the SC joint to dislocate.

- **Dislocation of the acromioclavicular joint:** It may occur following a severe blow on the superolateral part of the shoulder. In severe form, both acromioclavicular and coracoclavicular ligaments are torn. Consequently the shoulder separates from the clavicle and falls because of the weight of the limb. The acromioclavicular joint dislocation is often termed *shoulder separation*.

SCAPULOTHORACIC ARTICULATION/LINKAGE

The scapulothoracic articulation is not a true articulation but a functional linkage between the ventral aspect of the scapula and lateral aspect of the thoracic wall. The linkage is provided by serratus anterior muscle. The movements of scapula around the chest wall are facilitated by the presence of loose areolar tissue between the serratus anterior and subscapularis muscles.

SCAPULOHUMERAL RHYTHM

Most of the movements at the shoulder involve the movements of humerus and scapula simultaneously and not successively.

According to older concept, abduction of shoulder up to 90° occurs at the glenohumeral/scapulohumeral joint and beyond 90° the movement is essentially an upward rotation of the scapula.

But recently it has been established beyond doubt by fluoroscopic studies that there is rotation of scapula even from the initial stages of abduction at the shoulder. Thus there is rhythm between the scapular and humeral movements called *scapulo-humeral rhythm.* In abduction, there is 1° of lateral rotation of scapula for every 2° of movement at the scapulo-humeral joint. The paralysis of muscles, which interferes with this rhythm seriously affects the movements of the shoulder.

Golden Facts to Remember

- Primary articulation of shoulder girdle — Glenohumeral joint
- Most freely mobile joint in the body ⎫
- Most commonly dislocated joint in the body ⎬ Shoulder joint
- Most common joint to undergo recurrent dislocation ⎭
- Commonest dislocation of the shoulder joint — Inferior dislocation
- Largest synovial bursa in the body — Subacromial/subdeltoid bursa
- Most important factor to provide stability to the shoulder joint ⎫
⎬ Musculotendinous cuff/rotator cuff
- Guardian of the shoulder joint ⎭
- Most common cause of the shoulder pain — Disorders of the rotator cuff
- Chief anchor of the acromioclavicular joint — Coracoclavicular ligament
- Chief anchor of the sternoclavicular joint — Articular disc
- Strongest ligament of the upper limb — Coracoclavicular ligament

Clinical Case Study

A 54-year-old executive officer fell down from the stairs. He was feeling severe pain in his right shoulder. He was taken to the emergency OPD. On examination the doctors observed that the officer was sitting on the stool with right arm by the side of his body and he was supporting his right elbow with his left hand. The inspection of right shoulder revealed loss of its normal rounded contour and loss of skin sensations in the lower half of the deltoid region. Any attempt to perform active or passive movement was stopped by severe pain in shoulder. He was diagnosed as a case of **dislocation of right shoulder.**

Questions

1. Why shoulder joint is commonly dislocated?

2. What is the most common type of shoulder dislocation?
3. What is the cause of loss of normal rounded contour of the shoulder?
4. What is the cause for loss of skin sensation in the lower half of the deltoid region?

Answers

1. Because of the disproportionate size of articular surfaces and lax joint capsule.
2. Inferior (commonly called *anterior dislocation* by the clinicians).
3. Because the pull of pectoralis major and subscapularis muscles had displaced the upper end of humerus medially.
4. Injury to the axillary nerve.

CHAPTER 7

Cutaneous Innervation, Venous Drainage and Lymphatic Drainage of the Upper Limb

CUTANEOUS INNERVATION

The knowledge of cutaneous innervation is essential during physical examination of the patient. The sensory testing of skin of the upper limb is performed whenever a damage of nerves arising from C3 to T2 spinal segments is suspected. Light touch and pinprick are the main sensations tested routinely, but the temperature, two-point discrimination, and vibration are also tested in special cases. The area of anesthesia and paresthesia are mapped out and matched with the dermatomal distribution. In compression of nerve roots of spinal nerves arising from C3 to T2 spinal segments due to spondylitis, pain is referred to the respective dermatomes.

CUTANEOUS NERVES OF THE UPPER LIMB

The cutaneous nerves of the upper limb are derived from the ventral rami of spinal nerves derived from C3 to T2 spinal segments. These nerves are derived from the ventral rami because the upper limb buds develop from ventral half of the body opposite the C3–T2 spinal segments. During dissection, the cutaneous nerves are seen to arise from three sources, viz.

1. Cervical plexus.
2. Brachial plexus.
3. Intercostobrachial nerve.

The cutaneous nerves carry sensations of pain, touch, temperature, and pressure. In addition, they carry sympathetic fibres, which supply sweat glands, dermal arterioles, and arrector pili muscles. The effect of sympathetic stimulation on skin, therefore, is sudomotor, vasomotor, and pilomotor, respectively. The area of skin supplied by a single spinal nerve/segment is termed 'dermatome'. *The cutaneous nerves contain fibres from more than one spinal nerve and each spinal nerve provides fibres to more than one cutaneous nerve.*

As a result, skin areas supplied by the cutaneous nerves do not correspond with dermatomes.

CUTANEOUS NERVES SUPPLYING DIFFERENT REGIONS OF THE UPPER LIMB (Fig. 7.1)

These are as follows:

1. **Pectoral region:**
   Above the 2nd rib, this region is supplied by the **supraclavicular nerves** (C3, C4) and below the 2nd rib by the intercostal nerves (T2–T6).

2. **Axilla:**
   The skin of the armpit is supplied by:
   (a) intercostobrachial nerve (T2) and
   (b) small branches from T3.

3. **Shoulder:**
   (a) Upper half of the deltoid region is supplied by the **supraclavicular nerves** (C3, C4).
   (b) Lower half of the deltoid region is supplied by the **upper lateral cutaneous nerve** of the arm, which is a cutaneous branch of the axillary nerve.

4. **Arm (brachium):**
   (a) *Upper medial part* of the arm is supplied by the **intercostobrachial nerve** (T2) derived from 2nd intercostal.
   (b) *Lower medial part* of the arm is supplied by the **medial cutaneous nerve of the arm** (T1, T2) from medial cord of the brachial plexus.
   (c) *Upper lateral half* of the arm is supplied by the **upper lateral cutaneous nerve** of the arm from axillary nerve.
   (d) *Lower lateral half* of the arm is supplied by the **lower lateral cutaneous nerve** of the arm (C5, C6) from radial nerve.
   (e) *Posterior aspect* of the arm is supplied by the **posterior cutaneous nerve** of the arm (C5) from radial nerve.

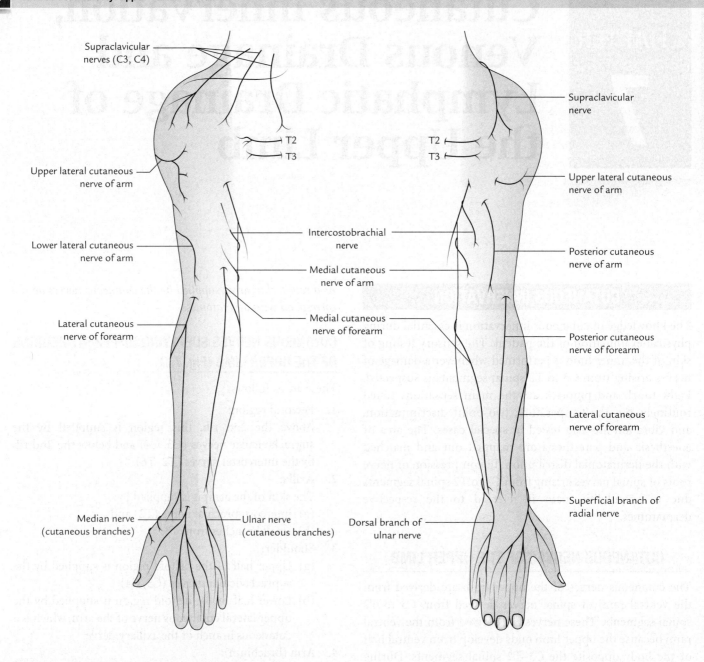

Fig. 7.1 Cutaneous innervation of the upper limb.

FOREARM (ANTEBRACHIUM)

It is supplied by *medial, lateral,* and *posterior cutaneous nerves* derived from the medial, lateral, and posterior cords of the brachial plexus, respectively.

- *Medial side* of the forearm is supplied by the **medial cutaneous nerve** of the forearm (C8, T1) from the medial cord of the brachial plexus. It becomes cutaneous halfway down the arm along the basilic vein.
- *Lateral side* of the forearm is supplied by the **lateral cutaneous nerve** of the forearm (C5, C6) from musculocutaneous nerve from the lateral cord of the brachial plexus. It is the continuation of the

musculocutaneous nerve. It emerges at the lateral border of the biceps and divides into anterior and posterior branches.
- *Posterior side* of the forearm is supplied by the **posterior cutaneous nerve** of the forearm (C6, C7, C8) from radial nerve, a branch from the posterior cord of the brachial plexus. It runs down the posterior aspect of forearm up to the wrist.

HAND

1. **Palm of the hand**
   (a) Lateral two-third of the palm is supplied by the palmar cutaneous branch of the median nerve.

(b) Medial one-third of the palm is supplied by the palmar cutaneous branch of the ulnar nerve.

2. **Dorsum of the hand**
   (a) *Lateral two-third of the dorsum of hand* is supplied by the superficial terminal branch of the radial nerve (superficial radial nerve).
   (b) *Medial one-third of the dorsum of hand* is supplied by the dorsal branch/posterior cutaneous branch of the ulnar nerve.

DIGITS

1. Palmar aspects of the lateral 3½ digits and their dorsal aspects up to distal half of the middle phalanges are supplied by the digital branches of median nerve.
2. Palmar aspects of the medial 1½ digit and their dorsal aspects up to distal half of the middle phalanges by the palmar digital branches of the ulnar nerve.
3. Dorsal aspects of the lateral 3½ digits up to proximal half of their middle phalanges are supplied by the digital branches of the radial nerve.
4. Dorsal aspects of the medial 1½ digit up to their middle phalanges are supplied by the digital branches of the ulnar nerve.

DERMATOMES OF THE UPPER LIMB
(Figs 7.2 and 7.3)

As already mentioned, the area of the skin supplied by a single spinal nerve is called **dermatome.**

In the trunk, the arrangement of dermatomes is simple (typical) because spinal nerves supplying it do not form plexuses and are arranged segmentally. A **typical dermatome** extends on the side of the trunk from the anterior median line to the posterior median line.

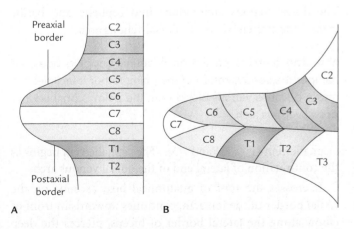

Fig. 7.2 Arrangement of dermatomes in the developing upper limb: **A**, simple dermatomal pattern to begin with C5 supplying the preaxial strip and T1 the postaxial strip; **B**, definitive dermatomal pattern of the upper limb bud.

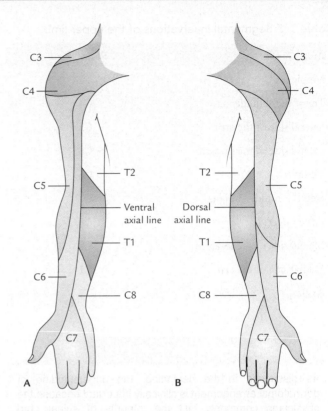

Fig. 7.3 Dermatomes of the upper limb: **A**, anterior aspect; **B**, dorsal aspect.

In the limbs, the arrangement of dermatomes is complicated because of the rotation of the limbs during their development. It becomes further complicated because spinal nerves supplying them form plexuses. (For details, see Chapter 5 of *Textbook of Clinical Neuroanatomy,* 2e by Vishram Singh.) During development, before rotation each limb has preaxial and postaxial borders with former being directed towards the head. The digits along the preaxial border are thumb in the upper limb and big toe in the lower limb. During rotation of the limbs, the upper limb rotates laterally. As a result its preaxial border and thumb lie on the lateral side. The lower limb rotates medially. Therefore, its preaxial border and big toe lie on the medial side. Consequently the dermatomes are arranged consecutively downwards on the lateral side of the upper limb and upwards on the medial side of the upper limb.

To be very precise, the dermatomes of the upper limb are arranged in a numerical sequence as follows:

1. From the shoulder to the thumb, along the preaxial border by C3–C6 spinal segments.
2. From the thumb to the little finger by C6–C8 spinal segments.
3. From the little finger to the axilla along the postaxial border by C8–T2 spinal segments.

The segmental innervation is summarized in Table 7.1.

Table 7.1 Segmental innervations of the upper limb

Area	Segment
Nipple	T4
Tip of the shoulder	C4
Lateral side of the arm	C5
Lateral side of the forearm	C6
Thumb	C6
Hand + middle 3 digits	C7
Little finger	C8
Medial side of the forearm	C8
Medial side of the arm	T1
Axilla	T2

Clinical correlation

As discussed in the beginning, the understanding of dermatomal arrangement is clinically important because the physicians commonly test the integrity of spinal cord segments from C3 to T2 by performing the sensory examination for touch, pain, and temperature. This is so because the sensory loss of the skin following injuries to the cord conforms to the dermatome.

N.B. The students must remember that there is varying degrees of overlapping of adjacent dermatomes. Consequently the area of sensory loss following damage to the cord segments is always less than the area of distribution of the dermatomes.

VENOUS DRAINAGE OF THE UPPER LIMB

The veins draining the upper limb, as elsewhere in the body, are divided into two sets/groups (a) superficial and (b) deep.

The **superficial veins** are located in the superficial fascia and are easily accessible. Being easily accessible, they are frequently used by the clinicians for drawing blood samples or for giving intravenous injections.

The **deep veins** lie deep to muscles and accompany arteries as *venae comitantes*.

SUPERFICIAL VEINS

Superficial veins have the following **general features**:

1. The superficial veins lie in the superficial fascia.
2. The superficial veins have a tendency to run away form the pressure sites, hence they are absent in the palm,

along the ulnar border of the forearm, and back of the elbow.
3. There are two major superficial veins, one along the preaxial border and the other along the postaxial border of the limb. The preaxial vein (cephalic vein) is longer than the postaxial vein (basilic vein), but the postaxial basilic vein drains more efficiently. The load of long cephalic vein is greatly relieved as a good amount of its blood is transferred to the efficient basilic vein by the median cubital vein (communicate channel).

The superficial veins are accompanied by the cutaneous nerves and superficial lymphatics.

Superficial veins comprise:

1. Dorsal venous arch
2. Cephalic vein
3. Basilic vein
4. Median cubital vein

Dorsal venous arch (Fig. 7.4): The dorsal venous arch is a network of veins on the dorsum of hand. It presents irregular arrangement of veins usually with its transverse element, which lies 2–3 cm proximal to the heads of metatarsals.

Tributaries

The tributaries of dorsal venous arch are:

1. Three dorsal metacarpal veins.
2. A dorsal digital vein from the medial side of little finger.
3. A dorsal digital vein from the lateral side of index finger.
4. Two dorsal digital veins of the thumb.
5. Veins draining palm of hand. These are (a) veins that pass around the margins of the hand and (b) perforating veins, which pass dorsally through the interosseous spaces.

The dorsal venous arch drains into cephalic and basilic veins—the efferent vessels of dorsal venous arch.

N.B. The pressure on the palm during gripping does not hamper the venous return of the palm, rather it facilities the return because venous blood from the palm is drained into dorsal venous arch.

Cephalic vein (Figs 7.4 and 7.5): The cephalic vein begins as the continuation of lateral end of the dorsal venous arch.

It crosses the roof of anatomical box, ascends on the radial border of the forearm, continues upwards in front of elbow along the lateral border of biceps, pierces the deep fascia at the lower border of the pectoralis major, runs in cleft between the deltoid and pectoralis major (deltopectoral groove) up to the infraclavicular fossa, where it pierces the clavipectoral fascia and drains into the axillary vein.

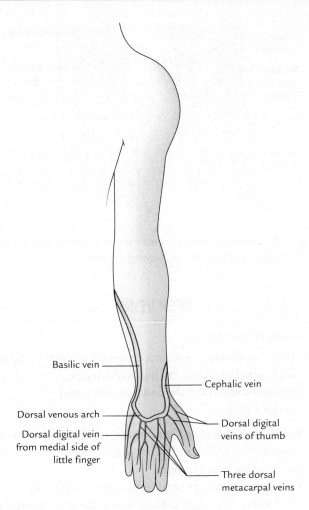

Fig. 7.4 Dorsal venous arch and initial parts of the courses of cephalic and basilic veins.

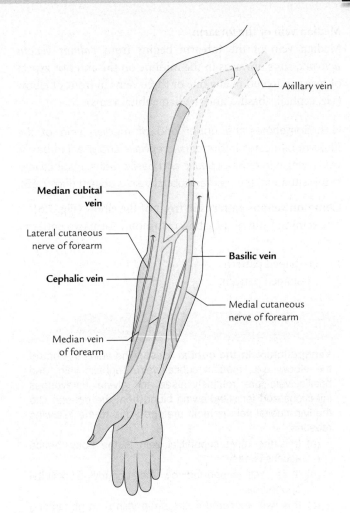

Fig. 7.5 Cephalic and basilic veins.

N.B.

- At elbow, greater amount of blood from the cephalic vein is shunted into the basilic vein through *median cubital vein*.
- Cephalic vein is accompanied by the *lateral cutaneous nerve of the forearm*.
- An accessory cephalic vein from back of the forearm (occasional) ends in the cephalic vein below the elbow.
- Cephalic vein is the *preaxial vein of the upper limb* and corresponds to the *great saphenous vein of the lower limb*.

Basilic vein (Figs 7.4 and 7.5): The basilic vein begins as the continuation of the medial end of the dorsal venous arch of the hand. It runs upwards along the back of the medial border of the forearm, winds round this border near the elbow to reach the anterior aspect of the forearm, where it continues upwards in front of the elbow along the medial side of the biceps brachii up to the middle of the arm, where it pierces deep fascia, unites with the brachial veins and runs along the medial side of the brachial artery to become continuous with the axillary vein at the lower border of the teres major.

N.B.

- Basilic vein is the postaxial vein of the upper limb and corresponds to the *short saphenous vein of the lower limb*.
- About 2.5 cm above the medial epicondyle of humerus, it is joined by the median cubital vein.
- It is accompanied by the *medial cutaneous nerve of the forearm*.

Median cubital vein (Fig. 7.5): It is a communicating venous channel between the cephalic and basilic veins, which shunts blood from the cephalic vein to the basilic vein.

It begins from the cephalic vein, 2.5 cm below the elbow bend, runs obliquely upwards and medially to end in the basilic vein, 2.5 cm above the bend of elbow.

The important features of median cubital vein are as follows:

- It is separated from brachial artery by the bicipital aponeurosis.
- It communicates with the deep veins through a perforator vein, which pierces the bicipital aponeurosis.
- It receives median vein of the forearm.
- It shunts blood from cephalic vein to the basilic vein.

Median vein of the forearm

Median vein of the forearm begins from *palmar venous network*, runs upwards in the midline on the anterior aspect of forearm to end in any one of three veins in front of elbow (viz. cephalic, basilic, and median cubital veins).

N.B. Sometimes the upper end of *median vein of the forearm* bifurcates into *median cephalic* and *median basilic veins*, which join the cephalic and basilic veins, respectively. In this situation, the median cubital vein is absent (Fig. 7.6B).

Common venous patterns in front of the elbow (Fig. 7.6)

The veins in front of the elbow commonly form two patterns, viz.

1. H-shaped pattern.
2. M-shaped pattern.

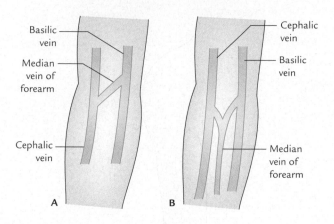

Fig. 7.6 Common venous patterns in front of the elbow: A, H-shaped pattern; B, M-shaped pattern.

Clinical correlation

Venepuncture in the cubital fossa: The veins in front of the elbow, e.g., median cubital vein, cephalic vein, and basilic vein are routinely used for giving intravenous injections and for withdrawing blood from the donors. The median cubital vein is most preferred due to the following reasons:

(a) It is the most superficial vein in the body, hence access is easy.

(b) It is well supported by the underlying bicipital aponeurosis.

(c) It is well anchored to the deep vein by a perforating vein, hence it does not slip during procedure.

- The cephalic vein is preferred for hemodialysis in the patients with chronic renal failure (CRF), to remove waste products from blood.
- The cut-down of cephalic vein in the deltopectoral groove is preferred when the superior vena cava infusion is necessary.
- The basilic vein is preferred for *cardiac catheterization* for the following reasons:

(a) The diameter of basilic *vein increases as it* ascends from cubital fossa to the axillary vein.

(b) It is in direct line with the axillary vein. To enter the right atrium the catheter passes in succession as follows:

Basilic vein → axillary vein → subclavian vein → brachiocephalic vein → superior vena cava → right atrium of the heart.

- The cephalic vein is not preferred for cardiac catheterization due to the following reasons:

(a) Its diameter does not increase as it ascends.

(b) It joins the axillary vein at a right angle hence it is difficult to maneuver the catheter around sharp cephaloaxillary angle.

(c) In deltopectoral groove, it frequently divides into small branches. One of these branches ascends over the clavicle and joins the external jugular vein.

DEEP VEINS

The deep veins comprise:

(a) venae comitantes, which accompany the large arteries, such as radial, ulnar, and brachial arteries,

(b) venae comitantes of the brachial artery, and

(c) axillary vein.

Venae comitantes of the radial and ulnar arteries accompany the radial and ulnar arteries, respectively, and join to form the brachial veins.

Venae comitantes are small veins, one on each side of the brachial artery. They join axillary vein at the lower border of the teres major muscle. The medial one often joins the basilic vein.

Axillary vein begins as a continuation of basilic vein at the lower border of the teres major muscle and runs through axilla, passes through its apex to continue as subclavian vein at the outer border of the first rib (for details see Chapter 4, page 52).

LYMPHATIC DRAINAGE OF THE UPPER LIMB (Fig. 7.7)

The lymphatic drainage of the upper limb follows the unnamed lymph vessels, which originate in the hand and run upwards towards the axilla. When they reach cubital fossa, the lymph passes through **cubital nodes**. From here lymph vessels run superiorly to drain into the axillary lymph nodes.

LYMPH VESSELS

The lymph vessels draining the lymph from the upper limb, as elsewhere in the body, are divided into two groups: superficial and deep.

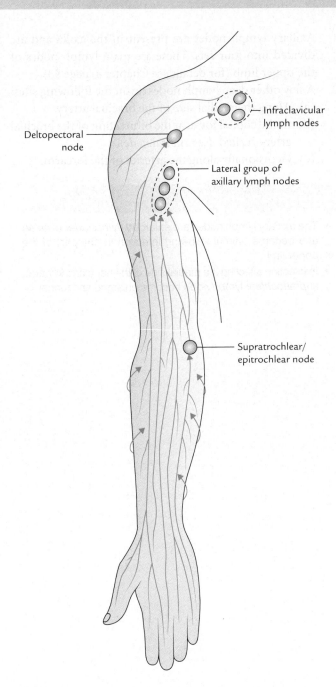

Fig. 7.7 Lymphatic drainage of the upper limb.

SUPERFICIAL LYMPH VESSELS

The superficial lymph vessels are located in the subcutaneous tissue. They are much more numerous than the deep lymph vessels. They generally accompany the superficial veins.

The superficial lymph vessels drain the lymph from skin and subcutaneous tissue. They course upwards towards the axilla. Most of them end in the axillary lymph nodes.

Those from lateral side of the limb and *lateral two digits* follow the cephalic vein and drain into the infraclavicular lymph nodes.

Those from medial side of the limb and *medial three digits* follow the basilic vein and drain into the lateral group of axillary nodes.

Some of the medial lymph vessels terminate in the **supratrochlear** or **epitrochlear nodes**, which are situated just above the medial epicondyle along the basilic vein.

A few lymph vessels drain the thumb end in the deltopectoral lymph nodes. The efferents from these nodes pierce the clavipectoral fascia to drain in the apical group of axillary nodes.

N.B.

- Almost all the superficial lymph vessels of the upper limb drain into *lateral group of axillary nodes*.
- Lymph from palm is drained into the lymph plexus on the dorsum of the hand.
- *Vertical area of lymph shed* is in the middle of the back of arm and forearm: The lymph vessels from the back of the arm and forearm curve around the medial and lateral borders of limb to reach the front of the limb, thus forming a vertical area of lymph shed.

DEEP LYMPH VESSELS

The deep lymph vessels are much less numerous than the superficial lymph vessels. They drain structures lying deep to deep fascia, viz. muscles. The deep lymph vessels course along the arteries and drain into the lateral group of the axillary lymph nodes.

Clinical correlation

- **Lymphangitis:** The inflammation of the lymph vessels is termed *lymphangitis*. It usually follows trivial injuries, e.g., cuts and pin-pricks, to any part of the upper limb. In acute lymphangitis, the lymph vessels may be seen underneath the skin as *red streaks*, which are tender (i.e., painful to touch).
- **Lymphedema:** The obstruction of lymph vessels may cause edema (i.e., swelling) in the area of drainage due to accumulation of tissue fluid.

LYMPH NODES

The lymph nodes draining the upper limb are divided into two groups: (a) superficial and (b) deep.

SUPERFICIAL LYMPH NODES

They lie in the superficial fascia, along the superficial vein. These are as follows:

1. Infraclavicular nodes, one or two in number, lie on the clavipectoral fascia along the cephalic vein. They drain

lymph from thumb including its web and upper part of the breast.

2. Deltopectoral node, lie in the deltopectoral groove along the cephalic vein just before it pierces the deep fascia. It is thought to be displaced infraclavicular node. It drains the lymph from the breast and adjoining small structures.

3. Superficial cubital/supratrochlear nodes lie 5 cm above the medial epicondyle along the basilic vein. They drain the lymph from the ulnar side of the hand and forearm.

DEEP LYMPH NODES

The deep lymph nodes are as follows:

1. Axillary lymph nodes are present in the axilla and are divided into four sets. These are main lymph nodes of the upper limb (for details see Chapter 4, page 53).

2. A few other deep lymph nodes lie on the following sites:
   (a) Along the medial side of the brachial artery.
   (b) In the cubital fossa, at the bifurcation of the brachial artery (called *deep cubital node*).
   (c) Occasionally along the arteries of the forearm.

Clinical correlation

- The axillary lymph nodes are enlarged (*lymphadenopathy*) and become painful following infection in any part of the upper limb.
- In infection affecting the medial side of the hand and forearm, *supratrochlear lymph node* become enlarged and tender.

Golden Facts to Remember

▶ Most prominent superficial vein in the body	Median cubital vein
▶ Most commonly used vein for venepuncture	
▶ Most preferred vein for cardiac catheterization	Basilic vein
▶ Commonest pattern of the superficial veins in front of elbow	H-shaped
▶ Most of the superficial lymph vessels of the upper limb drain into	Lateral group of the axillary lymph nodes
▶ Most distal superficial lymph node in the upper limb	Supratrochlear/epitrochlear node
▶ Commonest cause of lymphedema of the upper limb	Removal of the axillary lymph nodes during mastectomy
▶ Longest superficial vein of the upper limb	Cephalic vein
▶ Area of lymph shed in the arm and forearm	Vertical area in the middle of the back of arm and forearm

Clinical Case Study

A 38-year-old female went to the pathologist for routine blood examination. The pathologist asked the technician to collect the blood sample of the lady. While attempting to collect the blood sample from median cubital vein the technician noticed that the blood in the syringe is bright red. He immediately withdrew the needle.

In second attempt, he inserted the needle slightly medial to the previous puncture. The lady felt sharp pain, which radiated to the lateral three digits.

Questions

1. What is median cubital vein?

2. Name the fascial structure, which separates median cubital vein from brachial artery and median nerve.
3. Mention the cause of sharp pain that radiated to the lateral 3½ digits.
4. What does the bright red blood in syringe indicated during collection of the blood sample from the median cubital vein?

Answers

1. It is a communicating vein in front of elbow between the cephalic and basilic vein.
2. Bicipital aponeurosis.
3. Median nerve injury.
4. Puncture of the brachial artery.

Arm

The arm is the part of the upper limb between shoulder and elbow. The bone of the arm—the humerus articulates above with scapula to form shoulder joint and below with radius and ulna to form elbow joint. The humerus is almost entirely covered by muscles. The **primary neurovascular bundle of the arm** is located on the medial side of the arm, hence protected by the limb, which it serves. It consists of brachial artery, the basilic vein, and median, ulnar, and radial nerves.

SURFACE LANDMARKS

The following bony landmarks and soft tissue structures can be felt in the living individual:

1. **Greater tubercle of the humerus**—can be felt just below and lateral to the acromion, deep to deltoid with arm lying by the side of the trunk. It forms the most lateral bony point of the shoulder region.
2. **Shaft of the humerus**—can be felt indistinctly in thin individuals.
3. **Medial epicondyle of the humerus**—is the prominent bony projection felt on the medial side of the elbow. The projection is best seen and felt in midflexed elbow.
4. **Lateral epicondyle of the humerus**—can be felt in the upper part of the depression on the posterolateral aspect of the extended elbow.
5. **Medial and lateral supracondylar ridges**—can be felt in the lower one-fourth of the arm as the upward continuations of medial and lateral epicondyles, respectively.
6. **Deltoid muscle**—forms the rounded contour of the shoulder, which becomes prominent on abducting the arm. It covers the upper half of the humerus anteriorly, laterally, and posteriorly and its apex (i.e., tendon) is attached to the lateral side of the middle of humerus on deltoid tuberosity.

7. **Biceps muscle**—forms a conspicuous bulge on the front of arm, which becomes prominent on flexing the elbow. Its tendon can be felt on the front of the elbow.
8. **Brachial artery pulsations**—can be felt in front of the elbow just medial to the tendon of biceps muscle.
9. **Ulnar nerve**—can be rolled by the middle finger in the groove behind the medial epicondyle of the humerus.
10. The **superficial veins in front of elbow** (i.e., cephalic, basilic, and median cubital veins)—become visible when they are distended by applying tight pressure around the arm and then flexing and extending the elbow a few times with clenched fist.
11. **Head of radius**—can be felt in the depression on the posterolateral aspect of the elbow just distal to the lateral epicondyle. The rotation of the head of radius can be felt by supinating and pronating the forearm.
12. **Olecranon process of ulna** (proximal part of ulna)—is readily palpable on the back elbow between the medial and the lateral epicondyles.

COMPARTMENTS OF THE ARM (Fig. 8.1)

The deep fascia encloses the arm like a sleeve. The two fascial septa, one on the medial side and one on the lateral side extend inwards from the fascial sleeve and get attached to the medial and lateral supracondylar ridges of the humerus, respectively. These septa and fascial sleeve divide the arm into anterior and posterior compartments. Each compartment has its own muscles, nerve, and artery.

N.B. Some structures, however, pierce the intermuscular septa to shift from one compartment to the other, viz.

- Ulnar nerve and superior ulnar collateral artery pierce the medial intermuscular septum to enter the posterior compartment.
- Radial nerve and radial collateral artery pierce the lateral intermuscular septum to enter the anterior compartment.

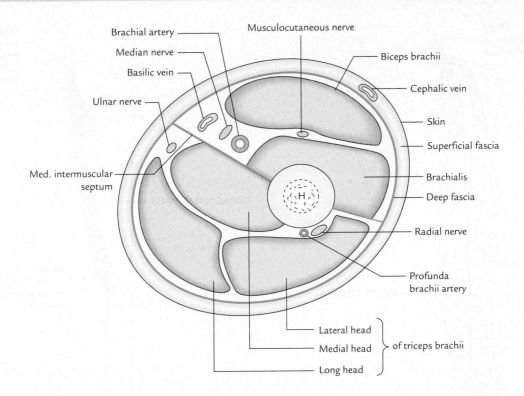

Fig. 8.1 Transverse section of the arm just below the level of insertion of deltoid muscle (H = humerus).

CONTENTS OF THE ANTERIOR COMPARTMENT OF THE ARM

- **Muscles:** Biceps brachii, coracobrachialis, and brachialis.
- **Nerve:** Musculocutaneous nerve.
- **Artery:** Brachial artery.

In addition to the above structures, the following large nerves also pass through the anterior compartment of arm:

- Median nerve.
- Ulnar nerve.
- Radial nerve.

Muscles

Biceps Brachii (Fig. 8.2)

Origin

The biceps brachii muscle arises from scapula by two heads: long and short:

1. **Long head** arises from **supraglenoid tubercle** within the capsule of shoulder joint. Its tendon runs above the head of humerus and emerges from the joint through intertubercular sulcus.
2. **Short head** arises along with coracobrachialis from the tip of the coracoid process.

The two heads join together in the distal third of the arm to form a belly that ends in a tendon, which gives off the *bicipital*

aponeurosis from its medial aspect, opposite the bend of elbow.

Insertion

The biceps muscle is inserted into:

(a) the posterior part of the radial tuberosity by its tendon. A bursa intervenes between the tendon and anterior part of the tuberosity, and
(b) the deep fascia on the medial aspect of forearm by its aponeurosis (bicipital aponeurosis). The aponeurosis protects the underlying brachial artery and median nerve.

Nerve supply

By musculocutaneous nerve (C5, C6, and C7).

Actions

1. It is strong supinator of the forearm, when elbow is flexed. This action is used in screwing movements such as tightening the screw with screw driver.
2. It is a powerful flexor of the forearm, when elbow is extended.
3. It is also a weak flexor of the shoulder joint.

Clinical testing

The biceps brachii is tested by asking the patient to flex the elbow against resistance when the forearm is supinated. In this act, the muscle forms a prominent bulge on the front of the arm.

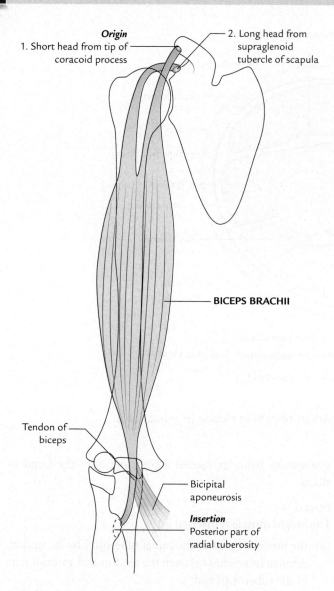

Origin
1. Short head from tip of coracoid process

2. Long head from supraglenoid tubercle of scapula

BICEPS BRACHII

Tendon of biceps

Bicipital aponeurosis

Insertion
Posterior part of radial tuberosity

Fig. 8.2 Origin and insertion of the biceps brachii.

Clinical correlation

Biceps reflex: It is tested during physical examination by tapping the tendon of biceps brachii by reflex hammer with forearm pronated and partially extended at elbow. The normal reflex is brief jerk-like flexion of the elbow. The normal reflex confirms the integrity of musculocutaneous nerve and C5 and C6 spinal segments.

Coracobrachialis (Fig. 8.3)
Origin
From the tip of coracoid process of the scapula along with short head of the biceps brachii.

Insertion
Into the middle of the medial border of the shaft of the humerus.

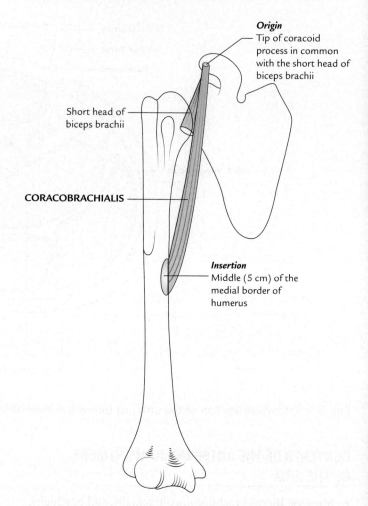

Origin
Tip of coracoid process in common with the short head of biceps brachii

Short head of biceps brachii

CORACOBRACHIALIS

Insertion
Middle (5 cm) of the medial border of humerus

Fig. 8.3 Origin and insertion of the coracobrachialis.

Nerve supply
By musculocutaneous nerve.

Actions
It is a weak flexor and adductor of the arm.

N.B.

• **Morphology of the coracobrachialis:** It represents the muscle of medial compartment of the forelimb of quadrupeds, which is not well-developed in human beings. In some animals, this muscle consists of three heads. In human beings, the upper two heads are fused and musculocutaneous nerve passes between the two fused heads. The lower third head has disappeared in humans. But, occasionally the lower head persists as a fibrous band **(ligament of Struthers)**, which extends between supratrochlear/trochlear spur and medial epicondyle of the humerus (Fig. 2.10). The median nerve and brachial artery then pass deep to the ligament and may be compressed.

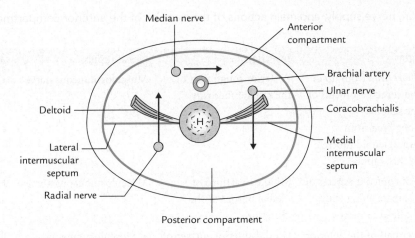

Fig. 8.4 Important events occurring at the level of insertion of the coracobrachialis.

- **Anatomical events at the insertion of coracobrachialis:**
  It is an important landmark as many anatomical events occur at this level (Fig. 8.4):

  1. Circular shaft of the humerus becomes triangular below this level.
  2. Brachial artery passes from medial side of arm to its anterior aspect.
  3. Basilic vein pierces the deep fascia.
  4. Median nerve crosses in front of the brachial artery from the lateral to medial side.
  5. Radial nerve pierces lateral intermuscular septum to pass from the posterior compartment to the anterior compartment.
  6. Ulnar nerve pierces medial intermuscular septum to go into the posterior compartment.
  7. Medial cutaneous nerve of the arm and forearm pierces the deep fascia.
  8. Nutrient artery pierces the humerus.

Brachialis (Fig. 8.5)

Origin

From the front of the lower half of the shaft of humerus. Superiorly the origin of brachialis embraces the insertion of deltoid.

Insertion

Into the anterior surface of the coronoid process of ulna including tuberosity of ulna.

Nerve supply

It has dual innervation:

1. Medial two-third by *musculocutaneous nerve*.
2. Lateral one-third by *radial nerve*.

Actions

It is the untiring strong flexor of the elbow joint hence it is often called 'work-horse of the elbow joint.'

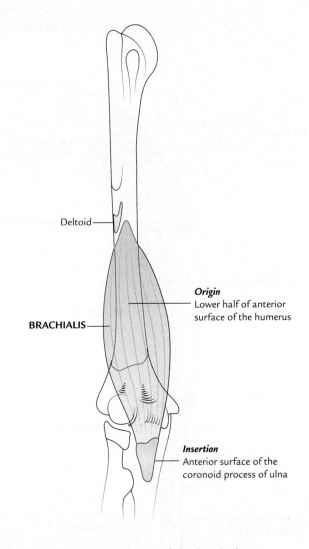

Fig. 8.5 Origin and insertion of the brachialis.

Table 8.1 summarizes the origin, insertion, nerve supply, and actions of muscles of the anterior compartment of the arm.

Table 8.1 Origin, insertion, nerve supply, and main actions of the muscles of the anterior compartment of the arm (i.e., front of the arm)

Muscle	Origin	Insertion	Nerve supply	Actions
Biceps brachii	• *Short head* from tip of the coracoid process of the scapula • *Long head* from supraglenoid tubercle of the scapula	Posterior rough part of the radial tuberosity	Musculocutaneous nerve	• Supination of the forearm when elbow is flexed • Flexion of the forearm when elbow is extended
Coracobrachialis	Tip of coracoid process of the scapula along with short head of biceps	Middle one-third of medial border of the humerus	Musculocutaneous nerve	Helps in flexion and adduction of the arm
Brachialis	Lower half of the anterior surface of the humerus	On the anterior surface of coronoid process of the ulna including ulnar tuberosity	• Musculocutaneous nerve (mainly) • Radial nerve	Flexion of the forearm in all positions

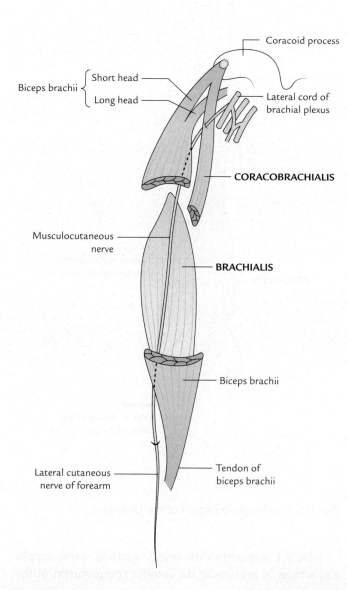

Fig. 8.6 Course and distribution of the musculocutaneous nerve.

Musculocutaneous Nerve (Figs 8.6 and 13.2)

Origin and course

The musculocutaneous nerve is the nerve of the front of arm. It arises from lateral cord of the brachial plexus in the axilla. It runs downwards and laterally, pierces the coracobrachialis which it supplies, then passes between the biceps and brachialis muscles. It appears at the lateral margin of the biceps tendon and pierces the deep fascia just above the elbow and descends over the lateral aspect of the forearm as the *lateral cutaneous nerve of the forearm*.

Branches and distribution

1. **Muscular branches** to the biceps brachii, coracobrachialis, and brachialis.
2. **Cutaneous branch** (the *lateral cutaneous nerve of forearm*) supplies the skin on the front and lateral aspect of the forearm.
3. **Articular branch** to elbow joint through its branch to the brachialis muscle.

Clinical correlation

Injury of the musculocutaneous nerve: Although, it is rare but if occurs it leads to the following signs and symptoms:
• Loss of strong flexion and supination.
• Loss of biceps tendon reflex.
• Loss of sensation along the lateral aspect of the forearm.

Brachial Artery (Fig. 8.7)

The brachial artery is the main artery of the arm. It begins at the lower border of the teres major muscle as a continuation of the axillary artery and terminates in front of the elbow at

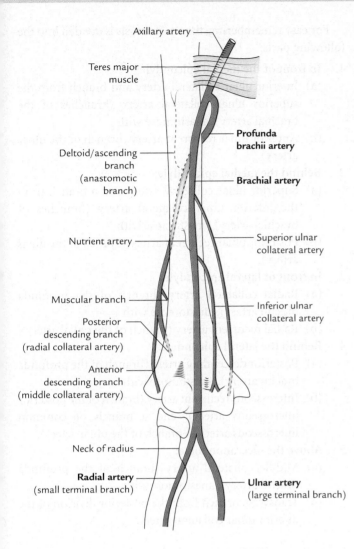

Fig. 8.7 Brachial artery.

N.B. The brachial artery is superficial throughout its course, being covered only by the skin and fasciae, hence easily accessible.

Branches

1. **Muscular branches** to the muscles of the anterior compartment of the arm.
2. **Profunda brachii artery** (largest and first branch). It arises from the posteromedial aspect of the brachial artery just below the lower border of the teres major. It accompanies the radial nerve with which it immediately leaves the *lower triangular intermuscular space* to enter the *spiral groove* on the posterior surface of the humerus.
3. **Nutrient artery to humerus** enters the nutrient foramen of humerus located near the insertion of coracobrachialis.
4. **Superior ulnar collateral artery** arises near the middle of the arm and accompanies the ulnar nerve.
5. **Inferior ulnar collateral (or supratrochlear artery)** arises near the lower end of humerus and divides into the anterior and posterior branches, which take part in the formation of arterial anastomosis around the elbow.
6. **Radial and ulnar arteries** (terminal branches).

Clinical correlation

- **Brachial pulse:** The brachial pulse is commonly felt in the cubital fossa medial to the tendon of biceps and its pulsations are auscultated for *recording the blood pressure.* The biceps tendon is easily palpable on flexing the elbow.

the level of neck of radius by dividing into radial and ulnar arteries.

Relations

Anteriorly   – *In the upper part,* it is related to medial cutaneous nerve of the forearm, which lies in front of it.

  – *In the middle part,* it is crossed by the median nerve from lateral to medial side.

  – *In the lower part,* in the cubital fossa, it is crossed by the bicipital aponeurosis.

Posteriorly   From above downwards, the brachial artery lies successively on long head of triceps, medial head of triceps, coracobrachialis, and brachialis muscles.

Medially   The ulnar nerve and basilic vein in the upper part of the arm; and median nerve in the lower part of the arm.

Laterally   The median nerve, coracobrachialis, and biceps in the upper part of arm and tendon of biceps in the lower part.

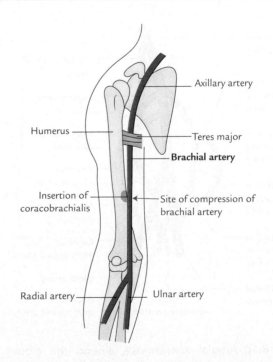

Fig. 8.8 Compression of the brachial artery against humerus.

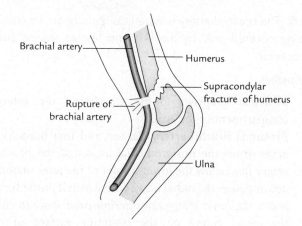

Fig. 8.9 Rupture of the brachial artery in supracondylar fracture of the humerus.

- **Compression of brachial artery:** The brachial artery can be effectively compressed against the shaft of humerus at the level of insertion of coracobrachialis to stop the hemorrhages in the upper limb occurring from any artery distal to the brachial artery, e.g., bleeding wounds of the palmar arterial arches (Fig. 8.8).
- **Rupture of the brachial artery in supracondylar fracture** of the humerus may lead to *Volkmann's ischemic contracture* (Fig. 8.9). For details see Chapter 9, p. 114.

Arterial Anastomosis around the Elbow (Fig. 8.10)

The arterial anastomosis around the elbow takes place between the branches of brachial artery and those from the upper ends of radial and ulnar arteries.

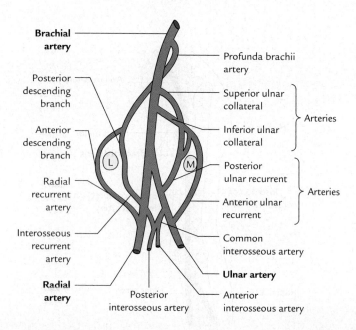

Fig. 8.10 Arterial anastomosis around the elbow joint (L = lateral epicondyle, M = medial epicondyle).

For easy remembering, the anastomosis is divided into the following parts:

1. **In front of the medial epicondyle:**
   (a) Inferior ulnar collateral artery and branch from the superior ulnar collateral artery (branches of the brachial artery), anastomose with
   (b) Anterior ulnar recurrent artery (branch of the ulnar artery).
2. **Behind the medial epicondyle:**
   (a) Superior ulnar collateral artery and a branch from the inferior ulnar collateral artery (branches of brachial artery), anastomose with
   (b) Posterior ulnar recurrent artery (branch of the ulnar artery).
3. **In front of lateral epicondyle:**
   (a) Radial collateral artery (branch of the profunda brachii artery), anastomose with
   (b) Radial recurrent artery (branch of the radial artery).
4. **Behind the lateral epicondyle:**
   (a) Posterior descending artery (branch of the profunda brachii artery), anastomose with
   (b) Interosseous recurrent artery (branch of the posterior interosseous artery); and a branch of common interosseous artery (a branch of the ulnar artery).
5. **Above the olecranon fossa:**
   (a) Middle collateral artery (branch of the profunda brachii artery), anastomose with
   (b) Transverse branch from the posterior division of the inferior ulnar collateral artery.

Large Nerves Passing Through the Arm

These are median, ulnar, and radial nerves:

Median Nerve

The median nerve arises from the lateral and medial cords of the brachial plexus in axilla. It is closely related to the brachial artery throughout its course in the arm. Therefore, it is like the brachial artery, it is superficially located except at elbow where it is crossed by the bicipital aponeurosis.

The relationship of median nerve with the brachial artery in the arm is as under (Fig. 8.11):

1. **In the upper part,** it is lateral to the artery.
2. **In the middle part,** it crosses in front of the artery from lateral to medial side.
3. **In the lower part,** it is medial to the artery up to elbow.

Branches

In the arm, the median nerve gives rise to the following branches:

1. **Nerve to pronator teres** just above the elbow.
2. **Vasomotor nerve** to the brachial artery.
3. **Articular branch** to the elbow joint at or just below the elbow.

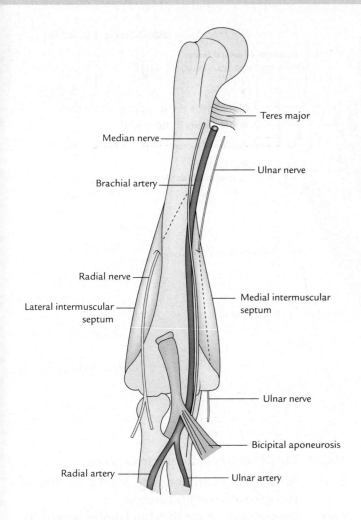

Fig. 8.11 Relations of the median nerve with the brachial artery in arm. The course of the radial and ulnar nerves in the arm is also shown.

Ulnar Nerve

The ulnar nerve arises from medial cord of the brachial plexus in the axilla. It then runs downwards on the medial side of the arm medial to the brachial artery up to the insertion of coracobrachialis. Here it pierces the medial intermuscular septum along with the superior ulnar collateral artery to enter the posterior compartment of the arm. At the elbow, the ulnar nerve passes behind the medial epicondyle of humerus where it can be easily palpated. *The ulnar nerve does not give any branch in the arm.*

Radial Nerve (Fig. 8.12)

Origin and course

The radial nerve arises from the posterior cord of the brachial plexus in the axilla. In the arm the nerve first lies posterior to the brachial artery. Then it winds around the back of the arm to enter the radial/spiral groove of humerus between the lateral and medial heads of the triceps; where it is accompanied by profunda brachii artery. At the lower end of the spiral groove, it pierces lateral intermuscular septum and enters the

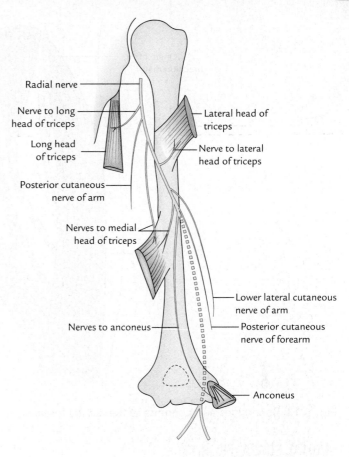

Fig. 8.12 Course, relations, and branches of the radial nerve in the arm.

anterior compartment of the arm. Here it continues downward in front of the elbow in the cubital fossa, between the brachialis and brachioradialis muscles. Then at a variable point it divides into two terminal branches: (a) a sensory branch, the *superficial radial nerve*, and (b) a motor branch, the *deep radial nerve*. The latter disappears into the substance of supinator muscle just below the elbow.

Branches

1. **In the axilla:**
   (a) Nerves to long and medial heads of triceps.
   (b) Posterior cutaneous nerve of the arm.
2. **In the spiral groove:**
   (a) Nerves to lateral and medial heads of triceps.
   (b) Nerve to anconeus.
   (c) Lower lateral cutaneous nerve of the arm.
   (d) Posterior cutaneous nerve of forearm.
3. **In the anterior compartment of the arm:**
   (a) Nerves to brachialis, brachioradialis, and extensor carpi radialis longus.
   (b) Articular branches to the elbow joint.
   (c) Deep radial nerve.
   (d) Superficial radial nerve.

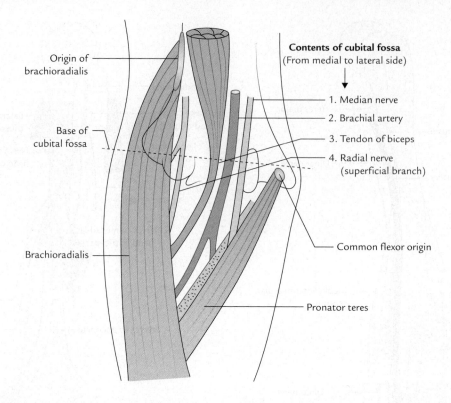

Contents of cubital fossa
(From medial to lateral side)

1. Median nerve
2. Brachial artery
3. Tendon of biceps
4. Radial nerve (superficial branch)

Origin of brachioradialis

Base of cubital fossa

Brachioradialis

Common flexor origin

Pronator teres

Fig. 8.13 Boundaries and contents of the cubital fossa.

CUBITAL FOSSA (Fig. 8.13)

The cubital fossa is a triangular hollow in front of the elbow. It corresponds (i.e., homologous) to the popliteal fossa of the lower limb.

Boundaries

Lateral: Medial border of brachioradialis muscle.

Medial: Lateral border of pronator teres muscle.

Base: An imaginary horizontal line, joining the front of two epicondyles of the humerus.

Apex: Meeting point of the lateral and medial boundaries. Here brachioradialis overlaps the pronator teres.

Floor: It is formed by two muscles, *brachialis* in the upper part and *supinator* in the lower part (Fig. 8.14).

Roof: It is formed from superficial to deep by (Fig. 8.15):

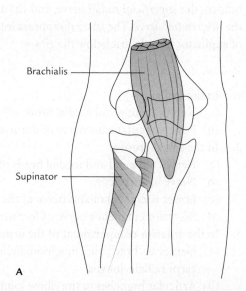

Brachialis

Supinator

A

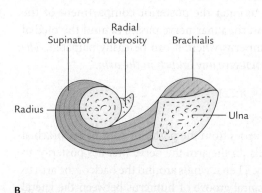

Supinator

Radial tuberosity

Brachialis

Radius

Ulna

B

Fig. 8.14 Muscles forming the floor of cubital fossa: **A**, anterior view; **B**, cross-sectional view.

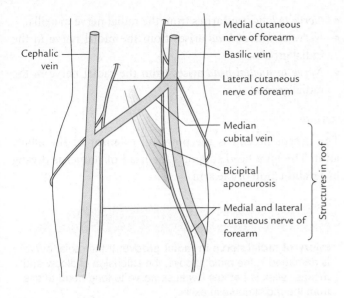

Cephalic vein

Medial cutaneous nerve of forearm

Basilic vein

Lateral cutaneous nerve of forearm

Median cubital vein

Bicipital aponeurosis

Medial and lateral cutaneous nerve of forearm

Structures in roof

Fig. 8.15 Structures in the roof of cubital fossa.

(a) *skin,*
(b) *superficial fascia* containing (i) median cubital vein connecting cephalic and basilic veins, and (ii) medial and lateral cutaneous nerves of the forearm, and
(c) *deep fascia,* strengthened by bicipital aponeurosis.

CONTENTS

The cubital fossa is actually narrow space, and therefore, its contents are displayed only if the elbow is flexed and its margins are pulled apart.

The contents of cubital fossa from the medial to lateral side are as follows (Fig. 8.13):

1. **Median nerve:** It leaves the fossa by passing between two heads of pronator teres.
2. **Brachial artery:** It terminates in the fossa at the level of neck of radius by dividing into radial and ulnar arteries. The radial artery is superficial and leaves the fossa at the apex. The ulnar artery is deep and passes deep to the pronator teres.
3. **Biceps tendon:** It passes backwards and laterally to be attached on the radial tuberosity.
4. **Radial nerve:** It lies in the gap between brachialis medially and brachioradialis laterally. At the level of lateral epicondyle it divides into two terminal branches: (a) superficial radial nerve and (b) deep radial nerve. The latter disappears in the substance of supinator muscle. The superficial radial nerve passes downwards under the cover of brachioradialis.

Mnemonic: The contents of cubital fossa from the medial to lateral side are easily remembered by the *mnemonic*—MBBS (M = Median nerve, B = Brachial artery, B = Biceps tendon, S = Superficial radial nerve; Fig. 8.13).

Clinical correlation

Clinical significance of cubital fossa: The knowledge of anatomy of the cubital fossa is clinically important for the following reasons:

(a) The **median cubital vein** in this region is the vein of choice for collecting blood samples and giving intravenous injections.
(b) The **brachial pulse** in this region is easily felt medial to biceps tendon, for **recording the blood pressure.**
(c) To deal with the fractures around elbow, viz. supracondylar fracture of the humerus. The contents of cubital fossa especially the brachial artery and median nerve are vulnerable in supracondylar fracture of the humerus.

CONTENTS OF THE POSTERIOR COMPARTMENT OF THE ARM

- **Muscle:** Triceps brachii.
- **Nerve:** Radial nerve.
- **Artery:** Profunda brachii artery.

In addition to these structures the following structures also pass through this compartment:

- Ulnar nerve.
- Ulnar collateral arteries.

Ulnar nerve and ulnar collateral arteries are described on page 99.

Muscles

Triceps Brachii (Fig. 8.16)

Triceps brachii is a large muscle, which forms most of the substance on the back of arm. As its name implies, it has three heads.

Origin

1. **Long head,** arises from the infraglenoid tubercle of the humerus.
2. **Lateral head,** arises from an oblique ridge above the spiral groove on the upper part of the posterior surface of the shaft of humerus.
3. **Medial head** arises from the posterior surface of the lower half of the shaft humerus below the spiral groove.

The medial head is actually deep to the other two heads but it is named medial because at the level of radial groove it lies medial to the lateral head.

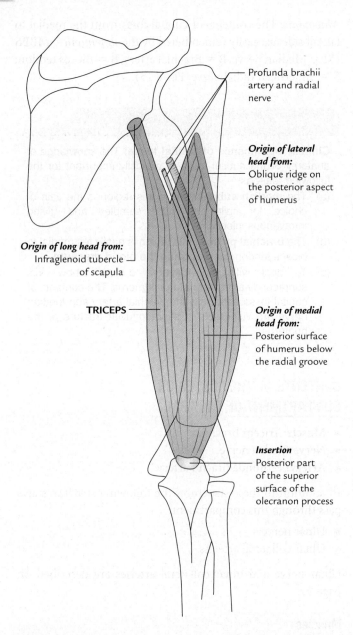

Fig. 8.16 Origin and insertion of the triceps brachii.

Insertion

The common tendon is inserted into the posterior part of the superior surface of the olecranon process of ulna.

N.B. A few fibres of deep head are inserted into the posterior aspect of the capsule of elbow joint and are referred to as **articularis cubiti** or **subanconeus muscle**. These fibres prevent the nipping of the capsule during extension of the arm.

Nerve supply

By radial nerve (C7, C8). Each head receives a separate branch from radial nerve in the following manner:

- *Nerve to long head* arises from the radial nerve in axilla.
- *Nerve to lateral head* arises from the radial nerve in the radial groove.
- *Nerve to medial head* arises from the radial nerve in the radial groove.

Actions

The triceps brachii is the powerful extensor of the elbow joint. The long head supports the head of humerus during hyperabduction of the arm.

Clinical correlation

Injury of radial nerve in radial groove: If the radial nerve is damaged in the radial groove, the extension of elbow and triceps reflex is not lost because nerve to long head arises from the radial nerve in axilla.

Radial Nerve

It is described on page 99.

Profunda Brachii Artery (Deep Artery of the Arm, Fig. 8.17)

The profunda brachii artery is the largest branch of the brachial artery. It arises from the posterolateral aspect of the brachial artery just below the teres major. It accompanies the radial nerve through the radial groove and then terminates by dividing into anterior and posterior descending branches, which take part in the arterial anastomosis around the elbow joint.

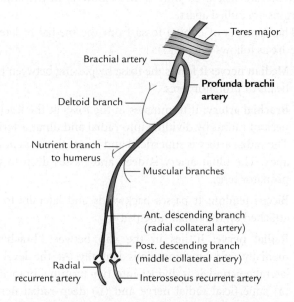

Fig. 8.17 Branches of the profunda brachii artery.

Branches

1. **Deltoid (ascending) branch:** It ascends between long and lateral heads of triceps and anastomoses with the descending branch of the posterior circumflex humeral artery.
2. **Nutrient artery to humerus:** It enters the shaft of humerus in the radial groove, just behind the deltoid tuberosity.
3. **Anterior descending (radial collateral) artery:** It is the smaller terminal branch, which accompanies the radial nerve and anastomoses with the radial recurrent artery in front of the lateral epicondyle of the humerus.
4. **Posterior descending (middle collateral) artery:** It is the larger terminal branch of the profunda brachii artery, which descends behind the shaft of humerus and anastomoses with the interosseous recurrent artery behind the lateral epicondyle of the humerus.

Golden Facts to Remember

- Most lateral bony point of the shoulder region

  Greater tubercle of the humerus

- Workhorse of the forearm flexion

  Brachialis muscle

- Most felt arterial pulse for recording blood pressure

  Brachial pulse in the cubital fossa

- Best place to compress the brachial artery to stop hemorrhage in the arm and hand

  Medial aspect of humerus near the middle of arm (site of insertion of coracobrachialis)

- Largest branch of the brachial artery

  Profunda brachii artery

- Neurovascular structures jeopardized in midshaft fracture of the humerus

  Radial nerve and profunda brachii artery

- Most preferred vein for venepuncture in the upper limb

  Median cubital vein

- Damage of the radial nerve in spiral groove causes only weakness in extension of elbow and not the total inability to extend elbow

  Because branches of the radial nerve supplying long and medial heads of triceps arise in axilla, i.e., above radial groove

- Ligament of Struthers

  Fibrous band extending between the supratrochlear spur and medial epicondyle of humerus

- Workhorse of the forearm extension

  Medial head of triceps

Clinical Case Study

A 45-year-old weight lifter while lifting the heavy weight in weight lifting competition suddenly felt a sudden snap and severe pain in his shoulder region. He dropped the weight and left the platform. He was taken to the hospital for check up. On examination the doctor noticed a ball-like bulge near the centre of the distal part of the anterior aspect of the arm. The patient was not able to supinate his arm and his forearm was pronated and flexed. A diagnosis of **rupture of tendon of long head of biceps** was made.

Questions

1. What are the causes of rupture of tendon of long head of biceps and which age group does it mostly affect?
2. What is origin of long and short heads of the biceps brachii?
3. What caused the ball-like bulge in the front of the arm and name this deformity?

Answers

1. (a) Rupture of tendon long head of biceps usually occurs from wear and tear of an inflamed tendon as it moves back and forth in the bicipital groove of the humerus. It may also result from forceful flexion of arm against excessive resistance as during weight lifting.

   (b) It usually occurs in individuals >35 years of age.

2. (a) *Long head* from the supraglenoid tubercle of the scapula.

   (b) *Short head* from the tip of coracoid process of the scapula.

3. (a) Detached belly of the biceps muscle.

   (b) Popeye deformity.

Forearm

The forearm extends from the elbow to the wrist and contains two bones, which are tied together by the thin strong fibrous membrane—the *interosseous membrane*. The head of radius is at the proximal end of the forearm whereas the head of ulna is at the distal end of the forearm. The radius and ulna at both their ends articulate with each other to form the superior and inferior radio-ulnar joints. All important movements of supination and pronation of the forearm occur at these joints. The upper ends of radius and ulna articulate with the lower end of humerus to form elbow joint. The main purpose of the movements of the forearm at elbow and radio-ulnar joints is to place the hand at the desired place. The muscles, nerves, and vessels are present both on the front and back of the forearm.

Surface Landmarks

A. On the Front of Forearm

1. **Medial and lateral epicondyles of the humerus** can be easily felt at the elbow; the medial epicondyle is more prominent than the lateral epicondyle. The ulnar nerve can be rolled behind the medial epicondyle (also see page 93).
2. **Tendon of biceps brachii** can be easily palpated in front of the elbow. The pulsations of the brachial artery can be felt just medial to the tendon.
3. **Head of radius and olecranon process of the ulna** have been described on page 97.

B. On the Back of Forearm

1. **Olecranon process of the ulna** is the most prominent bony elevation on the back of the elbow in the midline. In an extended elbow, the tip of olecranon process lies in a horizontal line with two epicondyles of the humerus and in flexed elbow the three points when joined, form an *equilateral triangle*.
2. **Posterior border of the ulna** is subcutaneous throughout its length. It can be felt in the longitudinal furrow on the back of forearm with elbow flexed. It separates the flexor and extensor muscles of the forearm.

3. **Styloid processes of the radius and ulna** can be easily felt on the lateral and medial sides of the wrist, respectively. *The styloid process of radius is located about 1.25 cm more distally.*
4. **Dorsal tubercle of the radius (Lister's tubercle)** can be palpated on the posterior aspect of the distal end of the radius in line with the cleft between index and middle fingers.

FASCIAL COMPARTMENTS OF THE FOREARM

The forearm is enclosed in sheath of deep fascia of the forearm (antebrachial fascia). It is attached to the posterior subcutaneous border of the ulna. From the deep surface fascia, septa pass between the muscles and some of these septa reach the bone.

This deep fascia, together with interosseous membrane and fibrous intermuscular septa divide the forearm into several compartments, each having its own muscles, nerves, and blood supply. Classically, the forearm is divided into the two compartments: (a) anterior compartment and (b) posterior compartment (Fig. 9.1).

The anterior compartment contains the structures on the front of the forearm and the posterior compartment contains the structure on the back of the forearm.

Near the wrist, the deep fascia presents two localized thickenings, the flexor and the extensor retinacula, which retain the digital tendons in position during hand movements.

Flexor Retinaculum (Fig. 9.2)

The flexor retinaculum is a strong fibrous band formed by the thickening of deep fascia in front of the carpus (anatomical wrist). It is rectangular in shape and has roughly the size and shape of a postage stamp. Like a postage stamp, it presents two surfaces and four borders. Medially it is attached to the pisiform and the hook of the hamate whereas laterally it is attached to the tubercle of scaphoid and crest of the trapezium. With carpus, it forms an osseofibrous tunnel called **carpal tunnel** for the passage of flexor tendons of the

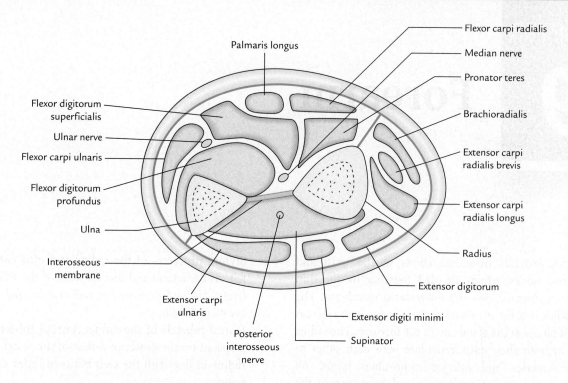

Fig. 9.1 Fascial compartments of the forearm. Cross section through the upper third of the forearm.

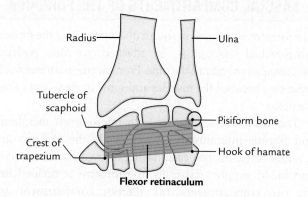

Fig. 9.2 Flexor retinaculum. (*Source*: Fig. 4.1, Page 33, *Selective Anatomy Prep Manual for Undergraduates*, Vol. I, Vishram Singh. Copyright Elsevier 2015, All rights reserved.)

digits. The flexor retinaculum is described in detail in Chapter 11, page 139.

FRONT OF THE FOREARM

The following muscles, vessels, and nerves are to be studied on the front of the forearm:

1. **Muscles:** Eight muscles, arranged in two groups.
2. **Arteries:** Two arteries, radial and ulnar.
3. **Nerves:** Three nerves, median, ulnar, and radial.

MUSCLES OF THE FRONT OF THE FOREARM

The muscles of the forearm are generally divided into two groups: superficial and deep.

Superficial Muscles of Front of Forearm (Fig. 9.3)

This group comprises five muscles. From lateral to medial side, these are:

1. Pronator teres.
2. Flexor carpi radialis.
3. Palmaris longus.
4. Flexor digitorum superficialis.
5. Flexor carpi ulnaris.

All these muscles are flexor of the forearm and have a common origin—from the front of the medial epicondyle of the humerus called common flexor origin.

Pronator Teres (Fig. 9.4)

Pronator teres is smallest and most lateral of the superficial flexors of the forearm. It forms the medial boundary of the cubital fossa.

Origin

It arises by two heads (a) *superficial (humeral) head* from the medial epicondyle of the humerus, and (b) *deep (ulnar) head* from the medial margin of the coronoid process of the ulna.

Insertion

Into the rough impression on the middle one-third of the lateral surface (most convex part) of the radius.

Nerve supply

By the median nerve.

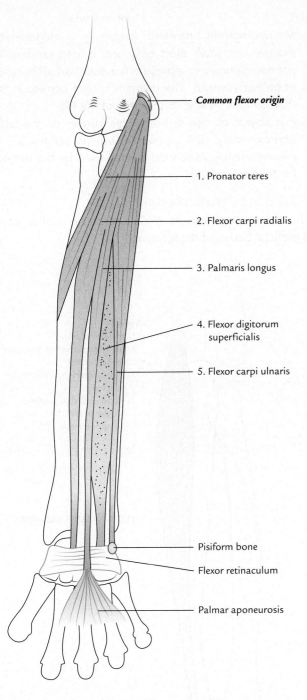

Fig. 9.3 Superficial muscles of the front of the forearm.

Actions
It is the main pronator of the forearm. It also helps in the flexion of elbow.

Clinical testing
The pronator teres is tested by asking the patient to pronate the forearm from supine position against resistance with elbow flexed.

N.B.
- *Median nerve* passes between the two heads of pronator teres.

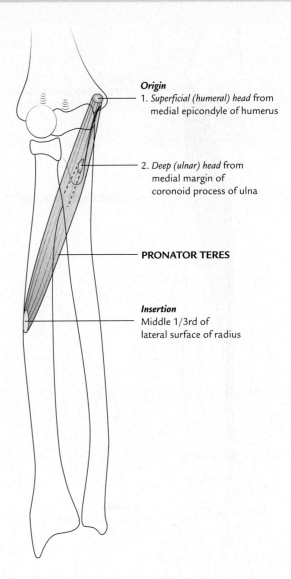

Fig. 9.4 Origin and insertion of the pronator teres.

- *Ulnar artery* passes deep to the deep head of pronator teres, thus ulnar artery is separated from the median nerve by the deep head of pronator teres in the region of cubital fossa.

Flexor Carpi Radialis (Fig. 9.5)
Origin
From the medial epicondyle of humerus by a common flexor origin.

Insertion
On to the anterior aspects of the bases of second and third metacarpals.

Nerve supply
By the median nerve.

Actions
1. Acting with flexor carpi ulnaris, it flexes the wrist.
2. Acting with brachioradialis, it abducts the wrist.

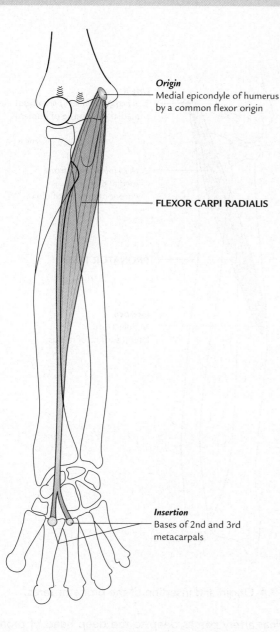

Fig. 9.5 Origin and insertion of the flexor carpi radialis.

N.B. The tendon of flexor carpi radialis (FCR) is a good guide to the radial artery, which lies just lateral to it at the wrist.

Palmaris Longus
Origin
From the medial epicondyle of humerus by a common flexor origin.

Insertion
Its long cord-like tendon crosses superficial to the flexor retinaculum and attaches to its distal part and joins the apex of palmar aponeurosis.

Nerve supply
By the median nerve.

Actions
It flexes the wrist and makes the palmar aponeuroses tense.

N.B.
- Morphologically, *palmaris longus* is a degenerating muscle with small short belly and a long tendon. The palmar aponeurosis represents the distal part of the tendon of palmaris longus. The palmaris longus corresponds to the *plantaris* muscle on the back of the leg.
- It is absent on one or both sides (usually on the left) in approximately 10% of people, but its actions are not missed. Hence, its tendon is often used by the surgeons for *tendon grafting*.

Flexor Carpi Ulnaris (Fig. 9.6)
The flexor carpi ulnaris (FCU) is most medial of the superficial flexors of the forearm.

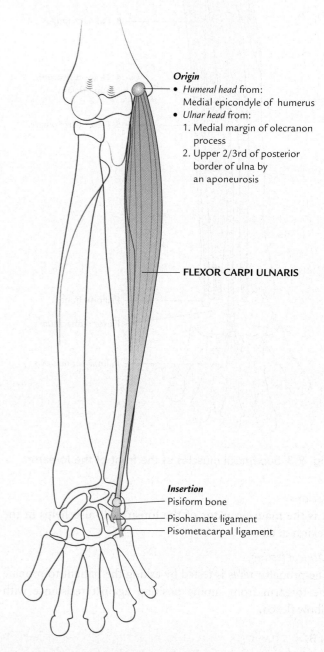

Fig. 9.6 Origin and insertion of the flexor carpi ulnaris.

Origin

It arises by two heads: a small humeral head and a large ulnar head.

(a) *humeral head* from the medial epicondyle of the humerus by a common flexor origin, and

(b) *ulnar head* from the medial margin of the olecranon process and by an aponeurosis from the upper two-third of the posterior border of the ulna.

Insertion

Into (a) pisiform bone and (b) hook of hamate and the base of fifth metacarpal bone (through *pisohamate* and *pisometacarpal ligaments*, respectively). The latter is the true insertion because a sesamoid bone (pisiform) develops in its tendon.

Nerve supply

By the ulnar nerve.

Actions

1. Acting with the extensor carpi ulnaris, it adducts the wrist joint.
2. Acting with the flexor carpi radialis, it flexes the wrist joint.

N.B.

- The *ulnar nerve* enters the forearm by passing between the two heads of flexor carpi ulnaris, which are connected to each other by a tendinous arch.
- The tendon of flexor carpi ulnaris is a good guide to ulnar nerve and ulnar artery, which lie on its lateral side at the wrist.

Flexor Digitorum Superficialis (sublimis; Fig. 9.7)

The flexor digitorum superficialis (FDS) is the largest muscle of the superficial group of muscles on the front of the forearm. Actually speaking, it forms the intermediate muscle layer between the superficial and deep groups of the forearm muscles.

Origin

It arises by two heads:

(a) *humero-ulnar head*, from the medial epicondyle of humerus, sublime tubercle on the medial margin of the coronoid process of ulna and medial (ulnar) collateral ligament of the elbow joint,

(b) *radial head*, from the anterior oblique line of the radius, extending from the radial tuberosity to the insertion of pronator teres (upper half of the anterior border of radius).

Insertion

Middle phalanges of medial four fingers. The mode of insertion is as follows. The muscles splits into two layers: superficial and deep. The superficial layer forms two

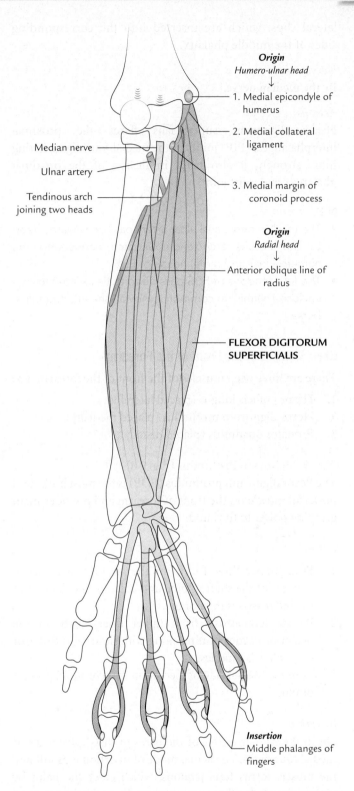

Origin
Humero-ulnar head
↓
1. Medial epicondyle of humerus
2. Medial collateral ligament
3. Medial margin of coronoid process

Origin
Radial head
↓
Anterior oblique line of radius

FLEXOR DIGITORUM SUPERFICIALIS

Median nerve
Ulnar artery
Tendinous arch joining two heads

Insertion
Middle phalanges of fingers

Fig. 9.7 Origin and insertion of the flexor digitorum superficialis.

tendons, which are inserted into middle phalanges of middle and ring fingers. The deep layer also forms two tendons, which are inserted into middle phalanges index and little fingers. Before insertion each of the four tendons splits, opposite the proximal phalanx, into medial and lateral slips, which are inserted into the corresponding sides of the middle phalanx.

Nerve supply
By the median nerve.

Actions
Flexor digitorum superficialis flexes the proximal interphalangeal (PIP) joints of the medial four digits. Acting more strongly, it also helps in flexion of the proximal phalanges and wrist joint.

N.B.
- The median nerve and ulnar artery pass downwards deep to the fibrous arch/tendinous arch connecting the humero-ulnar and radial heads of FDS.
- The four tendons of FDS pass deep to flexor retinaculum enclosed within a common synovial sheath, the *ulnar bursa*.

Deep Muscles of the Front of the Forearm

There are three deep muscles of the front of the forearm, viz.
1. Flexor pollicis longus (placed laterally).
2. Flexor digitorum profundus (placed medially).
3. Pronator quadratus (placed distally).

Flexor Digitorum Profundus (Fig. 9.8)

The flexor digitorum profundus (FDP) is the most bulky and powerful muscle on the front of forearm and provides main gripping power to the hand.

Origin
1. From upper three-fourth of the anterior and medial surfaces of the shaft of ulna and adjacent medial half of the interosseous membrane.
2. By an aponeurosis from upper three-fourth of the posterior border of ulna along with flexor and extensor carpi ulnaris muscles.
3. From the medial side of olecranon and coronoid process of ulna.

Insertion
On to the palmar aspect of the bases of distal phalanges of medial four digits. The actual mode of insertion is as follows: the muscle forms four tendons, which enter the palm by passing deep to the flexor retinaculum. Opposite the proximal phalanx of corresponding digit, the tendon perforates the tendon of flexor digitorum superficialis and passes forward to be inserted in palmar surface of the distal phalanx.

Nerve supply
1. Medial half by the ulnar nerve.

2. Lateral half by the anterior interosseous nerve – a branch of the median nerve.

Actions
FDP flexes the distal interphalangeal (DIP) joints of medial four digits. It also helps to flex the wrist joint.

N.B.

Flexor digitorum profundus—
(a) is most powerful and bulky muscle of the forearm,
(b) has dual innervation by median and ulnar nerves,
(c) provides most of the gripping power to hand,
(d) forms four tendons which enter the hand by passing deep to flexor retinaculum, posterior to the tendons of FDS in a common synovial sheath—ulnar bursa,
(e) forms most of the surface elevation medial to the palpable posterior border of the ulna, and
(f) provides origin to the lumbrical muscles in the palm.

Clinical testing
The flexor digitorum profundus is tested by asking the patient to flex the DIP joint, while holding the PIP joint in extension.

The integrity of the median nerve in forearm is tested in this way by using index finger and that of ulnar nerve by using little finger.

Flexor Pollicis Longus (Fig. 9.8)

The flexor pollicis longus lies lateral to the FDP and clothes the anterior aspect of the radius distal to the attachment of supinator muscle.

Origin
From upper two-third of the anterior surface of the radius below the anterior oblique line and adjoining part of the interosseous membrane.

Insertion
Into the anterior surface of the base of distal phalanx of the thumb.

Actions
It primarily flexes the distal phalanx of the thumb but secondarily it also flexes proximal phalanx and first metacarpal at the metacarpophalangeal (MP) and carpometacarpal (CM) joints respectively.

N.B.
- The *anterior interosseous nerve* and vessels descend on interosseous membrane between flexor pollicis longus and flexor digitorum profundus.
- The flexor pollicis longus is the only muscle, which flexes the interphalangeal joints of the thumb.

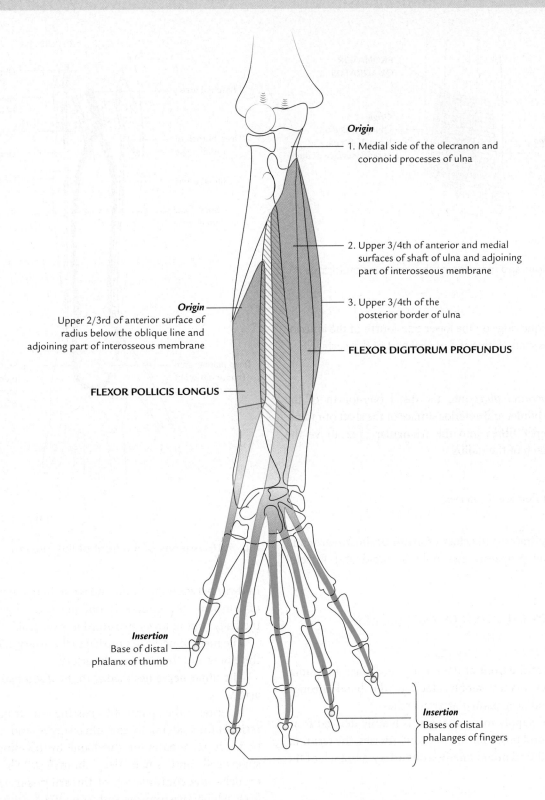

Origin
1. Medial side of the olecranon and coronoid processes of ulna

2. Upper 3/4th of anterior and medial surfaces of shaft of ulna and adjoining part of interosseous membrane

3. Upper 3/4th of the posterior border of ulna

FLEXOR DIGITORUM PROFUNDUS

Origin
Upper 2/3rd of anterior surface of radius below the oblique line and adjoining part of interosseous membrane

FLEXOR POLLICIS LONGUS

Insertion
Base of distal phalanx of thumb

Insertion
Bases of distal phalanges of fingers

Fig. 9.8 Origin and insertion of the flexor digitorum profundus and flexor pollicis longus.

Clinical testing

The flexor pollicis longus is tested by asking the patient to flex the interphalangeal joint of the thumb, while proximal phalanx of the thumb is held in extension.

Pronator Quadratus (Fig. 9.9)

It is a flat quadrilateral muscle, which extends across the front of the distal parts of the radius and ulna.

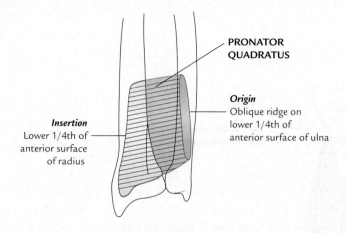

Fig. 9.9 Origin and insertion of the pronator quadratus.

Origin

From an oblique ridge on the lower one-fourth of the anterior surface of the shaft of ulna and medial part of this surface.

Insertion

1. The *superficial fibres* into the distal one-fourth of the anterior border and anterior surface of the shaft of radius.
2. The deeper fibres into the triangular area above the ulnar notch of the radius.

Nerve supply

By anterior interosseous nerve.

Actions

Pronator quadratus is the chief pronator of the forearm and is assisted by pronator teres only in rapid and forceful pronation.

ARTERIES OF THE FRONT OF THE FOREARM (Fig. 9.10)

The arteries of the front of the forearm are ulnar and radial arteries. They mainly supply blood to the hand through superficial and deep palmar arterial arches.

The blood supply to the forearm is mainly derived from the anterior and posterior interosseous arteries, the terminal branches of the common interosseous artery, a branch of the ulnar artery.

Ulnar Artery

Course

The ulnar artery is the larger terminal branch of the brachial artery. It begins in the cubital fossa at the level of the neck of the radius (or 1 cm distal to the flexion crease of the elbow). It runs downwards and reaches the medial side of the forearm

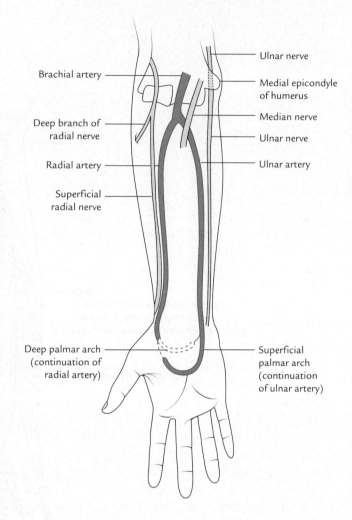

Fig. 9.10 Arteries of the front of the forearm.

midway between the elbow and wrist. In the upper one-third of forearm, the course is oblique (i.e., downwards and medially) but in lower two-third it is vertical.

The median nerve lies medial to the artery 2.5 cm distal to the elbow and then crosses the artery.

The ulnar nerve lies medial to the distal two-third of the artery.

It enters the palm by passing in front of flexor retinaculum lateral to the ulnar nerve and the pisiform bone. It terminates in the hand by dividing into large superficial and small deep branches. The superficial branch—the continuation of the artery *superficial palmar arch*, which anastomosis with superficial palmar branch of the radial artery.

Relations

In the upper part of its course, it lies deep to superficial flexor muscles. In the lower part of its course, it becomes superficial and lies between the tendons of flexor carpi ulnaris and flexor digitorum superficialis. The details are as under:

Anterior: The upper part of the ulnar artery is covered by five superficial muscles of the forearm, viz.
   (a) Pronator teres.
   (b) Flexor carpi radialis.
   (c) Palmaris longus.
   (d) Flexor digitorum superficialis.
   (e) Flexor carpi ulnaris.
The lower part of the ulnar artery is covered only by the skin and superficial and deep fasciae.

Posterior: Only the origin of ulnar artery lies on brachialis, while in the remaining whole part of its course it lies on flexor digitorum profundus.

Medial:
   (a) Ulnar nerve.
   (b) Flexor carpi ulnaris.

Lateral: Flexor digitorum superficialis.

Branches

1. **Muscular branches** to neighboring muscles.
2. **Anterior and posterior ulnar collateral (recurrent) arteries,** which take part in the arterial anastomosis around the elbow joint.
3. **Common interosseous artery,** which arises from the upper part of the ulnar artery and after a very short course at the upper border of interosseous membrane, it divides into *anterior* and *posterior interosseous arteries.*
4. **Anterior and posterior ulnar carpal branches,** which take part in the formation of anterior and posterior carpal arches.
5. **Terminal branches** are two, the larger superficial branch continues as the *superficial palmar arch,* while the smaller deep branch joins the *deep palmar arch.*

Clinical correlation

Aberrant ulnar artery: In about 3% of individuals, the ulnar artery may arise high in the arm and passes superficial to the flexor muscles of the forearm and is termed *superficial ulnar artery.* This variation should always be kept in mind while withdrawing blood samples or giving intravenous injections, because if superficial ulnar artery is mistaken for a vein it may be damaged and produce bleeding. Further, if an irritating drug is injected into the aberrant artery, the result could be fatal.

Anterior Interosseous Artery (Fig. 9.21)

It along with the posterior interosseous artery is the main source of blood supply to the forearm. It is also the deepest artery on the front of the forearm.

The *anterior interosseous artery* descends on the front of interosseous membrane in company with the anterior interosseous nerve (a branch of the median nerve). It pierces the membrane at the upper border of pronator quadratus to enter the posterior compartment of the forearm (*cf.* peroneal artery of the leg), where it anastomoses with the posterior interosseous artery and travels underneath the extensor retinaculum to reach the dorsal aspect of the wrist to join the dorsal carpal arch. The *posterior interosseous artery* is usually smaller than the anterior. It passes posteriorly between the oblique cord and proximal border of the interosseous membrane. It accompanies the posterior interosseous nerve (deep branch of the radial nerve). It gives rise to the interosseous recurrent artery, which takes part in the arterial anastomosis around the elbow joint.

Radial Artery

Origin and Course

The radial artery is the smaller terminal branch of the brachial artery. It begins in cubital fossa at the level of the neck of radius. It passes downwards to the wrist with lateral convexity. In the upper part, it lies beneath the brachioradialis on the deep muscles of the forearm. In the distal part of the forearm, it lies on the anterior surface of the radius and is covered only by the skin and fascia. The superficial radial nerve lies lateral to the middle one-third of the radial artery. The radial artery leaves the forearm by winding around the lateral aspect of the wrist to reach the anatomical snuff-box on the posterior surface of the hand. Its further course is described in the hand.

Relations

Anterior: The upper part of the radial artery is overlapped by brachioradialis, while its lower part is covered only by the skin, and superficial and deep fasciae.

Posterior: The radial artery from above to downward lies on the following structures:
   (a) Biceps tendon.
   (b) Supinator.
   (c) Pronator teres.
   (d) Flexor digitorum superficialis.
These structures together form the bed of the radial artery.

N.B. The radial artery is quite superficial throughout its whole course as compared to the ulnar artery.

Branches in the Forearm

1. **Muscular branches** to the lateral muscles of the forearm.
2. **Radial recurrent artery** arises in the cubital fossa and takes part in the formation of arterial anastomose around the elbow joint.

3. **Palmar carpal branch**, arises near the wrist and anastomosis with the palmar carpal branch of the ulnar artery.

4. **Superficial palmar branch** arises just above the wrist and enters the palm of the hand by passing in front of the flexor retinaculum. It joins the terminal part of the ulnar artery to complete the *superficial palmar arch.*

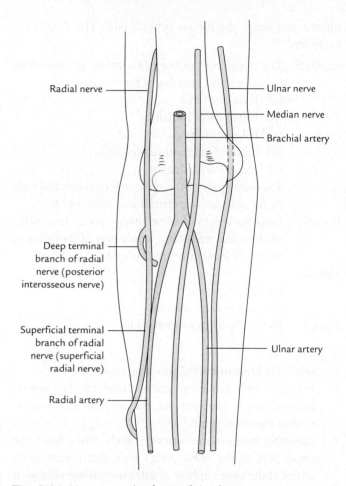

Fig. 9.11 Nerves on the front of the forearm.

Labels on figure:
- Radial nerve
- Ulnar nerve
- Median nerve
- Brachial artery
- Deep terminal branch of radial nerve (posterior interosseous nerve)
- Superficial terminal branch of radial nerve (superficial radial nerve)
- Ulnar artery
- Radial artery

Clinical correlation

- **Examination of radial pulse:** It is felt on the radial side of the front of wrist where the radial artery lies on the anterior surface of the distal end of radius, and covered only by the skin and fascia. At this site, the radial artery lies between the tendon of flexor carpi radialis medially and tendon of brachioradialis laterally. While examining the radial pulse, thumb should not be used because it has its own pulse, which may be mistaken for patient's pulse. The radial pulse is commonly used for examining the pulse rate.

- **Volkmann's ischemic contracture (ischemic compartment syndrome):** The sudden complete occlusion (e.g., due to tight plaster cast) or laceration (due to supracondylar fracture of the humerus) of the brachial artery can cause paralysis of flexor muscles of the forearm due to ischemia within a few hours. The muscles can tolerate ischemia up to 6 hours only. Thereafter they undergo necrosis and fibrous tissue replaces the necrotic tissue. As a result, muscles shorten permanently producing a flexor deformity characterized by flexion of the wrist, extension of the MP joints, and flexion of the IP joints, which leads to loss of hand power.

NERVES OF THE FRONT OF THE FOREARM (Fig. 9.11)

The nerves of the front of the forearm are median, radial, and ulnar.

The radial and ulnar nerves as their name indicates run along the radial and ulnar margins of the forearm inside the radial and ulnar nerves. The median nerve, according its name, runs in median region of the forearm.

Median Nerve

The median nerve is the **principal nerve of the front of the forearm** and supplies all the muscles of the front of the forearm except medial half of the flexor digitorum profundus and flexor carpi ulnaris, which are supplied by the ulnar nerve.

The median nerve leaves the cubital fossa by passing between the two heads of pronator teres. Here it crosses the ulnar artery (from medial to lateral side) from which it is separated by the deep head of pronator teres. Then along with ulnar artery, it passes beneath fibrous arch joining two heads of flexor digitorum superficialis and run deep to this muscle on the surface of flexor digitorum profundus.

At the wrist, about 5 cm proximal to flexor retinaculum, the median nerve emerges from behind the lateral border of the flexor digitorum superficialis and lies behind the tendon of palmaris longus. Note that in front of the wrist the median nerve becomes superficial lying between the tendons of FDS medially and FCR laterally and covered only partly by the tendon of palmaris longus.

The median nerve enters the palm of the hand by passing deep to the flexor reticulum through **carpal tunnel.**

Branches (Fig. 9.12)

1. **Muscular branches** in the cubital fossa to pronator teres, flexor carpi radialis (FCR), palmaris longus, and flexor digitorum superficialis (FDS).

2. **Articular branches** to the elbow and proximal radio-ulnar joint.

3. **Anterior interosseous** nerve arises in the upper part of the forearm and passes downwards on the anterior surface of the interosseous membrane between the

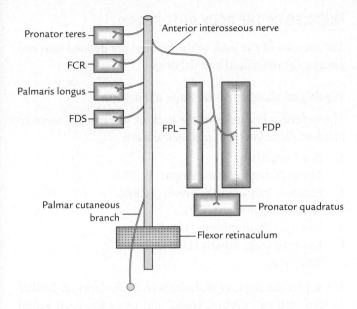

Fig. 9.12 Branches of the median nerve in the forearm.

flexor pollicis longus (FPL) and flexor digitorum profundus (FDP). It passes deep to pronator quadratus and ends on the anterior surface of the carpus. It supplies flexor pollicis longus, lateral half of the flexor digitorum profundus, and pronator quadratus. It also provides articular twigs to distal radio-ulnar and wrist joints.

4. **Palmar cutaneous branch** arises about 5 cm above the wrist and passes forward in front of flexor retinaculum to supply the skin over thenar eminence and central part of the palm.

For details see Chapter 13, page 175.

Ulnar Nerve

The ulnar enters the front of the forearm by passing through the gap between the two heads of flexor carpi ulnaris *(cubital tunnel)*. It then runs downward on the medial side of the forearm between the FCU and FDP. It enters the palm of the hand by passing in front of the flexor retinaculum lateral to the pisiform bone.

In the distal two-third of the forearm, the ulnar artery is lateral to the ulnar nerve.

Branches

1. **Muscular branches** to the flexor carpi ulnaris and medial half of the FDP.
2. **Articular branch** to the elbow joint.
3. **Palmar cutaneous branch** arises in the middle of the forearm and supplies the skin over the hypothenar eminence. It sometimes supplies palmaris brevis.

4. **Dorsal cutaneous branch** arises in distal third of the forearm. It passes medially between the tendon of flexor carpi ulnaris and ulna to reach the dorsum of the hand.

For details see Chapter 13.

Radial Nerve

The **radial nerve** enters the cubital fossa from behind the arm by descending between the brachioradialis and brachialis muscles. In front of lateral epicondyle, it divides into two terminal branches—deep and superficial.

The **deep branch of radial nerve** winds around the neck of radius between the two heads of supinator and enters the posterior compartment of the forearm as *posterior interosseous nerve.*

The **superficial branch of the radial nerve (superficial radial nerve)** is the main continuation of the radial nerve. It runs downwards under the cover of brachioradialis on the lateral side of the radial artery. About 7.5 cm above the wrist, the nerve leaves the artery, passes underneath the tendon of brachioradialis to reach the posterior aspect of the wrist and divides into terminal branches (four or five nerves), which supply the skin of lateral two-third of the posterior aspect of the hand and posterior surface of the proximal phalanges of lateral 3½ digits. The area of skin supplied by the radial nerve on the dorsum of hand is variable.

For details see Chapter 13, page 174.

Clinical correlation

Surgical safe-side of forearm: Lateral side of the anterior aspect of the forearm is considered to be the 'safe-side' by the surgeons because the branches of the median nerve, the main nerve of the front of the forearm are mostly directed medially to supply the muscles of the front of forearm. The major nerve on the lateral side is the superficial radial nerve. It is only a sensory branch of the radial nerve and runs deep to the brachioradialis muscle in the proximal forearm.

RELATIONSHIP OF STRUCTURES ON THE FRONT OF THE WRIST (Fig. 9.13)

The structures lying in front of the conventional wrist from lateral to medial side are:

1. Radial artery.
2. Tendon of flexor carpi radialis (FCR).
3. Tendon of palmaris longus.
4. Flexor digitorum superficialis.
5. Ulnar artery.
6. Ulnar nerve.
7. Tendon of flexor carpi ulnaris.

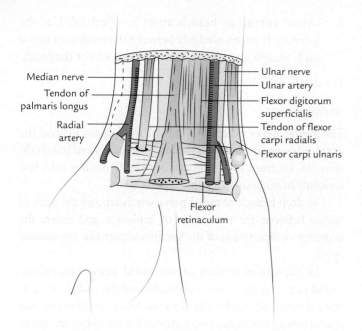

Median nerve

Tendon of
palmaris longus

Radial
artery

Ulnar nerve

Ulnar artery

Flexor digitorum
superficialis

Tendon of flexor
carpi radialis

Flexor carpi ulnaris

Flexor
retinaculum

Fig. 9.13 Structures lying in front of the wrist.

N.B. Median nerve lies deep to the tendon of palmaris longus.

Clinical correlation

Suicidal cuts of wrist
- A *deep laceration on the radial side of the wrist* as in a suicide attempt may cut the following structures, from lateral to medial side:
  – Radial artery.
  – Tendon of FCR.
  – Tendons of palmaris longus and flexor digitorum superficialis.
  – Median nerve.
- A *deep laceration on the ulnar side of the wrist* as in suicide attempt may cut the following structures; from medial to lateral side:
  – Tendon of flexor carpi ulnaris.
  – Ulnar nerve.
  – Ulnar artery.

BACK OF THE FOREARM

The following structures are to be studied on the back of the forearm:

1. Muscles of the back of the forearm.
2. Posterior interosseous nerve.
3. Posterior and anterior interosseous arteries.

MUSCLES OF THE BACK OF FOREARM

The muscles of the back of the forearm are divided into two groups: (a) superficial and (b) deep.

Superficial Muscles of the Back of Forearm

The superficial muscles of the back of forearm are seven in number. From lateral to medial these are:

1. Brachioradialis.
2. Extensor carpi radialis longus (ECRL).
3. Extensor carpi radialis brevis (ECRB).
4. Extensor digitorum (ED).
5. Extensor digiti minimi (EDM).
6. Extensor carpi ulnaris (ECU).
7. Anconeus.

The superficial muscles of the back of the forearm are further divided into two groups: lateral and posterior. Each group consists of three muscles:

Lateral group of superficial extensors

1. Brachioradialis.
2. Extensor carpi radialis longus.
3. Extensor carpi radialis brevis.

Posterior group of superficial extensors

1. Extensor digitorum.
2. Extensor digiti minimi.
3. Extensor carpi ulnaris.
4. Anconeus.

The arrangement of superficial muscles on the back of forearm is shown in Figure 9.14.

N.B.
- Four of the superficial muscles (extensor carpi radialis brevis, extensor digitorum, extensor digiti minimi, and extensor carpi ulnaris) arise by a common tendon from the tip of lateral epicondyle of the humerus called *common extensor origin*.
- All the seven muscles cross the elbow joint.

The origin, insertion, nerve supply, and actions of the superficial muscles of the back of forearm are presented in the Table 9.1.

The origin and insertion of superficial extensors of the forearm is shown in Figures 9.15–9.18.

Deep Muscles of the Back of Forearm (Fig. 9.19)

There are five deep muscles of the back of forearm, from above downwards these are:

1. Supinator.

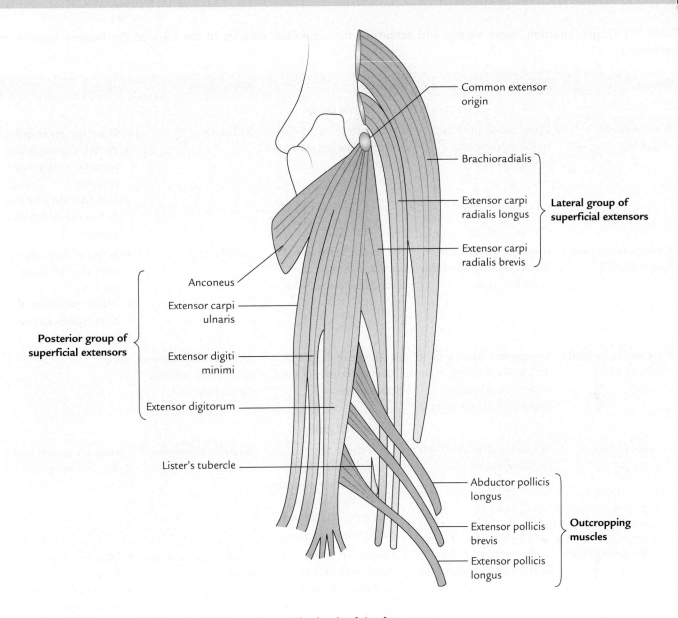

Fig. 9.14 Arrangement of the superficial muscles on the back of the forearm.

2. Abductor pollicis longus (APL).
3. Extensor pollicis brevis (EPB).
4. Extensor pollicis longus (EPL).
5. Extensor indicis.

The three deep extensors of the forearm, which act on thumb (*abductor pollicis longus, extensor pollicis brevis,* and *extensor pollicis longus*) lie deep to the superficial extensors and in order to gain insertion on the three short long bones of thumb '**crop out**' (emerge) from the furrow in the lateral part of the forearm between lateral and posterior groups of superficial extensor. These three muscles are therefore termed **outcropping muscles.**

The origin, insertion, nerve supply, and actions of deep muscles of the back of forearm are presented in Table 9.2.

N.B.

- None of the deep muscles of the back of forearm cross the elbow joint.
- All of them arise from the radius, ulna, and interosseous membrane.
- All of them are supplied by the *posterior interosseous nerve* (deep branch of the radial nerve).

Table 9.1 Origin, insertion, nerve supply, and actions of the superficial muscles of the back of the forearm (superficial extensors)

Muscle	Origin	Insertion	Nerve supply	Actions
Lateral group				
Brachioradialis (Fig. 9.15)	Upper two-third of the lateral supracondylar ridge of the humerus	Lateral surface of the distal end of radius just above the styloid process	Radial nerve	• Flexes the elbow joint. • Pronates the supinated forearm to midprone position • Supinates the pronated forearm to midprone position
Extensor carpi radialis longus (ECRL)	Lower one-third of the lateral supracondylar ridge of the humerus	Lateral side of the dorsal surface of the base of second metacarpal bone	Radial nerve	• Acting with extensor carpi ulnaris extends the wrist • Acting with flexor carpi radialis abducts the wrist
Extensor carpi radialis brevis (ECRB)	By a common tendon from the lateral epicondyle of the humerus and lateral ligament of the elbow joint	Lateral side of the dorsal surface of the base of third metacarpal bone	Posterior interosseous nerve before piercing the supinator	-do-
Posterior group				
Extensor digitorum	By a common tendon from the lateral epicondyle	• Gives rise to four tendons for medial four digits. • By the extensor expansion it is inserted into the dorsum of middle and terminal phalanges	Posterior interosseous nerve	Extends the medial four digits. Can also extend the wrist
Extensor digiti minimi	By the common tendon from the lateral epicondyle	• Lies medial to the extensor digitorum tendon for the little finger. • Through the extensor expansion, it is inserted into the dorsum of middle and terminal phalanges of little finger	Posterior interosseous nerve	• Extends the little finger • Helps in the extension of the wrist
Extensor carpi ulnaris (ECU)	By the common tendon from the lateral epicondyle and by an aponeurosis from the upper two-third of the posterior border of ulna along with flexor carpi ulnaris and flexor digitorum profundus	Into a tubercle on the medial side of the dorsal surface of the base of the fifth metacarpal	Posterior interosseous nerve	• Acting with extensor carpi radialis it extends the wrist • Acting with flexor carpi ulnaris it adducts the wrist
Anconeus	From the back of the lateral epicondyle	Lateral side of the olecranon process and upper one-fourth of the posterior surface of the ulna	Nerve to anconeus, which arises from radial nerve in spiral groove and descends through medial head of the triceps brachii	Weak extensor of the elbow joint

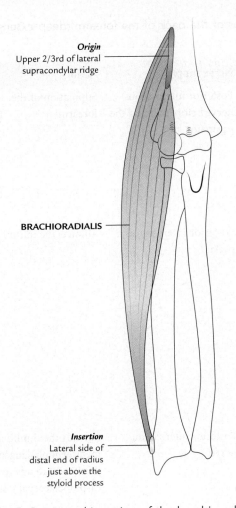

Origin
Upper 2/3rd of lateral
supracondylar ridge

BRACHIORADIALIS

Insertion
Lateral side of
distal end of radius
just above the
styloid process

Fig. 9.15 Origin and insertion of the brachioradialis.

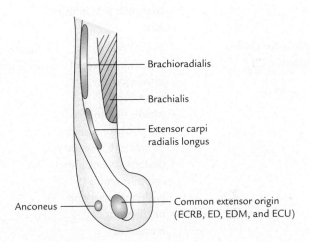

Brachioradialis

Brachialis

Extensor carpi
radialis longus

Anconeus

Common extensor origin
(ECRB, ED, EDM, and ECU)

Fig. 9.16 Lateral aspect of the lower end of humerus showing origin of seven superficial muscles of the back of forearm (ECRB = extensor carpi radialis brevis, ED = extensor digitorum, EDM = extensor digiti minimi, ECU = extensor carpi ulnaris).

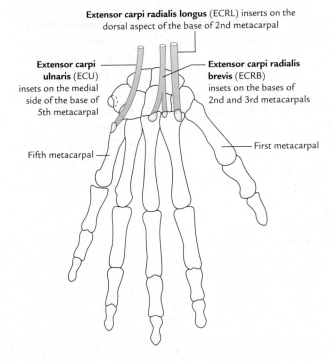

Extensor carpi radialis longus (ECRL) inserts on the
dorsal aspect of the base of 2nd metacarpal

Extensor carpi
ulnaris (ECU)
insets on the medial
side of the base of
5th metacarpal

Extensor carpi radialis
brevis (ECRB)
insets on the bases of
2nd and 3rd metacarpals

Fifth metacarpal

First metacarpal

Fig. 9.17 Insertion of the extensor carpi ulnaris, extensor carpi radialis longus, and extensor carpi radialis brevis.

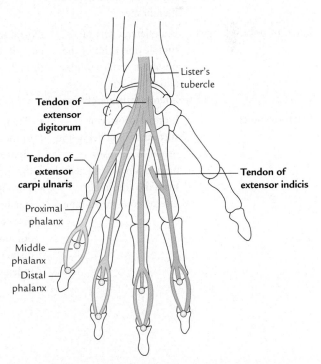

Lister's
tubercle

Tendon of
extensor
digitorum

Tendon of
extensor
carpi ulnaris

Tendon of
extensor indicis

Proximal
phalanx

Middle
phalanx

Distal
phalanx

Fig. 9.18 Insertion of the extensor digitorum, extensor carpi ulnaris, and extensor indicis.

Table 9.2 Origin, insertion, nerve supply, and actions of the deep muscles of the back of the forearm (deep extensors of forearm)

Muscle	Origin	Insertion	Nerve supply	Action
Supinator (Fig. 9.20)	• Lateral epicondyle • Lateral ligament of the elbow joint • Annular ligament • Supinator crest of ulna and from the triangular area in front of it	Upper one-third of the posterior, lateral, and anterior surfaces of the radius	Posterior interosseous nerve before piercing the supinator	Supination of the forearm
Abductor pollicis longus (APL)	• Lateral part of the posterior surface of ulna below the anconeus • Middle one-third of the posterior surface of radius (below the posterior oblique line) and intervening posterior surface of interosseous membrane	Lateral side of the base of first metacarpal	Posterior interosseous nerve	Abducts the thumb
Extensor pollicis brevis (EPB)	From a small area on the posterior surface of radius below the origin of abductor pollicis longus and from adjoining interosseous membrane	Dorsal surface of the base of proximal phalanx of thumb	Posterior interosseous nerve	Extends the thumb at metacarpophalangeal joint and extends the carpometacarpal joint
Extensor pollicis longus	From lateral part of middle one-third of the posterior surface of ulna and adjoining interosseous membrane	Dorsal surface of the base of distal phalanx of thumb	Posterior interosseous nerve	• Extends the joints of thumb • Helps in the extension of the wrist
Extensor indicis	From the posterior surface of ulna below the origin of extensor pollicis longus and also from the adjoining interosseous membrane	• The tendon lies medial to the extensor digitorum tendon for the index finger • Through the extensor expansion, it is inserted into the dorsum of middle and distal phalanges of the index finger	Posterior interosseous nerve	• Extends the index finger • Helps in the extension of the wrist

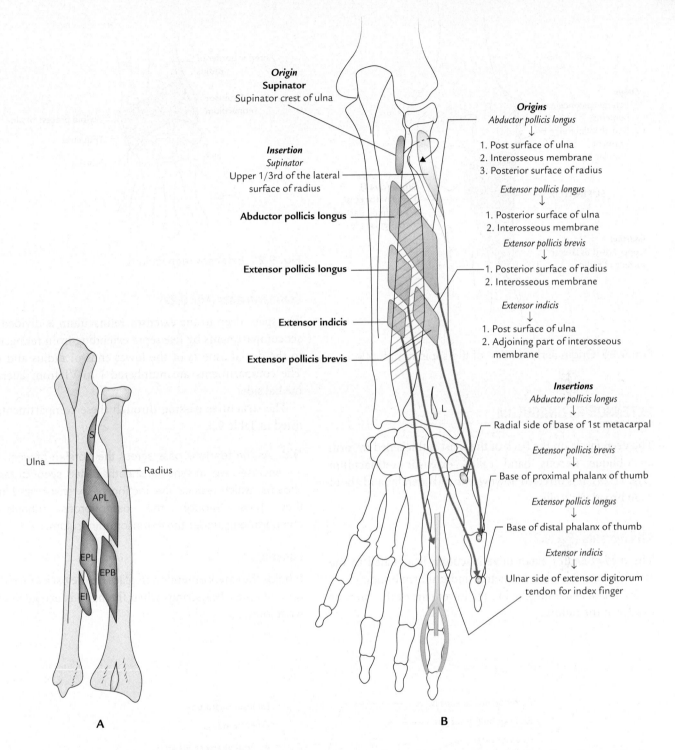

Origin
Supinator
Supinator crest of ulna

Insertion
Supinator
Upper 1/3rd of the lateral
surface of radius

Abductor pollicis longus

Extensor pollicis longus

Extensor indicis

Extensor pollicis brevis

Origins
Abductor pollicis longus
↓
1. Post surface of ulna
2. Interosseous membrane
3. Posterior surface of radius

Extensor pollicis longus
↓
1. Posterior surface of ulna
2. Interosseous membrane

Extensor pollicis brevis
↓
1. Posterior surface of radius
2. Interosseous membrane

Extensor indicis
↓
1. Post surface of ulna
2. Adjoining part of interosseous
membrane

Insertions
Abductor pollicis longus
↓
Radial side of base of 1st metacarpal

Extensor pollicis brevis
↓
Base of proximal phalanx of thumb

Extensor pollicis longus
↓
Base of distal phalanx of thumb

Extensor indicis
↓
Ulnar side of extensor digitorum
tendon for index finger

Ulna

Radius

S

APL

EPL

EPB

EI

L

A

B

Fig. 9.19 A, Origin of five deep muscles of the back of forearm from the posterior aspects of radius and ulna
(S = supinator, APL = abductor pollicis longus, EPL = extensor pollicis longus, EPB = extensor pollicis brevis, EI = extensor
indicis); **B,** Origin and insertion of the deep muscles on the back of the forearm (L = Lister's tubercle).

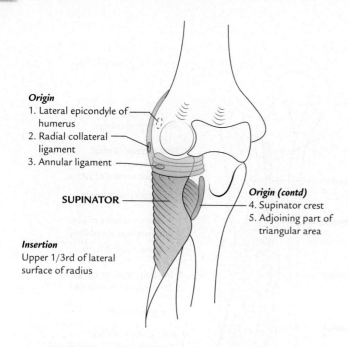

Origin
1. Lateral epicondyle of humerus
2. Radial collateral ligament
3. Annular ligament

SUPINATOR

Insertion
Upper 1/3rd of lateral surface of radius

Origin (contd)
4. Supinator crest
5. Adjoining part of triangular area

Fig. 9.20 Origin and insertion of the supinator muscle.

EXTENSOR RETINACULUM

The deep fascia on the back of the wrist is thickened to form an oblique fibrous band called **extensor retinaculum** (Fig. 11.29). It is directed downwards and laterally, and about 2 cm broad vertically.

Attachments (Fig. 9.21)

The *medial end* of extensor retinaculum is attached to the styloid process of ulna, triquetral, and pisiform bones.

Its *lateral end* is attached to the lower part of the anterior border of the radius.

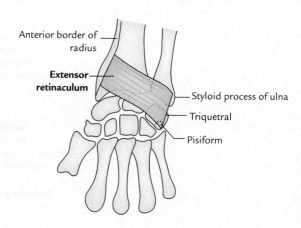

Anterior border of radius

Extensor retinaculum

Styloid process of ulna
Triquetral
Pisiform

Fig. 9.21 Extensor retinaculum.

Compartments (Fig. 9.22)

The space deep to the extensor retinaculum is divided into six compartments by five septa extending from retinaculum to the dorsal aspects of the lower ends of radius and ulna. The compartments are numbered I to VI from lateral to medial side.

The structures passing through these compartments are listed in Table 9.3.

N.B. As the tendons pass across the dorsum of wrist, they are enclosed within synovial sheaths called *synovial tendon sheaths*, which reduce the friction of extensor tendons as they pass through the osseofibrous tunnels—the compartments under the extensor retinaculum.

Functions

It holds the extensor tendon in place on the back of wrist and prevents their bowstrings when the hand is extended at the wrist joint.

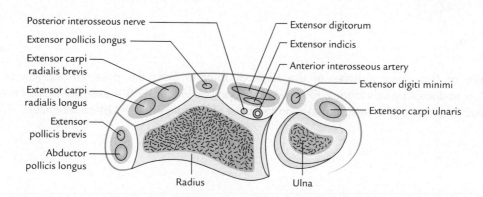

Posterior interosseous nerve
Extensor pollicis longus
Extensor carpi radialis brevis
Extensor carpi radialis longus
Extensor pollicis brevis
Abductor pollicis longus
Radius
Extensor digitorum
Extensor indicis
Anterior interosseous artery
Extensor digiti minimi
Extensor carpi ulnaris
Ulna

Fig. 9.22 Transverse section of the forearm just above the wrist showing structures passing deep to the extensor retinaculum.

Table 9.3 Structures passing through various compartments beneath the extensor retinaculum of wrist

Compartment	Structure/structures, passing through
I	• Abductor pollicis longus (APL) • Extensor pollicis brevis (APB)
II	• Extensor carpi radialis longus (ECRL) • Extensor carpi radialis brevis (ECRB)
III	Extensor pollicis longus (EPL)
IV	• Extensor digitorum (ED) • Extensor indicis (EI) • Posterior interosseous nerve • Anterior interosseous artery
V	Extensor digiti minimi (EDM)
VI	Extensor carpi ulnaris (EUC)

POSTERIOR INTEROSSEOUS NERVE (Fig. 9.23)

Origin and Course

The *posterior interosseous nerve* is the deep terminal branch of the radial nerve. It is **motor** and **chief nerve of the back of the forearm.** It begins in the cubital fossa as one of the two terminal branches of radial nerve at the level of lateral epicondyle of humerus. It leaves the cubital fossa by winding around the lateral side of the neck of radius in the substance of supinator. After emerging from supinator, it runs in the fascial plane between superficial and deep extensor muscles. At the lower border of extensor pollicis brevis, it passes deep to the extensor pollicis longus to lie on the posterior surface of interosseous nerve, on which it runs downwards up to the wrist where it ends into a **pseudoganglion.**

Branches (Fig. 9.23)

1. **Muscular branches**
   (a) *Before piercing supinator,* it gives branches to the extensor carpi radialis brevis and supinator.
   (b) *While passing through supinator,* it gives another branch to the supinator.
   (c) *After emerging from supinator,* it gives branches to three superficial extensors (extensor digitorum, extensor digiti minimi, and extensor carpi ulnaris) and all deep extensors.

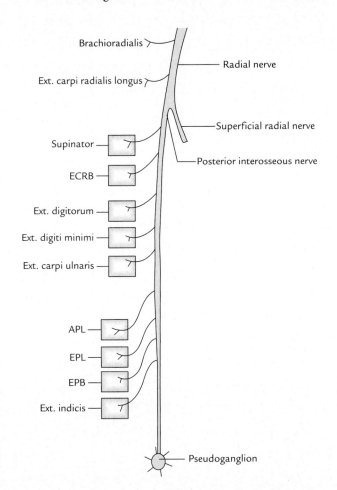

Fig. 9.23 Branches of the posterior interosseous nerve.

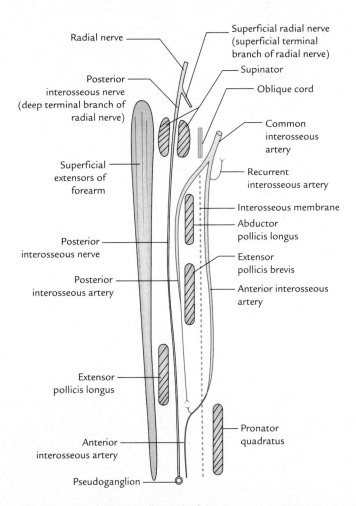

Fig. 9.24 Course and relations of the posterior interosseous artery.

2. **Articular branches** to the wrist joint, distal radio-ulnar joint, and carpal joints.

For details see Chapter 13, page 174.

N.B. All the muscles on the back of forearm are supplied by the posterior interosseous nerve except brachioradialis, extensor carpi radialis longus, and anconeus, which are supplied by the radial nerve directly.

Clinical correlation

Lesion of posterior interosseous nerve: The posterior interosseous nerve (i.e., deep terminal branch of the radial nerve) may be damaged during surgical exposure of the head of radius in fracture proximal end of radius. Since the extensor carpi radialis longus is spared wrist drop does not occur.

POSTERIOR INTEROSSEOUS ARTERY

The *posterior interosseous artery* (Fig. 9.24) is a smaller terminal branch of the common interosseous artery from ulnar artery. It begins in the cubital fossa, enters the back of the forearm by passing through the gap between the oblique cord and upper margin of the interosseous membrane. From here, it passes between supinator and abductor pollicis longus to accompany the posterior interosseous nerve. In the lower part of the forearm, it becomes markedly reduced and ends by anastomosing with the anterior interosseous artery. In the lower part of forearm, the anterior interosseous artery enters the back of the forearm by piercing interosseous membrane just above the pronator quadratus and supplies low one-fourth of the back of the forearm. The posterior interosseous artery in the cubital fossa gives **interosseous recurrent artery**, which takes part in the formation of anastomosis around the elbow joint.

Golden Facts to Remember

▶ All the flexor muscles of the forearm lie on the front of forearm *except*	Brachioradialis, which lies on the back of the forearm
▶ All the superficial flexors of the forearm are supplied by median nerve *except*	Flexor carpi ulnaris, which is supplied by the ulnar nerve
▶ Most powerful and most bulky muscle on the front of forearm	Flexor digitorum profundus
▶ Deepest muscle on the front of forearm	Pronator quadratus
▶ Deepest artery on the front of forearm	Anterior interosseous artery
▶ Principal nerve of the front of the forearm	Median nerve
▶ 'Safe side' on the anterior aspect of the forearm for surgeons	Lateral side of the front of the forearm
▶ Most superficial muscle along the radial side	Brachioradialis of the forearm
▶ Lister tubercle	Dorsal tubercle of radius
▶ Chief nerve of the back of the forearm	Posterior interosseous nerve
▶ All the muscles on the back of the forearm are extensors *except*	Brachioradialis, which is a flexor of the forearm
▶ Chief source of blood supply to the forearm	Ulnar artery
▶ Deepest artery on the front of the forearm	Anterior interosseous artery

Clinical Case Study

A 25-year-old girl, who was studying in the final MBBS, tried to commit suicide by slashing her wrist with a sharp knife. She was bleeding profusely and was immediately taken to the hospital, where the doctors, on examination, found a lacerated wound on the radial side of her wrist. Surgical procedure was performed and her life was saved.

Questions

1. Name the structures lying in front of the wrist.
2. Name the structures that are likely to be cut by deep lacerated wound on the radial side of wrist.
3. Injury of which structure leads to profuse bleeding?
4. Name the artery which lies in front of distal end of radius between the tendon of flexor carpi radialis and brachioradialis and mention its clinical importance.

Answers

1. From lateral to medial side these are: (a) radial artery, (b) tendon of flexor carpi radialis, (c) tendon of palmaris longus, (d) tendons of flexor digitorum superficialis, (e) ulnar artery, (f) ulnar nerve, and (g) tendon of flexor carpi ulnaris (Fig. 9.12).
2. Radial artery, tendon of flexor carpi radialis, tendon of palmaris longus, and median nerve.
3. Radial artery.
4. Radial artery. The 'radial pulse' is felt at wrist at this site.

Elbow and Radio-ulnar Joints

ELBOW JOINT

The elbow joint is a joint between the lower end of the humerus and upper ends of the radius and ulna. It actually includes two articulations: (a) **humero-ulnar articulation**, between the trochlea of the humerus and trochlear notch of the ulna, and (b) **humero-radial articulation**, between the capitulum of the humerus and the head of radius. On the surface, the joint line of elbow is situated 2 cm below the line joining the two epicondyles of humerus.

The complexity of elbow joint is further increased by its continuity with superior radio-ulnar joint. Thus there are three articulations in the elbow region, viz. (a) humero-ulnar, (b) humero-radial, and (c) superior (proximal) radio-ulnar. These are called **cubital articulations** (Fig. 10.1).

TYPE

It is a hinge type of synovial joint.

ARTICULAR SURFACES

The *upper articular surface* is formed by the capitulum and the trochlea of the lower end of the humerus.

The *lower articular surface* is formed by the upper surface of the head of the radius and trochlear notch of the ulna.

The **capitulum** is a rounded hemispherical eminence and possesses smooth articular surface only on its anterior and inferior aspects.

The **trochlea** is medial to capitulum and resembles a pulley. The medial flange of trochlea projects to a lower level than its lateral flange.

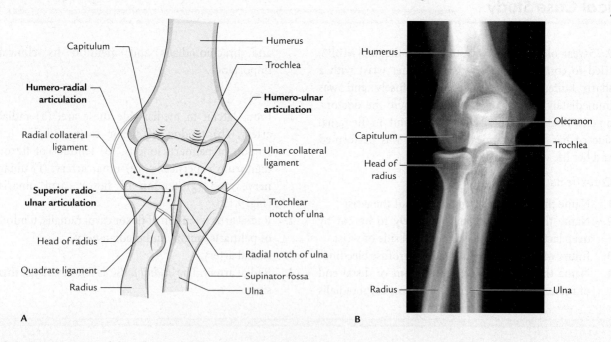

Fig. 10.1 Components of the elbow joint: **A**, schematic diagram; **B**, radiograph of normal elbow joint (anteroposterior view). (*Source*: Fig. 7.70D, Page 681, *Gray's Anatomy for Students*, Richard L Drake, Wayne Vogl, Adam WM Mitchell. Copyright Elsevier Inc. 2005, All rights reserved.)

The **trochlear notch** of ulna is formed by the upper surface of the coronoid process and anterior surface of the olecranon process.

The **upper end of radius** is circular in outline and slightly depressed in the center.

N.B. The distal end of humerus has *three non-articular fossae:* (a) *olecranon fossa,* a deep hollow above the posterior part of the trochlea. It lodges the tip of olecranon process of ulna during extension of the elbow, (b) *coronoid fossa,* a small hollow above the anterior surface of the trochlea. It lodges the anterior margin of coronoid process of ulna during flexion of the elbow, and (c) *radial fossa,* another small hollow lateral to the coronoid fossa, just above the capitulum. It lodges the anterior margin of the head of radius during flexion of the elbow.

LIGAMENTS (Figs 10.2 and 10.3)

CAPSULAR LIGAMENT (JOINT CAPSULE)

It is a fibrous sac enclosing the joint cavity (Fig. 10.2). The inner surface of the capsule is lined by the synovial membrane.

Attachment

Above, it is attached to the medial epicondyle, upper margins of radial, coronoid, and olecranon fossae, and lateral epicondyle of the humerus, i.e., it encloses all the non-articular fossae at the lower end of the humerus.

Below, it is attached to the anterior and medial margins of the coronoid process of ulna, upper margin of the annular ligament, and upper and medial margins of the olecranon process. Note, it is not attached to the radius.

To facilitate the movements of flexion and extension, the anterior and posterior aspects of the capsule are thinner than the sides. The inner surface of the joint capsule and non-articular bony parts inside the capsule are lined by synovial membrane (Fig. 10.3). The synovial membrane forms a crescentic fold between humero-radial and humero-ulnar parts, which contains an *extrasynovial fat.* Between the synovial membrane and joint capsule, there are *three other fat pads* occupying olecranon, coronoid, and radial fossae. The synovial membrane of elbow joint is continuous inferiorly with the synovial membrane of the superior radio-ulnar joint.

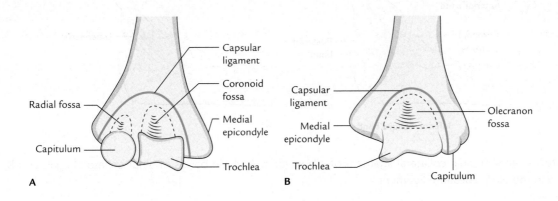

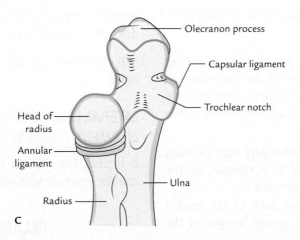

Fig. 10.2 Attachment of capsular ligament of elbow joint: **A**, anterior aspect; **B**, posterior aspect; **C**, anterosuperior aspect.

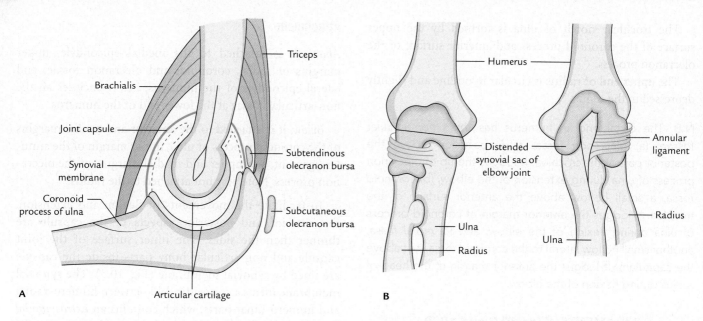

Fig. 10.3 Elbow joint: **A**, schematic sagittal section; **B**, synovial sac (distended).

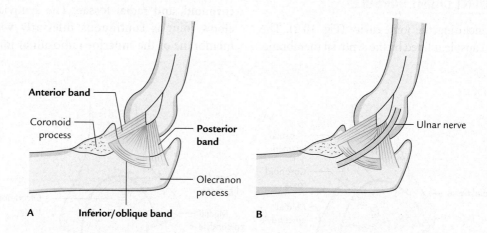

Fig. 10.4 Attachments of ulnar collateral ligament of elbow joint: **A**, three bands of ulnar collateral ligament; **B**, relation of ulnar nerve with the ulnar collateral ligament.

MEDIAL LIGAMENT (ULNAR COLLATERAL LIGAMENT; Fig. 10.4)

It is triangular in shape, with its apex attached to medial epicondyle of the humerus and base to the coronoid and olecranon processes of ulna. It is divided into three parts (or bands): anterior, posterior, and inferior—united by a thin region.

1. The strongest and stiffest *anterior part* extends from front of the medial epicondyle to a tubercle on the medial margin of the coronoid process.

2. The *posterior part* extends from back of the medial epicondyle of humerus to the medial margin of the olecranon process.

3. The *inferior part* or oblique band extends between the olecranon and the coronoid process.

Between anterior and posterior bands, intermediate fibres descend from medial epicondyle to the oblique band.

N.B. The medial collateral ligament is related to the ulnar nerve.

LATERAL LIGAMENT (RADIAL COLLATERAL LIGAMENT; Fig. 10.5)

It extends from lateral epicondyle of the humerus to the annular ligament with which it blends.

RELATIONS (Fig. 10.6)

Anterior: (a) Brachialis muscle, (b) median nerve, (c) brachial artery, (d) tendon of biceps

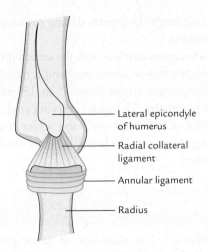

Fig. 10.5 Radial collateral ligament.

brachii. The last three structures are separated from joint capsule by brachialis.

Posterior: (a) Tendon of triceps (b) anconeus.

Medially: (a) Flexor carpi ulnaris, (b) ulnar nerve (posteromedially) (c) common flexor origin of the muscles of forearm (anteromedially).

Laterally (posterolateral): (a) Spinator (b) common extensor origin of muscles of forearm muscles, (c) extensor carpi radialis brevis.

BURSAE RELATED TO THE ELBOW JOINT

Four important bursae are related to the elbow joints—(a) two in relation to the triceps insertion and (b) two in relation to the biceps insertion:

1. **Subtendinous olecranon bursa**, a small bursa between triceps tendon and upper surface of the olecranon process.

2. **Subcutaneous olecranon bursa**, a large bursa between skin and subcutaneous triangular area on the posterior surface of the olecranon.

3. **Bicipitoradial bursa**, a small bursa separating biceps tendon from smooth anterior part of the radial tuberosity.

4. A small **bursa separating the biceps tendon from the oblique cord.**

STABILITY OF THE ELBOW JOINT

In adults, the elbow joint is quite stable due to the following two factors:

1. Pulley-shaped trochlea of humerus fits properly into jaw-like trochlear notch of ulna.
2. Strong ulnar and radial collateral ligaments.

BLOOD SUPPLY

The blood supply of elbow joints is by arterial anastomosis around the elbow formed by the branches of brachial, radial, and ulnar arteries.

NERVE SUPPLY

Nerve supply of elbow joint is by articular branches from:

(a) radial nerve (through its branch to anconeus),
(b) musculocutaneous nerve (through its branch to brachialis),
(c) ulnar nerve, and
(d) median nerve.

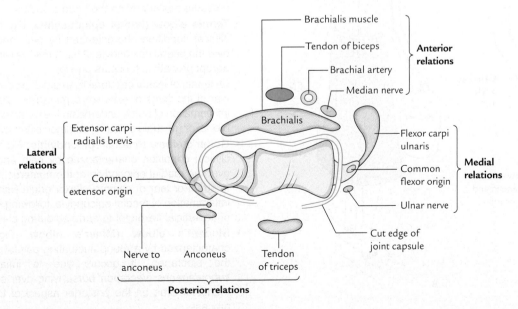

Fig. 10.6 Relations of the elbow joint.

Table 10.1 Movements of the elbow joint

Movements	Muscles producing movements
Flexion	• Brachialis • Biceps brachii • Brachioradialis*
Extension	• Triceps • Anconeus

*The brachioradialis acts most effectively in midprone position as when medical students walk by putting their aprons over their shoulders.

MOVEMENTS

Being an uniaxial joint, the elbow joint allows only flexion and extension. The range of flexion is about 140°. These movements and muscles producing them are presented in Table 10.1.

CARRYING ANGLE (Fig. 10.7)

The transverse axis of elbow joint is not transverse but oblique being directed downwards and medially. This is because medial flange of trochlea lies about 6 mm below its lateral flange. Consequently when the elbow is extended the arm and forearm do not lie in straight line, rather forearm is deviated slightly laterally. This angle of deviation of long axis of forearm from long axis of arm is termed **carrying angle**.

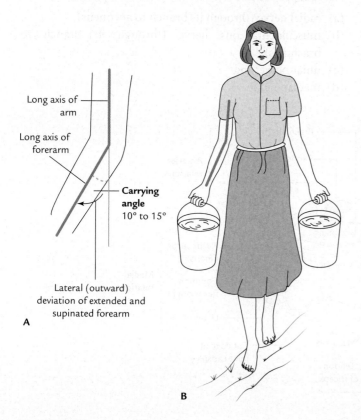

Long axis of arm

Long axis of forearm

Carrying angle 10° to 15°

Lateral (outward) deviation of extended and supinated forearm

A

B

Fig. 10.7 Carrying angle.

The carrying angle disappears during pronation and full flexion of forearm.

The forearm comes into line with the arm in the midprone position—the position in which the hand is mostly used.

The carrying angle varies from 5° to 15° and is more pronounced in females. The wider carrying angle in females avoids rubbing of forearms with the wider female pelvis while carrying loads, e.g., buckets filled with water from one place to another.

Clinical correlation

• **Elbow effusion:** The distension of elbow joint due to effusion within its cavity occurs posteriorly because capsule of the joint is thin posteriorly and covering fascia is also thin. The joint is aspirated by inserting a needle on the posterolateral side, above the head of radius with elbow at the right angle.

• **Dislocation of elbow:** Posterior dislocations of elbow are more common and are often associated with fracture of the coronoid process. The dislocation invariably occurs by falling on an outstretched hand. The triangular relationship between the olecranon and the epicondyles of humerus is lost. Note, in normal flexed elbow the tip of olecranon process and two epicondyles of humerus form an 'equilateral triangle' (Fig. 10.8).

  The reduction, if done early, is achieved fairly easily by first giving traction to overcome spasm and then flexing the forearm to lever joint back into the place.

• **Nursemaid's elbow/pulled elbow (subluxation of head of radius; Fig. 10.9)** occurs in preschool children, 1–3 years old when the forearm is suddenly pulled in pronation. The head of radius comes out of annular ligament and the elbow is kept slightly flexed and pronated. An attempt to supinate the forearm causes severe pain.

  The reduction is easily achieved by supinating and extending the elbow and simultaneously applying direct pressure posteriorly on the head of radius.

• **Tennis elbow (lateral epicondylitis; Fig 10.10):** It is a clinical condition characterized by pain and tenderness over the lateral epicondyle of the humerus with pain during abrupt pronation. It occurs due to:

  (a) sprain of lateral collateral ligament of elbow joint, or (b) a tear of the fibres of extensor carpi radialis brevis, or (c) an inflammation of bursa underneath the extensor carpi radialis brevis, or (d) strain or tear of common extensor origin.

• **Golfer's elbow (medial epicondylitis; Fig 10.10):** It is a clinical condition characterized by pain and tenderness over the medial epicondyle of the humerus. It occurs due to strain or tear of common flexor origin with subsequent inflammation of medial epicondyle, following repetitive use of superficial flexors of forearm as during playing golf.

• **Student's elbow (Miner's elbow; Fig 10.11)** is characterized by a round fluctuating painful swelling over the olecranon. It occurs due to inflammation of *subcutaneous olecranon bursa* lying over subcutaneous triangular area on the posterior aspect of the olecranon process.

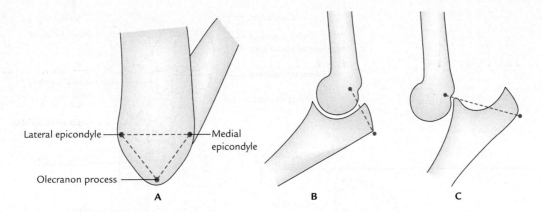

Fig 10.8 A, Formation of equilateral triangle by three bony points behind flexed elbow; **B,** elbow joint with normal relationship of three bony points of the elbow; **C,** posterior dislocation of the elbow joint causing disturbance in the relationship of three bony points of the elbow due to backward and upward displacement of the olecranon process. (*Source:* Fig. 2.2(A): B; Fig. 2.2(B): A; and B, Page 52, *Clinical and Surgical Anatomy,* 2e, Vishram Singh. Copyright Elsevier 2007, All rights reserved.)

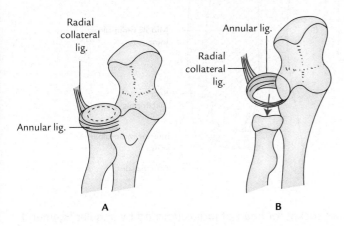

Fig. 10.9 Pulled elbow: **A,** head of radius within cup-shaped annular ligament; **B,** head of radius displaced down from the annular ligament.

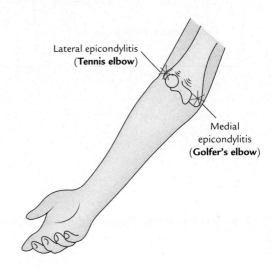

Fig. 10.10 Lateral and medial epicondylitis.

- **Nerve entrapments (compressions) around elbow:** The nerve entrapments around elbow are common and cause pain, muscle atrophy, and weakness in the area supplied by the entrapped nerve. The examples are:
  (a) *Median nerve entrapment:* The median nerve may be compressed: (a) where it passes between the two heads of pronator teres or (b) where it passes deep to fibrous arch between humero-ulnar and radial heads of flexor digitorum superficialis.
  (b) *Ulnar nerve entrapment:* The ulnar nerve may be compressed (a) where it passes posterior to the medial epicondyle of the humerus (commonest site) or (b) where it passes through cubital tunnel formed by tendinous arch joining the humeral and ulnar heads of flexor carpi ulnaris.
  (c) *Posterior interosseous nerve entrapment:* The posterior interosseous nerve may be compressed (a) where it passes deep to the arcade of Frohse, a musculoaponeurotic structure at the proximal edge of supinator muscle or (b) where it passes through the substance of supinator muscle.

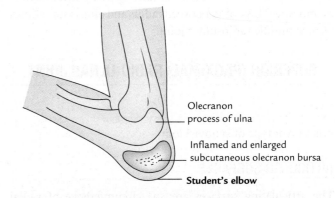

Fig. 10.11 Student's (Miner's) elbow.

RADIO-ULNAR JOINTS

The radius and ulna form two joints between them; one at their upper ends and one at their lower ends. They are called **superior** and **inferior radio-ulnar joints** (Fig. 10.12). Both these joints are **synovial joints of pivot variety.** They are

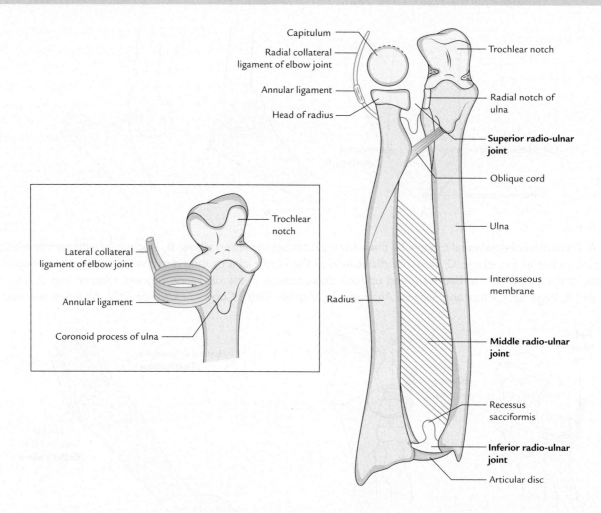

Fig. 10.12 Radio-ulnar joints. Figure in the inset on the left shows socket for head of radius (formed by annular ligament).

uniaxial joints permitting only rotation. The shafts of radius and ulna are also connected to each other by **interosseous membrane**. This union between radius and ulna is sometimes termed **middle radio-ulnar joint**.

SUPERIOR (PROXIMAL) RADIO-ULNAR JOINT

TYPE

It is a pivot type of synovial joint.

ARTICULAR SURFACES

The articulating surfaces are: (a) circumference of radial head and (b) fibro-osseous ring made by radial notch of ulna and annular ligament.

LIGAMENTS

1. **Capsular ligament (joint capsule):** The fibrous capsule surrounds the joint. It is continuous with that of elbow joint and is attached to the annular ligament.

2. **Annular ligament:** It is a strong fibrous band, which encircles the head of radius and holds it against the radial notch of ulna. It forms about four-fifth of the fibro-osseous ring within which the head of radius rotates. Medially the annular ligament is attached to the margins of radial notch of ulna. The upper margin of the ligament is continuous with the capsule of the shoulder joint and its lower part becomes narrow and embraces the neck of radius. The inner surface of annular ligament is covered by a thin layer of cartilage. Laterally, it blends with the radial collateral ligament.

3. **Quadrate ligament:** It is thin, fibrous ligament, which extends from neck of radius to the upper part of supinator fossa of ulna just below the radial notch.

Synovial membrane: It lines the inner aspect of the joint capsule and annular ligament of superior radio-ulnar joint and is continuous with the synovial membrane of the elbow joint. It is prevented from herniation by quadrate ligament.

RELATIONS

Anteriorly and laterally: Supinator muscle.
Posteriorly: Anconeus muscle.

BLOOD SUPPLY

By articular branches derived from arterial anastomosis on the lateral side of the elbow joint.

NERVE SUPPLY

By articular branches from musculocutaneous, median, radial, and ulnar nerves.

MOVEMENTS

Supination and pronation.

INFERIOR (DISTAL) RADIO-ULNAR JOINT

TYPE

Synovial joint of pivot variety.

ARTICULAR SURFACES

The articulating surfaces are (a) convex head of ulna, and (b) concave ulnar notch of radius.

LIGAMENTS

1. **Capsular ligament (joint capsule):** It is a fibrous sac which encloses the joint cavity and is attached to the margins of articular surfaces. The inner surface of the joint capsule is lined by synovial membrane. The synovial lining of the joint sends an upward prolongation in front of the lower part of the interosseous membrane called **recessus sacciformis**. The synovial cavity of joint does not communicate with the synovial cavity of the wrist joint.
2. **Articular disc:** It is a *triangular fibrocartilaginous* disc and is sometimes referred to by clinicians as **triangular ligament**. Its apex is attached to the base of the styloid process of ulna and its base to the lower margin of the ulnar notch of radius. The articular disc separates the inferior radio-ulnar joint from the wrist joint.
3. **Stability of elbow joint:** The main factors providing stability to elbow joint are:
   (a) Wrench-shaped articular surface of the olecranon process of ulna and pulley-shaped trochlea of humerus.
   (b) Strong medial and lateral collateral ligaments.

RELATIONS

Anteriorly: Flexor digitorum profundus.
Posteriorly: Extensor digiti minimi.

BLOOD SUPPLY

By anterior and posterior interosseous arteries.

NERVE SUPPLY

By anterior and posterior interosseous nerves.

A brief comparison of superior and inferior radio-ulnar joints is presented in Table 10.2.

MOVEMENTS

Supination and pronation.

INTEROSSEOUS MEMBRANE OF THE FOREARM (Fig. 10.8)

It is the fibrous sheet, which stretches between the interosseous borders of the radius and ulna. It holds these bones together and does not interfere with the movements, which take place between them. The **oblique cord** of fibrous tissue extending from lateral side of ulnar tuberosity to the lower end of radial tuberosity also helps to hold the radius and ulna together. This union between radius and ulna is sometimes termed **middle radio-ulnar joint**. This is a **syndesmosis type of fibrous joint**.

Table 10.2 Superior and inferior radio-ulnar joints

Features	Superior radio-ulnar joint	Inferior radio-ulnar joint
Type	Pivot type of synovial joint	Pivot type of synovial joint
Articular surfaces	• Circumference of head of radius • Fibro-osseous ring formed by annular ligament and radial notch of ulna	• Head of ulna • Ulnar notch of radius
Joint cavity	Communicates with the cavity of elbow joint	Does not communicate with the cavity of wrist joint
Prime stabilizing factor	Annular ligament	Articular disc
Movements	Supination and pronation	Supination and pronation

FEATURES OF THE INTEROSSEOUS MEMBRANE

1. Proximally it begins 2.3 cm below the tuberosity of the radius and distally it blends with the capsule of inferior radio-ulnar joint.
2. The fibres of the membrane run downwards and medially from radius to ulna.
3. The posterior interosseous vessels pass backwards through a gap between the upper border of interosseous membrane and oblique cord to reach the back of the forearm.
4. The anterior interosseous vessels enter the back of the forearm by piercing interosseous membrane 5 cm above its lower margin.

Relations

Anteriorly: Anterior interosseous artery and nerve.
Posteriorly: Anterior interosseous artery and posterior interosseous nerve.

Functions

1. Holds the radius and ulna together.
2. Transmits compression forces (applied to radius from hand) from radius to ulna. Such forces are then transferred to the humerus through stable humero-ulnar joint.
3. Provides attachments to muscles.

OBLIQUE CORD

It is a strong fibrous band which extends from medial side of the tuberosity of ulna to the lower part of the tuberosity of the radius. Its fibres are directed downwards and laterally, i.e., opposite to that of interosseous membrane.

N.B. Morphologically, the **oblique cord** between ulnar and radial tuberosities represent the degenerated (atrophied) part of the *flexor pollicis longus muscle.*

SUPINATION AND PRONATION (Fig. 10.13)

The movements of supination and pronation of forearm play an important role in performing the skilled movements of the hand. When elbow is semiflexed in midprone position, the palm is turned **upwards in supination** and **downward in pronation**. These actions can be easily remembered by a **mnemonic:** *Beggars supinate and kings pronate.* The supination and pronation are rotatory movements of forearm, which occur at superior and inferior radio-ulnar joints around a vertical axis. This axis is oblique and passes from center of head of radius above to the base of the styloid process of the ulna below. The axis of movement of supination and pronation is not stationary. It moves forwards and medially during supination; and backwards and laterally during pronation.

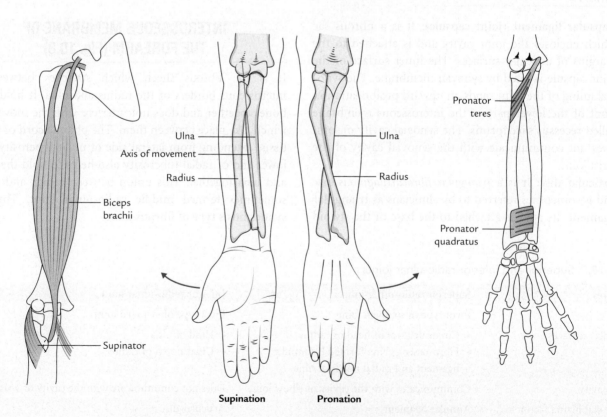

Fig. 10.13 Movements of supination and pronation.

Table 10.3 Movements of supination and pronation

Movements	Muscles producing movements
Supination	• Supinator • Biceps brachii supinates the forearm while the elbow is flexed • Brachioradialis supinates the pronated forearm to midprone position
Pronation*	• Pronator teres • Pronator quadratus • Brachioradialis, pronates the supinated forearm to midprone position

*The flexor carpi radialis, palmaris longus and gravity also help in pronation.

Morphologically, movements of supination and pronation are evolved for picking up the food and taking it to the mouth. *The food is picked up in pronation and put in mouth in supination.*

In **supination**, the radius and ulna lie parallel to each other. In **pronation**, there is rotation of lower end of radius along with articular disc on the head of ulna. As a result, the lower end of radius crosses in front of the lower end of ulna. Simultaneously the head of radius rotates within the fibro-osseous ring formed by the annular ligament and the radial notch of the ulna.

The movements of the supination and pronation, and muscle producing them are given in Table 10.3.

N.B. *The supination is more powerful than pronation* because: (a) it has antigravity movement, and (b) it is performed by powerful muscles, viz. biceps brachii. The *pronation is less powerful than supination* because it is performed by less powerful muscles, viz. pronator quadratus and pronator teres. Therefore, supination movements are used for tightening the nuts and bolts, whereas pronation movements are used for loosening/opening the nuts and bolts.

Golden Facts to Remember

▶ Cubital articulations — Humero-radial, humero-ulnar, and proximal radio-ulnar joints

▶ Student's elbow/Miner's elbow — Subcutaneous olecranon bursitis

▶ Most important bursa (clinically) around the elbow joint — Subcutaneous olecranon bursa

▶ Strongest band of ulnar collateral ligament of elbow joint — Anterior band

▶ Carrying angle (10°–15° in male and >15° in female) — Angle of deviation of long axis of forearm from long axis of arm when elbow is fully extended

▶ Commonest site of ulnar nerve entrapment (compression) — Behind the medial epicondyle of humerus

▶ Most important stabilizing factor of proximal radio-ulnar joint — Annular ligament

▶ Most important stabilizing factor of distal radio-ulnar joint — Articular disc (triangular ligament)

Clinical Case Study

A 35-year-old mother was crossing the road along with her 3-year-old son. After seeing a speeding car rushing towards them she suddenly pulled her son away by holding his left hand to avoid danger of being crushed by the car. The child cried out and later refused to use his left upper limb. The mother took the child to the doctor. On examination the doctor noticed that the child held his left forearm in a position with elbow semiflexed and forearm pronated. A diagnosis of 'pulled elbow' was made.

Questions

1. What is pulled elbow?
2. Why is pulled elbow common in preschool (1–3-year-old) children?
3. How can pulled elbow be reduced /treated?

Answers

1. In pulled elbow head of radius comes out of annular ligament of superior radio-ulnar joint (i.e., subluxation of radial head).
2. Because up to 3 years of age, the annular ligament is tubular and has large diameter, hence head of radius can be easily pulled out of the ligament by traction.
3. The reduction is easily achieved by pulling the forearm downward and then firmly supinating it. By doing so the subluxation of radius is reduced spontaneously. Finally the elbow is flexed and held in that position.

Hand

The hand (L. *Manus*) is the distal part/segment of the upper limb. It is a complex and highly evolved anatomic structure, which provides primary touch input to the brain and enables humans to perform complex fine motor tasks by way of its free movements, power grip, precision grip, handling, and pinching. The hand is man's great physical asset. It has enabled him to use various tools that his brain has invented. Therefore, good understanding of its structure and functions is essential. Everything that the doctors do to the hand should be aimed at restoring or maintaining its function. The movements of the hand occur primarily at the wrist joint or radio-carpal joint formed by the articulation of radius and first row of the carpal bones (e.g., scaphoid, lunate, and triquetral).

The hand consists of four functional units, viz.

1. Carpus.
2. Thumb.
3. Index finger.
4. A unit comprising middle, ring, and little fingers.

The carpus (first unit) provides a stabilizing platform for the three mobile units (2, 3, and 4).

The hand contains carpal bones, metacarpal bones, and phalanges.

N.B. Anatomically, the term *wrist* refers to carpus (carpal region) consisting of eight carpal bones and lies between forearm and hand but in general usage, *wrist* refers to distal end of forearm just proximal to distal ends of radius and ulna, around which the wrist watch is worn.

PALMAR ASPECT OF THE HAND

SURFACE LANDMARKS (Fig. 11.1)

1. **Tubercle of scaphoid**—can be felt at the base of thenar eminence, just lateral to the tendon of flexor carpi radialis. It is located deep to the lateral part of distal transverse crease of the wrist.
2. **Tubercle/crest of trapezium**—can be felt on deep palpation, distolateral to the tubercle of scaphoid.

3. **Pisiform bone**—can be felt at the base of hypothenar eminence medially. It lies deep to medial end of distal transverse crease of the wrist.
4. **Hook of hamate**—can be felt one finger's breadth distal to the pisiform bone.

SKIN OF THE PALM

The skin of the palm presents the following characteristic features:

1. It is thick to withstand wear and tear during work.
2. It is richly supplied by the sweat glands but contains no hair or sebaceous glands.
3. It is immobile as it is firmly attached to the underlying palmar aponeurosis.
4. It presents several longitudinal and transverse creases where the skin is firmly bound to the deep fascia.

N.B. To improve the grip the skin of the palm is ridged and furrowed and devoid of greasy sebaceous glands.

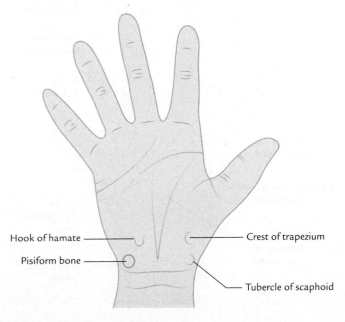

Hook of hamate

Pisiform bone

Crest of trapezium

Tubercle of scaphoid

Fig. 11.1 Surface landmarks.

Flexion Creases of the Wrist, Palm, and Fingers (Fig. 11.2)

1. **Flexion creases of the wrist (wrist creases):** The palmar aspect of the wrist presents two transverse flexion creases, viz.
   (a) *Proximal wrist crease.*
   (b) *Distal wrist crease.*

They are produced as a result of folding of the skin due to repeated flexion of the wrist. The distal wrist crease corresponds to the proximal border of the flexor retinaculum.

2. **Palmar flexion creases:** Usually there are four major palmar creases—two horizontal and two longitudinal which together roughly form an M-shaped pattern:
   (a) *Longitudinal palmar creases:*
      (i) **Radial longitudinal crease (lifeline of the palmistry):** It partly encircles the thenar eminence (ball of the thumb) and is formed due to action of short muscles of the thumb.
      (ii) **Midpalmar longitudinal crease (line of fate in palmistry):** It indicates the lateral limit of the hypothenar eminence (ball of the little finger). It is formed due to the action of short muscles of the little finger.
   (b) *Transverse palmar creases:*
      (i) **Distal transverse palmar crease:** It begins at or near the interdigital cleft between the index and little fingers and crosses the palm (with slight distal convexity) superficial to the shafts of the third, fourth, and fifth metacarpals.
      (ii) **Proximal transverse palmar crease:** It commences at the lateral border of the palm in common with the radial longitudinal crease, superficial to the head of the second metacarpal. It extends medially and slight proximally across the palm, superficial to the shafts of the third, fourth, and fifth metacarpals.

3. **Digital flexion creases:** Each of the medial four digits have three transverse flexion creases, while the thumb has two transverse creases:
   (a) *Proximal flexion crease:* It lies at the root of the finger about 2 cm distal to the metacarpophalangeal (MP) joint.
   (b) *Middle flexion crease:* It lies over the proximal interphalangeal (PIP) joint.
   (c) *Distal flexion crease:* It lies on or just proximal to the distal interphalangeal (DIP) joint.

The digital flexion creases become deeper when the digits are flexed.

Friction Ridges

The friction skin ridges are present on the finger pads called **fingerprints**. These have basic similarities but are not identical in any two individuals including identical twins. The four basic types of fingerprints are (Fig. 11.3): (a) arch, (b) whorl, (c) loop, and (d) composite (combination of first three). They are produced due to the pull of elastic fibres within the dermis. The friction ridges prevent the slippage when grasping the objects. The science of classification and identification of fingerprints is called **dermatoglyphics**.

> ### Clinical correlation
>
> - The person with Down syndrome (trisomy-21) usually has only one transverse palmar crease called *simian crease*.
> - Since the fingerprints are not identical in any two individuals including identical twins, they are used in criminal investigations to identify criminals.

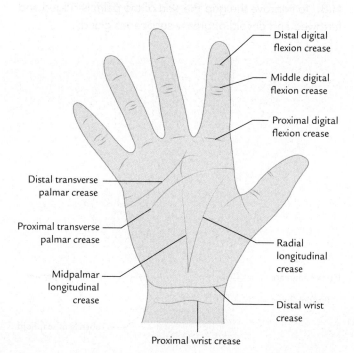

Distal digital flexion crease
Middle digital flexion crease
Proximal digital flexion crease
Distal transverse palmar crease
Proximal transverse palmar crease
Midpalmar longitudinal crease
Radial longitudinal crease
Distal wrist crease
Proximal wrist crease

Fig. 11.2 Flexor creases on the palmar aspect of wrist, palm, and digits.

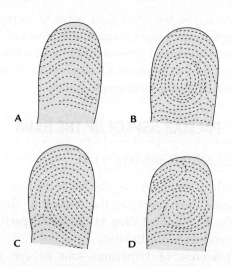

A   B

C   D

Fig. 11.3 Types of finger prints: A, arch; B, whorl; C, loop; D, composite.

SUPERFICIAL FASCIA OF THE PALM

The superficial fascia of the palm is made up of dense fibrous bands, which anchor the skin to the deep fascia of the palm. The superficial fascia of the palm presents two important features:

1. It contains a subcutaneous muscle, the **palmaris brevis** on the ulnar side of the palm, which probably helps to improve the grip.
2. It thickens to form a **superficial metacarpal ligament**, which stretches across the roots of fingers over the digital nerve and vessels.

Palmaris Brevis Muscle

It is subcutaneous muscle in the superficial fascia of the medial part of the palm. Morphologically, it represents the panniculus carnosus.

Origin

From flexor retinaculum and palmar aponeurosis.

Insertion

Into the skin along the medial border of the hand.

Nerve supply

Superficial branch of the ulnar nerve.

Actions

When an object is grasped tightly in the hand, it causes wrinkling of the medial palmar skin and helps to prevent the ulnar displacement of the hypothenar eminence.

DEEP FASCIA OF THE PALM

The deep fascia on the palmar aspect of hand is specialized to form three structures:

1. Flexor retinaculum.
2. Palmar aponeurosis.
3. Fibrous flexor sheaths of digits.

Flexor Retinaculum (Transverse Carpal Ligament)

It is a strong fibrous band which bridges the anterior concavity of carpus and converts it into an osseofibrous tunnel called **carpal tunnel** for the passage of flexor tendons of the digits.

The flexor retinaculum is rectangular and is formed due to thickening of the deep fascia in front of carpal bones.

Attachments (Fig. 11.4)

Medially: It is attached to the pisiform and the hook of hamate.

Laterally: It is attached to the tubercle of scaphoid and the crest of trapezium.

N.B.

On either side, the flexor retinaculum gives a slip (Fig. 11.4).

- A *superficial slip on the medial side* (called **volar carpal ligament**) is attached to the pisiform bone. The ulnar nerve and vessels pass deep to this slip.
- A *deep slip on the lateral side* is attached to the medial lip of groove of trapezium, converting it into a osseofibrous tunnel for the passage of the tendon of flexor carpi radialis.

Relations

Structures passing superficial to flexor retinaculum

From medial to lateral side these are (Fig. 11.5):

1. Ulnar nerve.
2. Ulnar artery.
3. Palmar cutaneous branch of ulnar nerve.
4. Tendon of palmaris longus.
5. Palmar cutaneous branch of median nerve.
6. Superficial palmar branch of radial artery.

Structures passing deep to the flexor retinaculum (i.e. through carpal tunnel)

These are as follows (Fig. 11.5):

1. Tendons of flexor digitorum superficialis (FDS).
2. Tendons of flexor digitorum profundus (FDP).

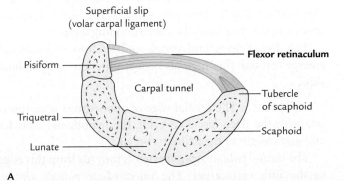
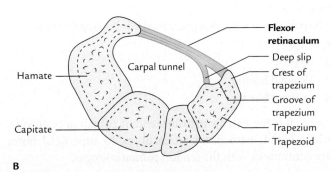

Fig. 11.4 Attachment of additional medial and lateral slips of the flexor retinaculum. **A,** at the level of proximal row of carpal bones; **B,** at the level of distal row of carpal bones.

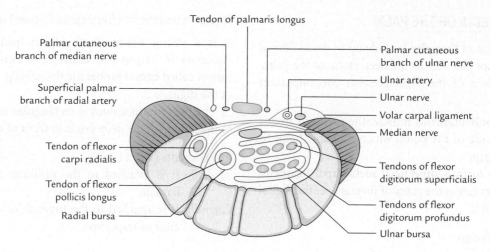

Fig. 11.5 Transverse section of wrist across the carpal tunnel showing structures passing superficial and deep to the flexor retinaculum.

3. Tendon of flexor pollicis longus (FPL).
4. Median nerve.

N.B.

- The flexor tendons of fingers (i.e., tendons of FDS and FDP) are enclosed in a synovial sheath called *ulnar bursa*.
- The tendon of flexor pollicis longus is on the radial side and enclosed in a separate synovial sheath called *radial bursa*.
- The tendon of flexor carpi radialis pass through a separate canal in the lateral part of the flexor retinaculum.

Palmar Aponeurosis

The deep fascia of the palm is thin over thenar and hypothenar eminences and thick in the central part of the palm where it forms the *palmar aponeurosis.*

The palmar aponeurosis (Fig. 11.6) is strong well-defined part of the deep fascia of the palm which covers the long flexor tendons and superficial palmar arch. It is triangular in shape and made up mainly of longitudinal fibres and few transverse fibres intersecting the former.

Its apex is directed proximally towards the wrist and its base is directed distally towards the roots of the fingers.

Features

The palmar aponeurosis presents the following features:

1. Apex.
2. Base.
3. Medial border.
4. Lateral border.

Apex: It is the narrow proximal end of palmar aponeurosis, which blends with flexor retinaculum. Its superficial fibres are continuous with the tendon palmaris longus.

Base: It is the broad distal end of palmar aponeurosis. Just proximal to the heads of metacarpals, the base divides into

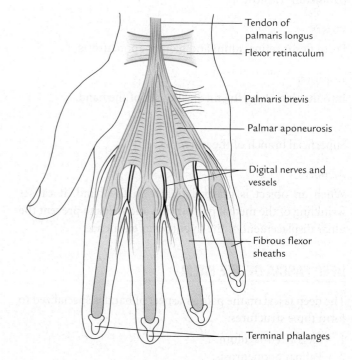

Fig. 11.6 Palmar aponeurosis.

four longitudinal slips, one each of medial four digits. Each slip, further divides into two slips, which blend with the fibrous flexor sheaths of the corresponding digits.

The digital nerve and vessels and tendons of lumbrical emerge through the intervals between the four longitudinal slips.

Medial border: The medial edge of aponeurosis is continuous with the deep fascia covering the hypothenar muscles and gives origin to the palmaris brevis.

The *medial palmar septum* extends inwards from this edge to the fifth metacarpal. The *intermediate palmar septum* extends inwards from near this edge obliquely to the third metacarpal.

Lateral border: The lateral edge of the aponeurosis is continuous with the deep fascia covering the thenar muscles. *Lateral palmar septum* extends inwards from this edge to the first metacarpal.

N.B. Morphologically, palmar aponeurosis represents the degenerated tendons of *palmaris longus muscle*.

Functions

1. Helps to improve the grip of hand by fixing the skin.
2. Protects the underlying tendons, nerves, and vessels.

Clinical correlation

Dupuytren's contracture (Fig. 11.7): It is a progressive fibrosis (interstitial increase in the fibrous tissue) in the medial part of the palmar aponeurosis. Consequently the medial part of the aponeurosis may undergo progressive thickening to form permanent contracture resulting in the flexion deformity of the little and ring fingers. The ring finger is most commonly affected. The proximal and middle phalanges are acutely flexed but distal phalanges remain unaffected. A surgical fasciectomy is required if the hand function is grossly impaired.

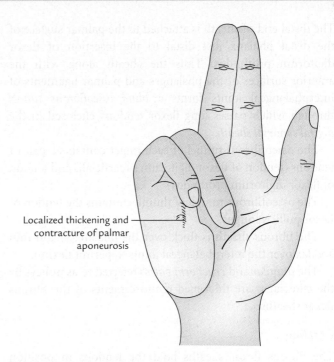

Fig. 11.7 Dupuytren's contracture.

FIBROUS FLEXOR SHEATHS OF THE FINGERS (Fig. 11.8)

The deep fascia on the anterior surface of each digit thickens and arches over the long flexor tendon to form the *fibrous sheath of the finger,* which extends from the head of the metacarpal to the base of distal phalanx.

Attachments

The arched fibrous sheath is attached to the margins of the phalanges and palmar ligaments of interphalangeal joints. The proximal end of sheath is open. Here its margins are continuous with the distal slips of the palmar aponeurosis.

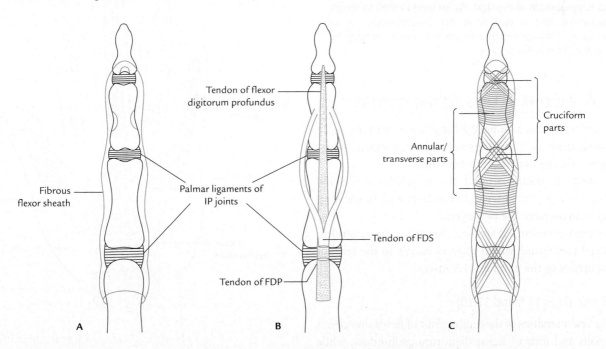

Fig. 11.8 Fibrous flexor sheaths of the fingers: **A,** attachment of the sheath; **B,** tendons passing through the sheath; **C,** arrangement of fibres within sheath—cruciate fibres in front of joints and transverse fibres in front of bones (FDS = flexor digitorum superficialis, FDP = flexor digitorum profundus).

The distal end of sheath is attached to the palmar surface of the distal phalanx just distal to the insertion of flexor digitorum profundus. Thus the sheath along with the anterior surfaces of the phalanges and palmar ligaments of interphalangeal joints forms a *blind osseofibrous tunnel* through which passes long flexor tendons enclosed in the *digital synovial sheath.*

The osseofibrous tunnel of each finger contains a pair of tendons (tendon of flexor digitorum superficialis and tendon of flexor digitorum profundus).

The osseofibrous tunnel of thumb contains the tendon of flexor pollicis longus.

The fibrous sheath is thick over the phalanges, and thin and lax over the interphalangeal joints to permit flexion.

The *annular* and *cruciform parts* (referred to as pulleys by the clinicians) are thickened reinforcements of the fibrous flexor sheaths.

Function

The fibrous flexor sheaths hold the tendons in position during flexion of digits.

Clinical correlation

Trigger finger: It is a clinical condition, in which a finger gets locked in full flexion and can be extended only after excessive voluntary effort or with the help of the other hand. When extension begins it occurs suddenly and with a click, hence the name—*trigger finger*. This condition is caused by the presence of a localized thickening of a long flexor tendon, preventing movement of the tendon within the fibrous flexor sheath of the digit. When tendon tries to move, its thickened part is caught in the osseofibrous tunnel momentarily. This condition can be relieved surgically by incising the fibrous flexor sheath.

SYNOVIAL SHEATHS OF LONG FLEXOR TENDONS

The synovial sheaths around the long flexor tendons serve as a lubricating device to prevent their friction, while moving within the osseofibrous tunnels.

The synovial sheath around the tendon(s) is double layered consisting of an outer and inner layer with lubricating synovial fluid between the two layers.

Every tendon within the synovial sheath has a mesotendon of synovial membrane which conveys vessels to the tendon (*cf.* mesenteries of the gut; Fig. 11.9 inset).

Ulnar Bursa (Figs 11.9 and 11.10)

The long flexor tendons of the fingers (four of flexor digitorum superficialis and four of flexor digitorum profundus), while passing through the osseofibrous carpal tunnel are enclosed in a common synovial sheath called *ulnar bursa*. The tendon invaginates the sheath from the lateral side.

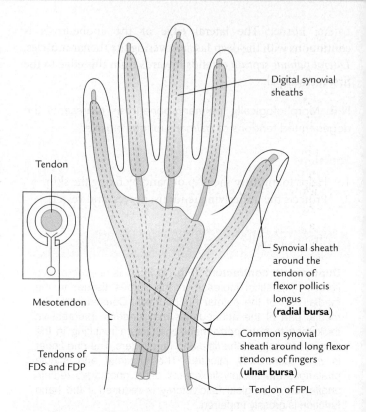

Fig. 11.9 Synovial sheaths around the long flexor tendons. Figure in the inset shows two layers of synovial sheath and mesotendon (FDS = flexor digitorum superficialis, FDP = flexor digitorum profundus, FPL = flexor pollicis longus).

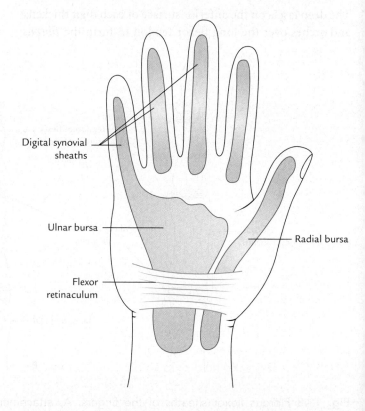

Fig. 11.10 Ulnar bursa, radial bursa, and digital synovial sheaths.

The *ulnar bursa* extends proximally into the forearm about a finger breadth (5 cm) proximal to the flexor retinaculum. Distally it extends in the palm up to the middle of the shafts of the metacarpal bones.

The distal medial end of ulnar bursa is continuous with the digital synovial sheath of the little finger.

Radial Bursa (Figs 11.9 and 11.10)

The tendon of flexor pollicis longus while passing through osseofibrous carpal tunnel is enclosed in a synovial sheath called **radial bursa**. Proximally it extends into the forearm about a finger breadth proximal to the flexor retinaculum. Distally it is continuous with digital synovial sheath of the thumb.

N.B.

The *radial bursa* is usually a separate from that of ulnar bursa but may communicate with *ulnar bursa* deep to flexor retinaculum.

Digital Synovial Sheaths (Figs 11.9 and 11.10)

The flexor tendons of digits while passing through the fibrous flexor sheaths are enclosed in the synovial sheath. The digital synovial sheath extends from head of metacarpals to the distal phalanges of the digits.

N.B.

- The digital synovial sheath of the little finger is continuous with the *ulnar bursa*.
- The digital synovial sheath of the thumb is continuous with the *radial bursa*.
- Parts of long flexor tendons of the index, middle, and ring fingers between the ulnar bursa and digital synovial sheaths are devoid of synovial sheaths.

Functions

Function of the ulnar and radial bursae, and digital synovial sheaths is to allow the long tendons of digits to move freely/ smoothly with minimum friction beneath flexor retinaculum and fibrous flexor sheaths.

Vincula Longa and Vincula Brevia (Fig. 11.11)

As the tendons lie within the fibrous flexor sheaths, they are connected to the phalanges by the thin bands of connective tissue, called **vincula**. *In each digital sheath, there are five vincula—two short and three long.* The short ones are called **vincula brevia** and long ones **vincula longa**. The vincula brevia are small triangular bands attached to the palmar aspect of the IP joints and distal part of adjoining proximal phalanx. The vincula longa are long, narrow band, which extend from the dorsal aspect of the tendon to the proximal part of the palmar surface of the proximal phalanx. The blood vessels reach the tendons through these vincula.

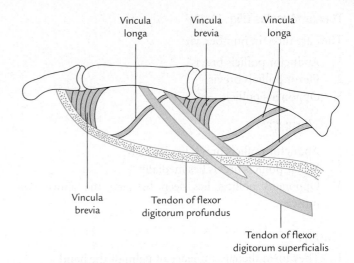

Fig. 11.11 The long flexor tendons of fingers showing vincula longa and brevia.

Clinical correlation

Tenosynovitis of the synovial sheaths of the flexor tendons: It is the infection and inflammation of the synovial sheaths of long flexor tendons, which mostly result from small penetrating wounds caused by pin prick or insertion of thorn. The infection of digital synovial sheaths results in the distension of sheath with pus. The digit gets swollen and becomes very painful due to stretching of sheath by pus. The infection may extend from digital synovial sheaths to the palmar spaces.

In case of infection of digital synovial sheaths of little finger and thumb, the infection may quickly reach into ulnar and radial bursae due to their continuity, if these bursae are involved and neglected. The proximal ends of these bursae may burst and pus may enter into the fascial space of forearm (*space of Parona*) between flexor digitorum profundus anteriorly and interosseous membrane and pronator quadratus posteriorly.

INTRINSIC MUSCLES OF THE HAND

These are short muscles whose origin and insertion is confined within the territory of the hand. They are responsible for skilled movements of the hand and also help the hand in adjusting for proper gripping. There are 20 intrinsic muscles in hand. They have small motor units; hence can act with precision to carry out skilled movements.

The intrinsic muscles of the hand are arranged into the following five groups:

1. Thenar muscles.
2. Adductor of thumb.
3. Hypothenar muscles.
4. Lumbricals.
5. Interossei.

Thenar Muscles (Fig. 11.12)

They are three in number, viz.

1. Abductor pollicis brevis.
2. Flexor pollicis brevis.
3. Opponens pollicis.

Relationship

1. Abductor pollicis brevis lies laterally.
2. Flexor pollicis brevis lies medially.
3. Opponens pollicis lies deep between the above two muscles.

Features

1. They form thenar eminence of palm of the hand.
2. They are chiefly responsible for opposition of thumb.
3. All of them are supplied by the recurrent branch of the median nerve (C8, TI).

N.B. The actions of thenar muscles are indicated by their names to some extent; but they all are involved in opposition providing pincer-like grip between the thumb and index finger.

Hypothenar Muscles (Fig. 11.12)

They are also three in number, viz.

1. Abductor digiti minimi.
2. Flexor digiti minimi.
3. Opponens digiti minimi.

Some authorities also consider palmaris brevis (see page 139) as one of the hypothenar muscles.

Relationship

1. Abductor digiti minimi lies medially.
2. Flexor digiti minimi lies laterally.
3. Opponens digiti minimi lies deep to the above two muscles.

Features

1. They form hypothenar eminence of the palm of the hand.
2. All of them are supplied by the deep branch of ulnar nerve. The origin, insertion, and actions of the thenar and hypothenar muscles are presented in Table 11.1.

N.B.
- The *flexor pollicis* brevis has dual nerve supply: superficial head by the median nerve and deep head by the deep branch of the ulnar nerve.
- Tendons of insertion of the flexor digiti minimi along with the abductor digiti minimi on the medial side of the base of first phalanx contain a sesamoid bone.

Adductor Pollicis Muscle (Fig. 11.13)

This fan-shaped muscle is located deep in the palm in contact with metacarpal and interossei. It consists of two heads: (a) oblique and (b) transverse.

Origin

1. *Oblique head* arises from anterior aspects of capitate bone and bases of second and third metacarpal bones—forming a crescentic shape.
2. *Transverse head* arises from ridge on distal two-third of the anterior surface of the shaft of the third metacarpal.

Insertion

Into the medial side of the base of proximal phalanx of the thumb.

Nerve supply

Deep branch of the ulnar nerve (C8, TI).

Actions

Adduction of the thumb to provide power to the grip.

N.B.
- The tendons of insertion of adductor pollicis on the medial side of the base of proximal phalanx of the thumb contain a *sesamoid bone.*
- The *deep palmar arch* and deep branch of *ulnar nerve* pass between the two heads of adductor pollicis.

Clinical testing (Foment's sign)

Give the patient a thin book and ask him to grasp it firmly between the thumbs and index fingers of both hands. If the muscle is healthy and acting normally, the thumbs will be straight. But if the muscle is paralyzed and not acting, the thumbs are flexed at IP joints (Fig. 13.4). This occurs because when adductors are not acting, flexor pollicis compensates for it.

Lumbrical Muscles (Fig. 11.14)

There are four lumbrical muscles and numbered first, second, third, and fourth from lateral to medial side. They are small slender muscles one for each digit. They are named *lumbricals* because of their elongated worm-like shape (L. lumbrical = earthworm).

Origin

1. **Lumbricals 1 and 2:** From lateral side of lateral two tendons of the flexor digitorum profundus.
2. **Lumbricals 3 and 4:** From adjacent sides of medial three tendons of the flexor digitorum profundus.

Insertion

The tendons cross the radial side of metacarpophalangeal (MP) joints to be inserted into the lateral side of dorsal digital expansion of the corresponding digit from second to fifth.

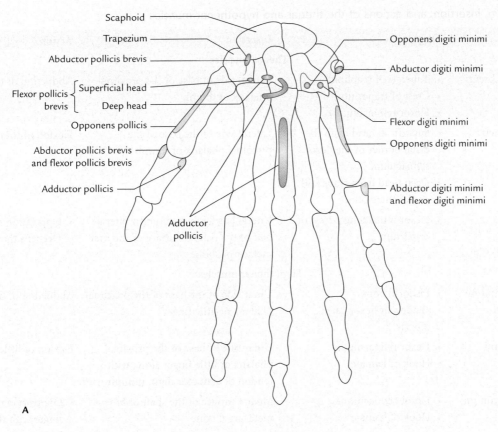

Scaphoid

Trapezium

Abductor pollicis brevis

Flexor pollicis brevis { Superficial head

Deep head

Opponens pollicis

Abductor pollicis brevis and flexor pollicis brevis

Adductor pollicis

Adductor pollicis

Opponens digiti minimi

Abductor digiti minimi

Flexor digiti minimi

Opponens digiti minimi

Abductor digiti minimi and flexor digiti minimi

A

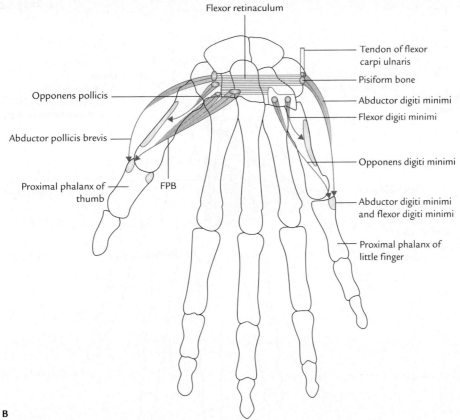

Flexor retinaculum

Opponens pollicis

Abductor pollicis brevis

Proximal phalanx of thumb

FPB

Tendon of flexor carpi ulnaris

Pisiform bone

Abductor digiti minimi

Flexor digiti minimi

Opponens digiti minimi

Abductor digiti minimi and flexor digiti minimi

Proximal phalanx of little finger

B

Fig. 11.12 Thenar and hypothenar muscles: **A,** bony attachment; **B,** origin and insertion (FPB = flexor pollicis brevis).

Table 11.1 Origin, insertion, and actions of the thenar and hypothenar muscles

Muscles	Origin	Insertion	Action
Thenar muscles			
Abductor pollicis brevis	• Tubercle of scaphoid • Crest of trapezium • Flexor retinaculum	Lateral side of base of the proximal phalanx of thumb	Abduction of thumb
Flexor pollicis brevis	• Superficial head from the distal border of the flexor retinaculum • Deep head from trapezoid and capitate bones	Lateral side of the base of the proximal phalanx of thumb	Flexion of thumb
Opponens pollicis	• Flexor retinaculum crest of trapezium	Lateral border and adjoining lateral half of the palmar surface of the first metacarpal bone	• Opposition of thumb • Deepens the hollow of palm
Hypothenar muscles			
Abductor digiti minimi	• Pisiform bone • Tendon of flexor carpi ulnaris	Ulnar side of the base of the proximal phalanx of little finger	Abduction of little finger
Flexor digiti minimi	• Flexor retinaculum • Hook of hamate	Ulnar side of base of the proximal phalanx of little finger along with tendon of abductor digiti minimi	Flexion of little finger
Opponens digiti minimi	• Flexor retinaculum • Hook of hamate	Medial surface of the shaft of 5th metacarpal bone	• Opposition of the tip of little finger with the tip of thumb • Deepens the hollow of palm

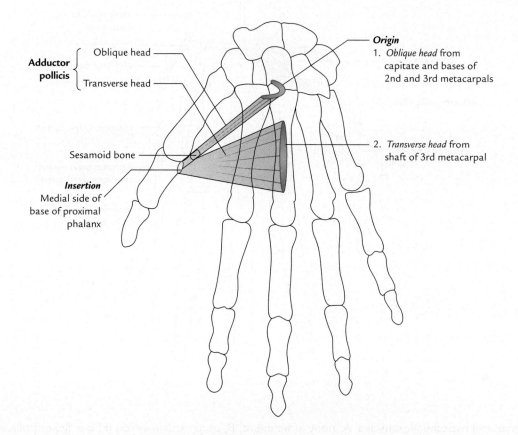

Fig. 11.13 Origin and insertion of the adductor pollicis muscles.

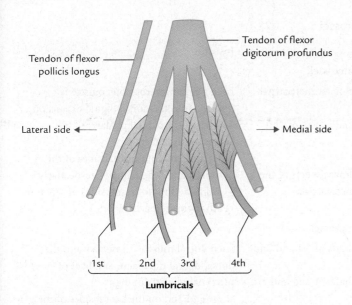

Tendon of flexor pollicis longus

Tendon of flexor digitorum profundus

Lateral side ←

→ Medial side

1st 2nd 3rd 4th

Lumbricals

Fig. 11.14 Lumbrical muscles.

Nerve supply

- First and second lumbricals by the median nerve (C8, T1).
- Third and fourth lumbricals by the deep branch of the ulnar nerve (C8, T1).

Actions

Lumbricals flex the metacarpophalangeal (MP) joints and extend the proximal and distal interphalangeal (PIP and DIP) joints.

Interossei (Fig. 11.15)

The eight small interosseous muscles, as their name indicates, are located between the metacarpals bones. They are arranged into two groups: palmar and dorsal.

Palmar Interossei

Palmar interossei are four small muscles, located between the palmar surfaces of the metacarpals. They are numbered 1–4 from lateral to medial side.

Dorsal Interossei

Dorsal interossei are four small muscles located between the shafts of the metacarpals and numbered from 1 to 4 from lateral to medial side.

N.B. There is one muscle each for first, second, fourth, and fifth digits but not for the third digit.

The origin and insertion of palmar and dorsal interossei is presented in Table 11.2.

The insertion of lumbricals and interossei in dorsal digital expansion is shown in Figure 11.16.

Nerve supply

All the palmar and dorsal interossei are supplied by the deep branch of the ulnar nerve.

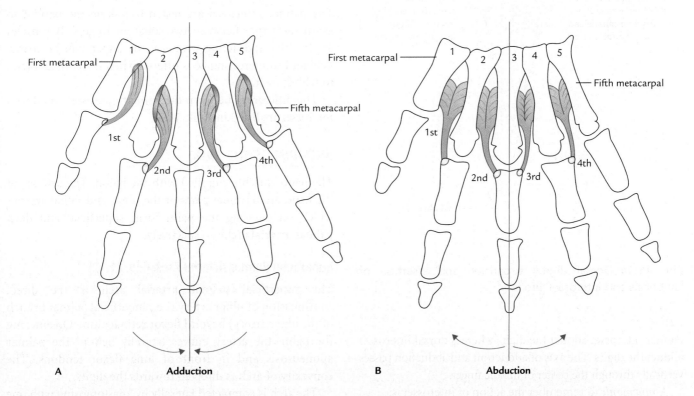

First metacarpal

Fifth metacarpal

1st 2nd 3rd 4th

A **Adduction**

First metacarpal

Fifth metacarpal

1st 2nd 3rd 4th

B **Abduction**

Fig. 11.15 Interosseous muscles: **A**, palmar interossei; **B**, dorsal interossei.

Table 11.2 Origin and insertion of the palmar and dorsal interossei

Muscles	Origin	Insertion
Palmar interossei		
• First palmar interosseous	Medial side of the base of 1st metacarpal	Each palmar interosseous muscle is inserted into the dorsal digital expansion and base of proximal phalanx of the corresponding digit
• Second palmar interosseous	Medial half of the palmar aspect of 2nd metacarpal	– 1st and 2nd into medial sides of the thumb and index fingers, respectively
• Third and fourth palmar interossei	Lateral parts of the palmar aspects of the shafts of 4th and 5th metacarpals	– 3rd and 4th into lateral sides of 4th and 5th digits, respectively
Dorsal interossei		
• First dorsal interosseous	Adjacent sides of the shafts of 1st and 2nd metacarpals	Each dorsal muscle is inserted into the dorsal digital expansion and base of proximal phalanx of digit
• Second dorsal interosseous	Adjacent sides of the shafts of 2nd and 3rd metacarpals	– 1st and 2nd on the lateral sides of the index and middle fingers, respectively
• Third dorsal interosseous	Adjacent sides of the shafts of 3rd and 4th metacarpals	– 3rd and 4th on the medial sides of the middle and ring fingers, respectively
• Fourth dorsal interosseous	Adjacent sides of the shafts of 4th and 5th metacarpals	

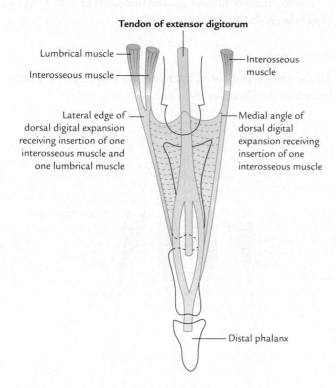

Fig. 11.16 Dorsal digital expansion and insertion of lumbricals and interossei into it.

Actions

Palmar interossei adduct the digits whereas dorsal interossei abduct the digits. The axis of adduction and abduction passes vertically through the center of middle finger.

A *mnemonic* to remember the action of interossei is:
Palmar ADduct (PAD); Dorsal ABduct (DAB).

N.B. Acting together, the palmar and dorsal interossei and the lumbricals produce flexion of metacarpophalangeal (MP) joints and extension of proximal and distal interphalangeal (PID and DIP) joints, this action is termed *Z-movement*.

Clinical testing

The palmar interossei are tested by asking the patient to grasp the paper between two adjacent fingers. If muscles are healthy and acting properly the paper will be firmly held and some resistance is offered when the clinician tries to withdraw it.

The differences between the palmar interossei and dorsal interossei are listed in Table 11.3.

ARTERIES OF THE HAND

The hand is richly supplied with the blood. The arteries of the hand are terminal parts of the ulnar and radial arteries which on entering the palm form **superficial** and **deep palmar arterial arches** respectively.

Superficial Palmar Arterial Arch (Fig. 11.17)

The superficial palmar arterial arch is the direct continuation of ulnar artery (i.e., superficial palmar branch of the ulnar artery) beyond flexor retinaculum. On entering the palm, the artery curves laterally behind the palmar aponeurosis and in front of long flexor tendons. The convexity of arch is directed towards the digits.

The arch is completed laterally by anastomosing with one of the following branches of the radial artery:

Table 11.3 Differences between the palmar and dorsal interossei

Features	Palmar interossei	Dorsal interossei
Location	On the palmar surface between the metacarpals	Between the metacarpals
Type	Unipennate	Bipennate
Origin	From palmar aspects of the metacarpals	From side of metacarpals
Action	Adduction of digits	Abduction of digits

1. Superficial palmar branch of the radial artery (most common).
2. Radialis indicis artery.
3. Princeps pollicis artery.

Branches

1. *Three common palmar digital arteries* go to the interdigital clefts between the fingers and each divides into two proper digital arteries, which supply their adjacent sides. In the interdigital clefts, they are joined by the palmar metacarpal arteries.
2. *One proper digital artery* runs along the medial side of the little finger which it supplies.
3. *Cutaneous branches to the palm*, which supply the skin and superficial fascia of the palm.

Relations
Superficial: Palmar aponeurosis.
Deep: 1. Long flexor tendons of FDS and FDP.
    2. Lumbricals.
    3. Digital branches of the median and ulnar nerves.

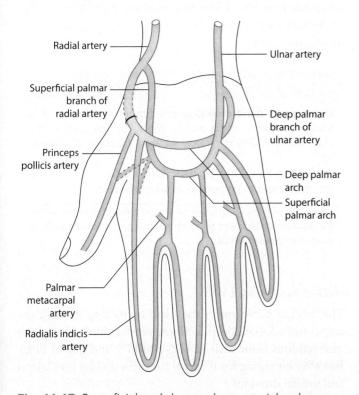

Fig. 11.17 Superficial and deep palmar arterial arches.

Surface Anatomy
The superficial palmar arch lies across the centre of the palm at the level of the distal border of the fully extended thumb.

Deep Palmar Arch (Fig. 11.17)
The deep palmar arch is the direct continuation of radial artery. The arch is completed medially (at the base of the fifth metacarpal) by anastomosing with the deep palmar branch of the ulnar artery.

The radial artery enters the palm from dorsal aspect of the hand by passing between the two heads of first dorsal interosseous muscle. Immediately after entering the palm, the radial artery gives off two branches: *arteria radialis indicis* and *arteria princeps pollicis*. In the palm, it passes between the two heads of adductor pollicis.

Branches

1. **Three palmar metacarpal arteries**, which join the common palmar digital arteries, the branches of the superficial palmar arch.
2. **Three perforating arteries**, which pass through the 2nd, 3rd, and 4th interosseous spaces to anastomose with dorsal metacarpal arteries.
3. **Recurrent branch/branches** run proximally in front of carpus to end in the *palmar carpal arch*.

Relations
Deep:
(a) Proximal parts of shafts of the metacarpals.
(b) Interosseous muscles.

Superficial:
(a) Long flexor tendons of the fingers.
(b) Lumbricals.

N.B. The deep branch of the ulnar nerve lies in the concavity of deep palmar arch.

Surface Anatomy
The deep palmar arch lies about 1 cm proximal to the superficial palmar arch.

The differences between the superficial and deep palmar (arterial) arches are given in Table 11.4.

Table 11.4 Differences between the superficial and deep palmar arches

	Superficial palmar arch	Deep palmar arch
Formation	By anastomosis between direct continuation of the ulnar artery (i.e., superficial palmar branch) with the small superficial branch of the radial artery	By anastomosis between direct continuation of the radial artery with the small deep palmar branch of the ulnar artery
Location	Superficial to long flexor tendons	Deep to long flexor tendons
Branches	• Three common palmar digital arteries • One proper digital artery • Cutaneous branches	• Three palmar metacarpal arteries • Three perforating arteries • Recurrent branches

---

Clinical correlation

Laceration of palmar arterial arches: The lacerated wounds of palmar arterial arches usually cause profuse and uncontrollable bleeding. The compression of brachial artery against humerus is the most effective method to control the bleeding.

The ligation or clamping of the radial artery or ulnar artery or both proximal to wrist fails to control the bleeding because of connections of these arches with the palmar and dorsal carpal arches.

NERVES IN THE PALM OF THE HAND

There are two nerves in the palm of the hand, viz.

1. Ulnar nerve.
2. Median nerve.

N.B. The *ulnar nerve* is the main motor nerve of the hand, whereas *median nerve* is the main sensory nerve of the hand.

Ulnar Nerve (Figs 11.18 and 11.19)

The ulnar nerve enters the palm by passing superficial to the flexor retinaculum between the pisiform bone and ulnar artery. At the distal border of flexor retinaculum it divides into superficial and deep terminal branches.

Superficial Branch

It enters the palm deep to palmaris brevis, which it supplies and then divides into digital branches. The digital nerves supply the skin of the medial 1½ finger. The digital nerves cross over the tips of digits and supply the skin on the dorsum of distal phalanges. The superficial branch of the ulnar nerve is accompanied by the superficial branch of the ulnar artery.

Deep Branch

It dips in the interval between abductor digiti minimi and flexor digiti minimi muscles, then pierces opponens digiti minimi to reach the deep part of the palm. It turns laterally

within the concavity of the deep palmar arch to end by supplying the adductor pollicis.

The deep branch supplies:

- **Muscular branches** to
  - three hypothenar muscles,
  - adductor pollicis,
  - four dorsal interosseous muscles,
  - four palmar interosseous muscles, and
  - medial two lumbricals.
- **Articular branches** to intercarpal, carpometacarpal, and intermetacarpal joints.

The distribution of ulnar nerve in the hand is summarized in Table 11.5.

N.B. The ulnar nerve supplies all the intrinsic muscles of the hand (except thenar muscles and lateral two lumbricals), which are concerned with fine movements of the hand as performed by musicians. Hence ulnar nerve is also termed **musician's nerve**.

Clinical correlation

Ulnar canal syndrome/Guyon's tunnel syndrome: It is clinical condition, which occurs due to compression of the ulnar nerve in Guyon's canal* at wrist. Clinically it presents as:

(a) Hypoesthesia in medial 1½ fingers, and
(b) Weakness of intrinsic muscles of hand.

---

*Ulnar tunnel/Guyon's canal is an osseofibrous tunnel formed by the pisohamate ligament bridging the concavity between pisiform bone and hook of hamate.

Median Nerve (Fig. 11.19)

The median nerve enters the hand by passing through the carpal tunnel, (i.e., deep to flexor retinaculum) along with nine tendons (four each of FDS and FDF and one of FPL). Just after emerging from carpal tunnel it divides into lateral and medial divisions.

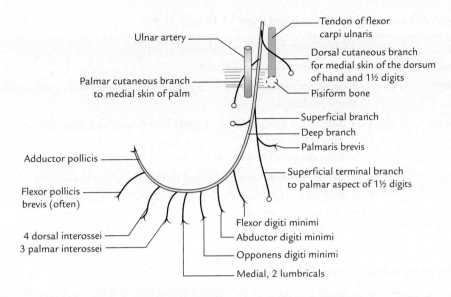

Fig. 11.18 Course and distribution of the ulnar nerve in hand.

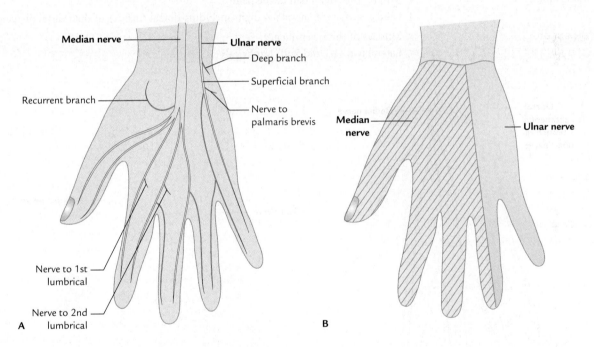

Fig. 11.19 Median and ulnar nerves in hand: A, branches; B, areas of sensory innervation of the palmar aspect of the hand.

Lateral division gives off:

(a) *recurrent branch*, which curls upwards to supply thenar muscles (e.g., abductor pollicis brevis, flexor pollicis brevis, and opponens pollicis) and

(b) *three proper palmar digital branches*, which provides sensory innervation to thumb and lateral side to the index finger. The digital branch to the index finger sends a twig to the first lumbrical.

Medial division gives off:

Two common digital nerves, which provides sensory innervation to the medial side of the index finger, middle finger, and lateral side of the ring finger. The lateral common digital nerve sends a twig to second lumbrical.

The distribution of median nerve in hand is summarized in Table 11.6.

FASCIAL SPACES OF THE HAND

By virtue of the arrangement of various fascia and fascial septa, many fascial spaces are formed in the region of the hand. Normally they are potential spaces filled with loose connective tissue but they become obvious only when fluid or pus collects in them. These spaces are of great sur-

Table 11.5 Distribution of the ulnar nerve in the hand (Figs 11.19 and 11.20)

Branches	Distribution
Palmar cutaneous branch*	Skin on the medial side of palm
Dorsal cutaneous branch**	Skin on the medial half of the dorsum of hand and dorsal aspect of medial 1½ fingers except distal phalanges
Superficial terminal branch	• Skin of the palmar aspect of medial 1½ fingers including skin on the dorsal aspect of the distal phalanges • Palmaris brevis muscle
Deep terminal branch	• All the intrinsic muscles of hand except lateral two lumbricals • Intercarpal, carpometacarpal, and intermetacarpal joints

*Palmar cutaneous branch of the ulnar nerve arises just proximal to wrist.
**Dorsal cutaneous branch of the ulnar nerve arises 5 cm proximal to wrist.

Table 11.6 Distribution of the median nerve in the hand

	Median nerve
Sensory distribution	• Skin on the lateral half of the palm • Palmar surface of lateral 3½ digits including dorsal surfaces of their distal phalanges
Motor distribution	• Muscles of thenar eminence • Lateral two (1st and 2nd) lumbricals

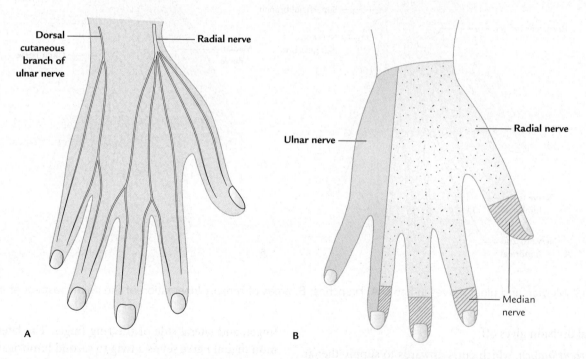

Fig. 11.20 Dorsum of the hand: A, nerves of dorsum of the hand; B, areas of sensory innervation of the dorsum of the hand.

gical importance because they may get infected and distended with pus. The knowledge of their boundaries is essential because they may limit the spread of infection in the palm.

The various spaces of hand are as follows:

A. Palmar spaces

1. Midpalmar space.

2. Thenar space.

3. Pulp spaces of digits.

B. Dorsal spaces

1. Dorsal subcutaneous space

2. Dorsal subaponeurotic space

C. Space of Parona

Midpalmar Space (Fig. 11.21)

The triangular midpalmar space is located under the medial half of hollow of the palm.

Boundaries

Anterior: From superficial to deep, it is formed by:
1. Palmar aponeurosis.
2. Superficial palmar arch.
3. Digital nerve and vessels supplying medial 3½ fingers.
4. Ulnar bursa enclosing flexor tendons of medial three fingers.
5. Medial three (2nd, 3rd, and 4th) lumbricals.

Posterior: Fascia covering interossei and medial three metacarpals.

Lateral: Intermediate palmar septum extending obliquely from near the medial edge of the palmar aponeurosis to the third metacarpal bone. This septum separates the midpalmar space from the thenar space.

Medial: Medial palmar septum extending from medial edge of palmar aponeurosis to the fifth metacarpal. This septum separates the midpalmar space from hypothenar space occupied by the hypothenar muscles.

Proximal: Midpalmar space is continuous with the forearm space of Parona.

Distal: Midpalmar space is continuous with the medial three web-spaces through **medial three lumbrical canals.**

N.B.

Web spaces: The web space is a subcutaneous space in each interdigital cleft and is filled with loose areolar tissue. It contains lumbrical tendon, interosseous tendon, digital nerve, and vessels.

The web space extends from the free margin of the web, as far proximally as the level of transverse metacarpal ligaments.

Clinical correlation

Infection of midpalmar space: The ulnar bursa is considered as the inlet for infection and lumbrical canals as the outlets of infection in midpalmar space. The pus form this space is drained by incisions in the medial two web spaces.

Thenar Space (Fig. 11.21)

The triangular thenar space is located under the outer half of the hollow of the palm.

Boundaries

Anterior: From superficial to deep, it is formed by:
1. Palmar aponeurosis (lateral part).
2. Digital nerve and vessels of lateral 1½ digits.
3. Radial bursa enclosing tendon of flexor pollicis longus.
4. Flexor tendons of the index finger.
5. First lumbrical.

Lateral: Lateral palmar septum extending from lateral edge of palmar aponeurosis to the first metacarpal.

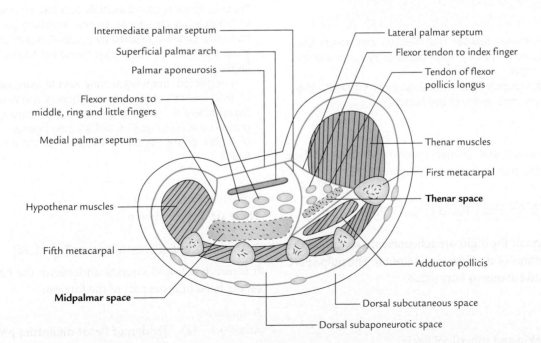

Fig. 11.21 Cross section of the hand showing palmar spaces and spaces on the dorsum of the hand.

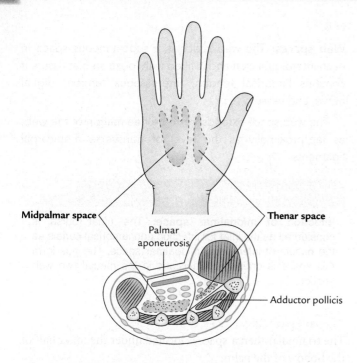

Fig. 11.22 Midpalmar and thenar spaces of the hand and their surface projections in the palm.

Medial: Intermediate palmar septum.
Posterior: Fascia covering the transverse head of adductor pollicis.
Proximal: The space is limited by the fusion of anterior and posterior walls in the carpal tunnel.
Distal: The space communicates with the first web space through the **first lumbrical canal**.

Clinical correlation

Infection of thenar space: The infection may reach the thenar space from infected radial bursa or synovial sheath of the index finger.

The pus from thenar space is drained by an incision in the first web space (web space of the thumb).

The midpalmar and thenar spaces and their surface projection in the palm are shown in Figure 11.22.

PULP SPACES OF THE DIGITS (Fig. 11.23)

The pulp spaces of the digits are subcutaneous spaces on the palmar side of tips of the fingers and thumb. The pulp space is filled with subcutaneous fatty tissue.

Boundaries

Superficially: Skin and superficial fascia.
Deeply: Distal two-third of distal phalanx.

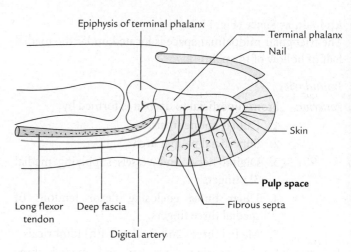

Fig. 11.23 Pulp space of the finger.

Features

1. The space is traversed by numerous fibrous septa extending from skin to the periosteum of the terminal phalanx, dividing it into many loculi.
2. The deep fascia of pulp of each finger fuses with the periosteum of terminal phalanx distal to the insertion of long flexor tendon.
3. The digital artery that supplies the diaphysis of phalanx runs through this space. The epiphysis of distal phalanx receives its blood supply proximal to the pulp space.

Clinical correlation

Pulp space infection: Being the most exposed parts of the digits the pulp spaces are prone for infection. An abscess in the pulp-space is called **whitlow** or **felon**. The rising tension in the pulp space causes severe throbbing pain. The pus from pulp space is drained by a lateral incision, opening all loculi and avoiding tactile skin sensation on the front of the finger.

If neglected, the whitlow may lead to avascular necrosis of distal four-fifth of the terminal phalanx due to occlusion of digital artery as result of pressure. The proximal one-fifth phalanx (i.e., epiphysis) is not affected because the branch of digital artery supplying it does not traverse the pulp space.

Dorsal Surfaces

These are described on p. 172.

Space of Parona (Forearm space; Fig. 11.24)

It is merely a fascial interval underneath the flexor tendons on the front of distal part of the forearm.

Boundaries

Anterior: (a) Tendon of flexor digitorum profundus and flexor digitorum superficialis surrounded by a synovial sheath (ulnar bursa).

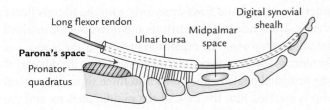

Fig. 11.24 Forearm space (Parona's space) as seen in section along the long axis of the hand.

(b)   Tendon of flexor pollicis longus surrounded by a synovial bursa (radial bursa).

Proximal: Proximally, it is continuous with the inter-muscular spaces of the forearm.

Distal: Distally it reaches the level of wrist.

Lateral: Outer border of the forearm.

Medial: Inner border of the forearm.

Clinical correlation

The forearm space (Parona's space) becomes infected from infected ulnar bursa. Pus collects behind the long flexor tendons.

Surgical Incisions on the Front of Wrist and Hand (Fig. 11.25)

The surgical incisions in the palm should be well-planned and given carefully to avoid contractures:

- Incisions should be parallel to major skin creases of the hand as far as possible.
- An incision should not cross the skin crease at a right angle.

Guidelines for some incisions are as follows (Fig. 11.25):

- To drain abscess of the *thenar space,* a vertical incision is given in first web space (A).
- To drain abscess from *midpalmar space,* small vertical incision should be given in the medial two web spaces (B).
- To drain abscess from *ulnar bursa,* incision should be given along the radial margin of hypothenar eminence (C).
- To drain abscess from *radial bursa,* incision should be given along the medial margin of thenar eminence (D).
- To drain pus from *digital synovial sheath,* vertical incisions should be given along the side of proximal and middle phalanges (E).
- To drain pus from pulp space, vertical incision should be given along the sides of pulp (F).
- To drain pus from space of Parona, vertical incisions should be given on the distal part of forearm (G).

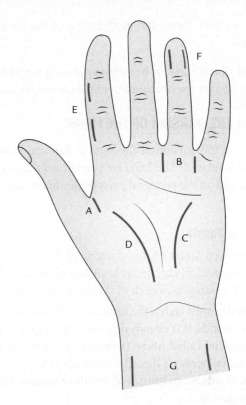

Fig. 11.25 Incisions on the front of wrist and hand for draining abscess from: **A**, thenar space; **B**, midpalmar space; **C**, ulnar bursa; **D**, radial bursa; **E**, digital synovial sheath; **F**, pulp space; **G**, space of Parona.

DORSUM OF THE HAND

Surface Landmarks

1.   **Knuckles,** the bony prominences at the junction of hand and digits, which become visible prominently when a fist is made. They are produced by the heads of metacarpals.
2.   **Anatomical snuff-box,** a triangular depression, which appears on the dorsolateral aspect of the hand when the thumb is hyperextended. The pulsations of radial artery can be felt in this box. The beginning of cephalic vein can also be seen at this site. The tendon of extensor pollicis longus forming its posterior boundary and tendons of abductor pollicis longus and extensor pollicis brevis forming its anterior boundary are clearly visible.
3.   **Extensor tendons of fingers** stand out clearly when the wrist is extended and digits are abducted. These tendons are not visible far beyond knuckles because they flatten here to form extensor expansions.
4.   **Dorsal venous network** is clearly visible and forms the prominent feature of the dorsum of hand.
5.   **Base of first metacarpal (thumb)** can be readily felt in the angle between the tendons of abductor pollicis longus and extensor pollicis longus.
6.   Whole of the **radial border** and most of the **dorsal surface of the second (index) metacarpal** can be readily

felt. Its base forms the prominence of the back of the hand.

N.B. The dorsal surfaces of *metacarpals* of the middle, ring, and little fingers are obscured by the extensor tendons.

SKIN ON THE DORSUM OF THE HAND

The skin on the dorsum of the hand is thin and loose when the hand is relaxed. The hairs are present on the dorsum of the hand and on the proximal parts of the digits, especially in males.

Superficial Fascia

The superficial fascia on the dorsum of the hand contains dorsal venous arch, cutaneous branches of the radial nerve, and dorsal cutaneous branch of the ulnar nerve (Fig. 11.20):

1. **Dorsal venous arch** is the network of veins on the dorsum of the hands. It is already described in Chapter 7, P. 86.
2. **Superficial radial nerve** (terminal cutaneous branch of the radial nerve) is described on page 158.
3. **Dorsal cutaneous branch of the ulnar nerve** is described on page 158.

Deep Fascia

The deep fascia on the back of the wrist is thickened to form thick fibrous band—the extensor retinaculum, which holds the extensor tendons in place (for details see pages 120 and 122).

EXTENSOR TENDONS ON THE DORSUM OF THE HAND

The extensor tendons on the dorsum of the hand are as follows:

1. **Tendons of the thumb:** They are three in number; one for each bone of the thumb:
   (a) Tendon of *abductor pollicis longus* (APL) is inserted on the base of 1st metacarpal.
   (b) Tendon of *extensor pollicis brevis* (EPB) is inserted on the base of proximal phalanx.
   (c) Tendon of *extensor pollicis longus* (EPL) is inserted on the base of distal phalanx.
2. **Tendons of extensor digitorum:** These are four in number, which diverge across the dorsum of the hand, where they are usually connected to one another by three oblique fibrous intertendinous bands. The tendons are united in such a way as to form with deep fascia an aponeurotic sheath, which is attached to the borders of the second and fifth metacarpals.

DORSAL DIGITAL EXPANSIONS (Fig. 11.16)

Each tendon of extensor digitorum expands over the metacarpophalangeal joint to cover its dorsal aspect and

sides like a hood and fuses anteriorly with the fibrous flexor sheath. The tendons of lumbricals and interossei are inserted into this expansion. The expansion narrows as the tendons of lumbricals and interossei converge towards it on the dorsum of the proximal phalanx and splits into three slips. The central slip is inserted into the base of the middle phalanx and the lateral slips to the base of terminal phalanx.

N.B.

- The dorsal digital expansion forms a *functional unit* to coordinate the actions of long extensors, long flexors, lumbricals and interossei on the digit.
- On the index finger and little finger, the expansion is strengthened by extensor indicis and extensor digiti minimi, respectively, which blends with it.

Clinical correlation

- **Mallet finger/baseball finger/cricketer's finger** (Fig. 11.26): The insertion of extensor tendon into the base of the terminal phalanx may be torn by a forceful blow on the tip of the finger, which causes sudden and strong flexion of the phalanx. Occasionally, small flakes of the bone may be avulsed. Consequently the distal phalanx assumes a flexed position with swan neck deformity and voluntary extension is impossible. This condition commonly occurs in *cricketers* and *baseball players*.
- **Boutonnière (button-hole) deformity** (Fig. 11.27): It is opposite to mallet finger deformity. It is characterized by flexion of proximal interphalangeal (PIP) joint and hyperextension of distal phalanx. It occurs when the flexed PIP joint pokes through the extensor expansion following rupture of its central portion of dorsal digital expansion due to a direct end on trauma to the finger.

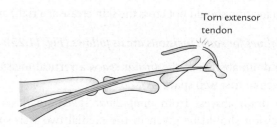

Torn extensor tendon

Fig. 11.26 Mallet finger with swan neck deformity.

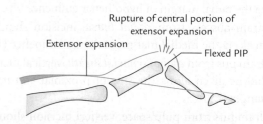

Rupture of central portion of extensor expansion

Extensor expansion

Flexed PIP

Fig. 11.27 Boutonniere (button-hole) deformity. Note proximal interphalangeal (PIP) joint is poking through the extensor expansion.

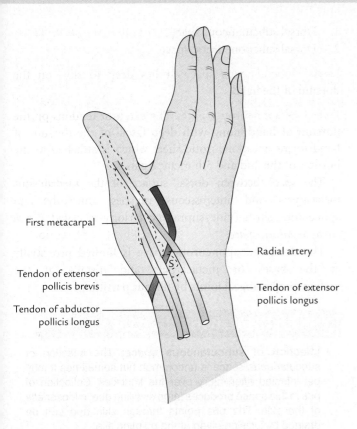

Fig. 11.28 Boundaries and contents of the anatomical snuffbox (S = scaphoid).

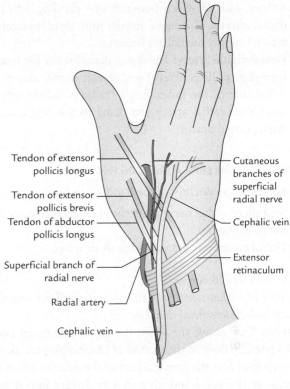

Fig. 11.29 Structures crossing the roof of anatomical snuffbox.

ANATOMICAL SNUFF-BOX (Figs 11.28 and 11.29)

The **anatomical snuff-box** is an elongated triangular depression seen on the lateral side of the dorsum of hand when the thumb is hyperextended.

Boundaries (Fig. 11.28)

Anterolaterally:

1. Tendon of abductor pollicis longus.
2. Tendon of extensor pollicis brevis.

Posteromedially: Tendon of extensor pollicis longus.
Floor: It is formed by

1. scaphoid and
2. trapezium.

Roof: It is formed by

1. skin and
2. superficial fascia.

Contents: Radial artery.
Structures crossing the roof deep to skin (Fig. 11.29):

1. Cephalic vein, from medial to lateral side.
2. Terminal branches of the superficial radial nerve, from lateral to medial side.

Clinical correlation

Clinical significance of anatomical snuff box:
- The pulsations of radial artery can be felt in the anatomical box.
- The tenderness in the anatomical box indicates fracture of scaphoid bone.
- The cephalic vein at this site is often used for giving intravenous fluids.
- The superficial branches of the radial nerve can be rolled over the tendon of extensor pollicis longus.

ARTERIES ON THE DORSUM OF THE HAND

1. **Radial artery:** The radial artery on leaving the forearm, winds round the radial side of the wrist lying on the radial collateral ligament. It passes through anatomical box, on the dorsal surface of scaphoid and trapezium and then passes forward into the palm of the hand by passing between the proximal ends of first and second metacarpals and two heads of the first dorsal interosseous muscle.
2. **Dorsal carpal arch:** It is an arterial arch lying on the dorsal aspect of the carpus. It is formed by the posterior carpal branches of the radial and ulnar arteries, respectively.

The dorsal carpal arch gives off *three dorsal metacarpal arteries,* each of which terminates by dividing into two digital arteries. The digital arteries from three metacarpal arteries supply medial 3½ fingers.

3. **Dorsal digital artery:** The dorsal digital artery for thumb (**princeps pollicis artery**) and dorsal digital artery for radial side of the index finger (**radialis indicis artery**) arise from radial artery just distal to the origin of its dorsal carpal branch.

Nerves of the Dorsum of the Hand (Fig. 11.27)

The nerves of the dorsum of the hand are two, viz.

1. Superficial radial nerve (superficial cutaneous branch of the radial nerve).
2. Dorsal cutaneous branch of the ulnar nerve.

Superficial Radial Nerve

The part of radial nerve in hand is its superficial terminal branch called *superficial radial nerve.*

About 7 cm above the wrist, the superficial radial nerve passes laterally deep to the tendon of brachioradialis, pierces the deep fascia on the dorsal aspect of the wrist to reach the dorsum of the hand and immediately divides into 4 or 5 dorsal digital nerves, which cross the roof of anatomical snuff-box and supply the skin over the lateral two-third of the dorsum of hand and dorsal aspects of lateral 3½ digits except the skin over their distal phalanges.

Dorsal Cutaneous Branch of Ulnar Nerve

It arises from ulnar nerve about 5 cm about the wrist. On reaching the hand, it divides into two branches which supply the skin of the medial 1½ finger except their distal phalanges.

Sensory innervation of the hand

Palmar aspect (Fig. 11.19)

1. Medial one-third of palm and medial 1½ digit except dorsal aspect of their distal phalanges by the ulnar nerve.
2. Lateral two-third of palm and lateral 3½ digits including dorsal aspect of their distal phalanges by the median nerve.

Dorsal aspect (Fig. 11.20)

1. Lateral two-third of dorsum of the hand and lateral 3½ digits except distal phalanges by the radial nerve.
2. Medial one-third of dorsum of the hand and medial 1½ digit except their distal phalanges by the ulnar nerve.

SPACES ON THE DORSUM OF THE HAND

These are two potential spaces on the dorsum of the hand (Fig. 11.29), viz.

1. Dorsal subcutaneous space.
2. Dorsal subaponeurotic space.

Dorsal subcutaneous space: It lies deep to skin on the dorsum of the hand.

Dorsal subaponeurotic space: The extensor tendons on the dorsum of hand along with deep fascia of the dorsum of hand forms an aponeurotic sheet which is attached to the borders of the 2nd and 5th metacarpals.

The space between dorsal surface of the medial four metacarpals and interosseous muscles anteriorly and aponeurotic sheet (vide supra) posteriorly is called *dorsal subaponeurotic space.*

The dorsal subaponeurotic space is limited proximally at the bases of metacarpals and distally at the metacarpophalangeal joints by fibrous partitions.

Clinical correlation

- **Infection of subcutaneous space:** The infection of subcutaneous space is uncommon but sometimes it may get infected after injury over the knuckles. Collection of pus in this space produces large swelling due to looseness of the skin. The pus points through skin and can be drained by incision given at the pointing site.
- **Infection of subaponeurotic space:** The septic infection of subaponeurotic space is generally *primary,* following wounds on the dorsum of the hand. It may, however, get involved *secondarily* to the infection of the midpalmar space. The pus collected in the subaponeurotic space is limited proximally at the bases of metacarpal bones and distally at the metacarpophalangeal joints. On each side, it is limited opposite the borders of second and fifth metacarpal bones. To drain the pus from this space, incisions are made in the aponeurosis between the tendons distally. Alternatively, two incisions may be made, one on the radial side and one along the ulnar side of extensor tendons.

ARCHES OF THE HAND

Like foot, the hand also has arches. The hand is composed of a series of three flexible **bony arches.** Their preservation following an injury is of supreme functional importance to the hand.

The arches of the hand are as follows:

1. **Transverse carpal arch:** It is formed by the concavity of the carpus with flexor retinaculum stretching between its pillars.
2. **Transverse metacarpal arch:** It is formed by the heads of the metacarpal bones, which are bound together by the deep metacarpal ligaments.
3. **Longitudinal arch:** It is formed by the palmar concavity of the metacarpals and normal slightly flexed posture of the digits.

FUNCTION OF ARCHES

The arches of the hand provide room for grasping objects in the hollow of palm.

The more accentuated the arches are, the more secure is the grip. The thenar and hypothenar muscles and palmaris brevis play an important role in providing adjusting power of the arches.

Clinical correlation

Abnormalities of arches of the hand: The disturbances of palmar arches result in *flat hand* with impairment of gripping power. The *flattening of carpal arch* seriously affects the gripping power of the thumb. It occurs due to surgical division of flexor retinaculum or injury to the carpus.

Golden Facts to Remember

▶ All the intrinsic muscles of the hand are supplied by the ulnar nerve *except*	Muscles of thenar eminence and first two lumbricals
▶ *Life line* of palmistry in the hand	Radial longitudinal palmar crease
▶ Digit to which maximum number of muscles are attached	Thumb (8 muscles)
▶ Musician's nerve	Ulnar nerve
▶ Most prominent feature on the dorsum of hand	Dorsal venous network
▶ Cricketer's finger/baseball finger	Flexion deformity of the finger
▶ Trigger finger	Locking of finger in full flexion
▶ Eye of the hand/peripheral eye	Median nerve

Clinical Case Study

A 27-year-old dental student while going to the college fell from the motorcycle with an outstretched right hand. He got up and went to the college to attend his classes. In the class, he felt pain in his right wrist. He went to emergency department for check-up. The Resident doctor over there, on examination, noticed tenderness in the region of anatomical snuff box of his right hand. The X-ray of hand did not reveal any fracture. The doctor made a diagnosis of sprained wrist. The elastic bandage was applied around the wrist and sent back. Three weeks later the student was still experiencing pain on moving his hand. He went to a senior orthopaedic surgeon, who after careful examination, made a diagnosis of fracture of the right scaphoid bone.

Questions

1. Name the carpal bones which form the floor of anatomical snuff-box.
2. Why fracture of scaphoid bone was wrongly diagnosed as sprained wrist?
3. The scaphoid bone is prone to avascular necrosis after its fracture. Why?
4. Why scaphoid bone is difficult to immobilize?

Answers

1. Scaphoid and trapezium.
2. In fracture of scaphoid, the X-ray examination often does not reveal fracture immediately after injury because displacement of fractured segments does not occur.
3. The scaphoid bone most commonly fractures through its narrow part called *waist*. The proximal segment undergoes avascular necrosis because it receives its arterial supply through the distal part of the bone, which is severed during fracture.
4. Because of its position and small size.

Joints and Movements of the Hand

JOINTS OF WRIST, HAND, AND FINGERS

The hand is the region of the upper limb distal to the wrist joint. It consists of three parts: (a) wrist, (b) metacarpus, and (c) digits.

The study of joints of hand is essential to understand the various movements of the hand. Of these, radio-carpal (wrist) and first carpometacarpal joints need to be studied in detail as they execute wide range of movements.

WRIST JOINT (RADIO-CARPAL JOINT; Fig. 12.1)

Type

The wrist joint is a **synovial joint of ellipsoid variety** between lower end of radius and carpus.

Articular surfaces

1. **Proximal articular surface** is formed by inferior surface of the lower end of radius and inferior surface of the triangular articular disc of inferior radio-ulnar joint.

    This articular surface is almost elliptical in shape and concave from side to side.

2. **Distal articular surface** is formed by the proximal surfaces of scaphoid, triquetral, and lunate bones. It is smooth and convex.

N.B.

• Although wrist joint is an articulation between forearm and hand, the medial bone of forearm — the **ulna** is excluded from this articulation by an articular disc.

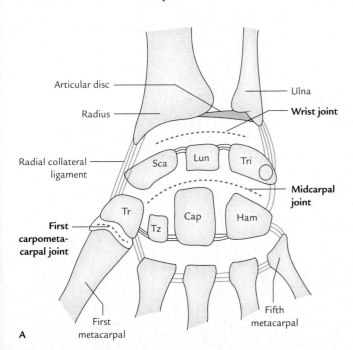

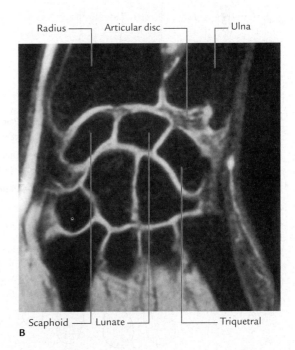

Fig. 12.1 Coronal section through wrist region: **A**, schematic diagram; **B**, as seen in magnetic resonance imaging, showing wrist joint, midcarpal joint, intercarpal joints, carpometacarpal joints. (*Source B:* Fig. 7.91C, Page 710, *Gray's Anatomy for Students*, Richard L Drake, Wayne Vogl, Adam WM Mitchell. Copyright Elsevier Inc. 2005, All rights reserved.)

- In the neutral position of the wrist, only the scaphoid and lunate are in contact with the radius and articular disc; the triquetral comes into contact with the articular disc only in the full adduction of the wrist.

The pisiform bone also does not participate in this articulation because it acts primarily as a sesamoid bone to increase the leverage of the flexor carpi ulnaris and lies in a plane anterior to the other carpal bones.

Ligaments (Fig. 12.2)

1. **Capsular ligament (joint capsule):** It is the fibrous covering of the joint and is attached above to the distal ends of radius and ulna, and below to the proximal row of carpal bones.

   The *synovial membrane* lines the inner surface of the fibrous capsule and extends up to the margins of the articular surfaces.
2. **Radial collateral ligament:** It extends from the tip of styloid process of radius to lateral aspects of the scaphoid and trapezium. It is related to the radial artery.
3. **Ulnar collateral ligament:** It extends from the tip of styloid process of ulna to the medial aspects of the triquetral and pisiform bones.
4. **Palmar radio-carpal ligament:** It extends from anterior margin of the lower end of radius to the anterior surfaces of the scaphoid, lunate, and triquetral bones. It is formed due to thickening of the lateral part of the anterior aspect of the fibrous capsule.

5. **Palmar ulnocarpal ligament:** It extends vertically downwards from the base of styloid process and adjoining part of articular disc to the anterior surface of the lunate and triquetral. It is formed due to thickening of the medial part of the anterior aspect of the fibrous capsule.
6. **Dorsal radio-carpal ligament:** It extends downwards and medially from the posterior margin of the lower end of radius to the dorsal surface of the scaphoid, lunate, and triquetral bones.

N.B. The strongest bonds of union of wrist joint are ulnar and radial collateral ligaments.

Relations (Fig. 12.3)

Anterior

1. Tendons of flexor digitorum superficialis (FDS), flexor digitorum profundus (FDP) and associated synovial sheath (ulnar bursa).
2. Tendon of flexor pollicis longus (FPL) and associated synovial sheath (radial bursa).
3. Median nerve.
4. Tendon of flexor carpi radialis and associated synovial bursa.
5. Ulnar nerve and vessels

Posterior

1. Extensor tendons of wrist and fingers, and associated synovial sheaths.

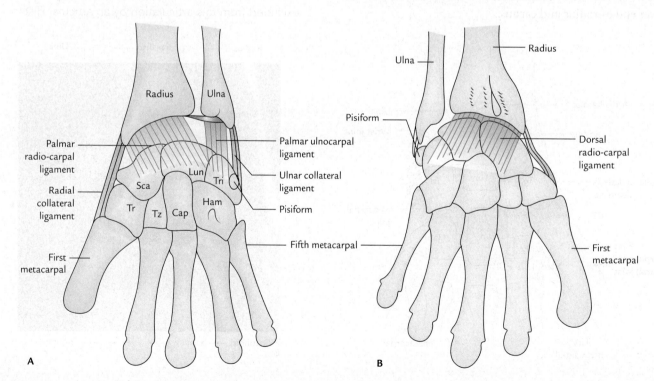

Fig. 12.2 Ligaments of the radio-carpal (wrist) joint: A, palmar radio-carpal and ulnocarpal ligaments; B, dorsal radio-carpal ligaments.

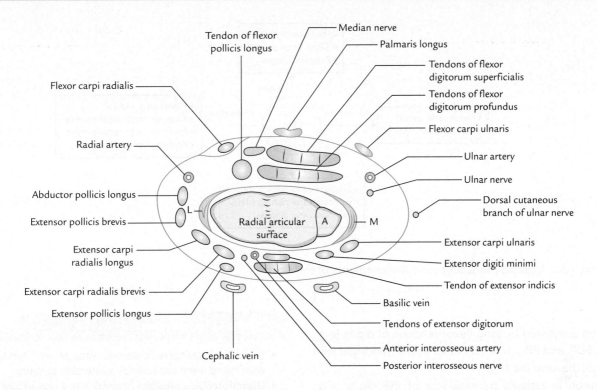

Fig. 12.3 Relations of the right wrist joint (A = articular disc, M = medial (ulnar) collateral ligament, L = lateral (radial) collateral ligament).

2. Anterior interosseous artery.
3. Anterior interosseous nerve.

Lateral
1. Radial artery (across the radial collateral ligament).
2. Tendon of abductor pollicis longus (APL).
3. Tendon of extensor pollicis brevis (EPB).

Medial: Dorsal cutaneous branch of ulnar nerve.

Movements
It is a biaxial joint and permits the following movements:

1. Flexion.
2. Extension.
3. Abduction.
4. Adduction.
5. Circumduction.

Flexion and extension occur along the *transverse axis,* and abduction and adduction occur along the *anteroposterior axis.*

N.B.
- The movements at the wrist joint are usually associated with movements at the midcarpal joint (joint between the proximal and distal rows of carpal bones). The wrist and midcarpal joints together are considered as *link joint.*
- Rotation is not possible at the wrist joint because the articular surfaces are ellipsoid in shape. The lack of rotation at wrist is compensated by the movements of pronation and supination of the forearm.
- The **wrist complex** consists of radio-carpal joint and midcarpal joint.

The movements at the wrist joint and muscles producing them are listed in Table 12.1 (also see Flowchart 12.1).

Table 12.1 Movements at the wrist joint and muscles producing them

Movement	Muscles
Flexion (upward bending of the wrist)	• Flexor carpi radialis (FCR) • Flexor carpi ulnaris (FCU) • Palmaris longus (PL)
Extension (backward bending of the wrist)	• Extensor carpi radialis longus (ECRL) • Extensor carpi radialis brevis (ECRB) • Extensor carpi ulnaris (ECU)
Abduction (lateral bending of the wrist)	• Flexor carpi radialis (FCR) • Extensor carpi radialis longus (ECRL) • Extensor carpi radialis brevis (ECRB) • Abductor pollicis longus (APL)
Adduction (medial bending of the wrist)	• Flexor carpi ulnaris (FCU) • Extensor carpi ulnaris (ECU)

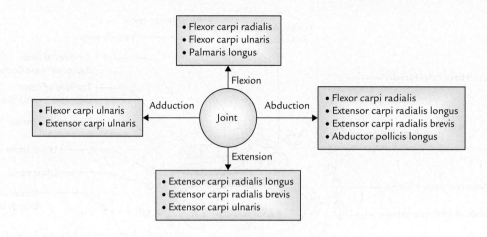

Flowchart 12.1 Muscles producing various movements of the wrist.

N.B.

- Flexion is assisted by long flexor tendons of digits (e.g., FDS, FDP, and FPL). It occurs more at the midcarpal joint than at the wrist joint.
- Extension is assisted by extensors of the digits (e.g., extensor digitorum, extensor digiti minimi, and extensor indicis). It occurs more at wrist than at midcarpal joint.
- Abduction occurs more at midcarpal joint than the wrist joint.
- Adduction mainly occurs at wrist joint.
- Flexion and extension of the hand are actually initiated at the midcarpal joint.

Range of movements (Fig. 12.4)

The range of movements (ROM) of the wrist joint is given in the box below:

Range of movements of the wrist joint	
Movement	Range
Flexion	0–60°
Extension	0–50°
Abduction	0–15°
Adduction	0–50°

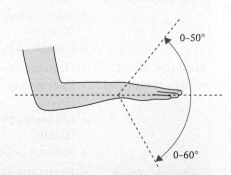

Fig. 12.4 Range of movements of the wrist joint.

Clinical correlation

- Superficial positions of nerves, vessels, and tendons at wrist make them exceedingly vulnerable to injury.
- **Ganglion** *(Gk = swelling or knot)*: It is a non-tender cystic swelling, which sometimes appears on wrist most commonly on its dorsal aspect. Its size varies from a small grape to a plum. It usually occurs due to mucoid degeneration of synovial sheath around the tendon. The cyst is thin walled and contains clear mucinous fluid. The flexion of wrist makes the cyst to enlarge and it may become painful.
- **Aspiration of the wrist joint:** It is usually done by introducing the needle posteriorly, immediately below the styloid process of ulna between the tendons of extensor pollicis longus and extensor indicis.
- **Immobilization of the wrist joint:** The wrist joint is immobilized in its optimum position of 30° dorsiflexion.

JOINTS OF THE HAND

The joints of hand are:

1. Intercarpal joints.
2. Midcarpal joint.

3. Carpometacarpal joints.
4. Intermetacarpal joints.

Intercarpal joints: These are plane type of synovial joints, which interconnect the carpal bones. They include the following joints:

1. Joints between the carpal bones of the proximal row.
2. Joints between the carpal bones of the distal row.
3. **Midcarpal joint** between the proximal and distal rows of the carpal bones.
4. **Pisotriquetral joint** formed between pisiform and palmar surface of triquetral bone.

Carpometacarpal joints: The carpometacarpal joints are plane type of synovial joints except for the carpometacarpal joint of the thumb, which is a saddle joint. The distal surfaces of the carpals of distal row articulate with the bases of metacarpals. Functionally and clinically, first carpometacarpal joint is the most important carpometacarpal joint and hence described in detail latter.

Intermetacarpal joints: These are plane type of synovial joints and formed by the articulation of the bases of adjacent metacarpals of the fingers.

N.B. Joint cavities of intercarpal, carpometacarpal, and intermetacarpal joints: There are the following three joint cavities among the above-mentioned joints (Fig. 12.1):

1. A continuous common cavity of all intercarpal and meta-carpal joints, except that of first carpometacarpal joint.

2. Cavity of first carpometacarpal joint.

3. Cavity of pisotriquetral joint.

Movements of the intercarpal and carpometacarpal joints are listed in Table 12.2.

First Carpometacarpal Joint (Fig. 12.1)

Type
It is synovial joint of saddle variety.

Table 12.2 Movements at the intercarpal, carpometacarpal (except first), metacarpophalangeal, and interphalangeal joints

Joints	Movements
Intercarpal (IC) joints	Gliding movements
Carpometacarpal (CM) joints	
• CM joint of thumb	Freely mobile
• CM joints of second and third fingers	Almost no moment
• CM joint of fourth finger	Slightly mobile
• CM joint of fifth finger	Moderately mobile

Articular surfaces
Proximal: Distal surface of the trapezium.
Distal: Proximal surface of the base of 1st metacarpal.

Both proximal and distal articular surfaces are reciprocally concavo-convex; hence permit wide range of movements at this joint.

Ligaments

1. **Capsular ligament (joint capsule):** It is thick loose fibrous sac, which encloses the joint cavity. It is attached proximally to the margins of articular surface of the trapezium and distally to the circumference of the base of first metacarpal bone. The inner surface of the capsule is lined by the *synovial membrane.*
2. **Lateral ligament:** It is a broad fibrous band stretching from lateral surface of the trapezium to the lateral side of the base of 1st metacarpal bone.
3. **Anterior (palmar) ligament:** It extends obliquely from palmar surface of trapezium to the ulnar side of the base of 1st metacarpal.
4. **Posterior (dorsal) ligament:** It also extends obliquely from dorsal surface of trapezium to the ulnar side of the base of 1st metacarpal.

Relations
The joints are surrounded by various muscles and tendons of the thumb. In addition, it is related to:

(a) radial artery on its posteromedial sides.
(b) First dorsal interosseous muscle on its medial side.

Blood supply
By radial artery.

Nerve supply
By median nerve.

Movements
The various movements, which take place at the first carpometacarpal joint are as follows:

1. Flexion and extension.
2. Abduction and adduction.
3. Opposition.
4. Medial and lateral rotation.
5. Circumduction.

The various movements of thumb at first carpometacarpal joint are described in detail on pages 168 and 169.

JOINTS OF THE DIGITS (Fig. 12.5)

The joints of digits are:

1. Metacarpophalangeal joints.
2. Interphalangeal joints.

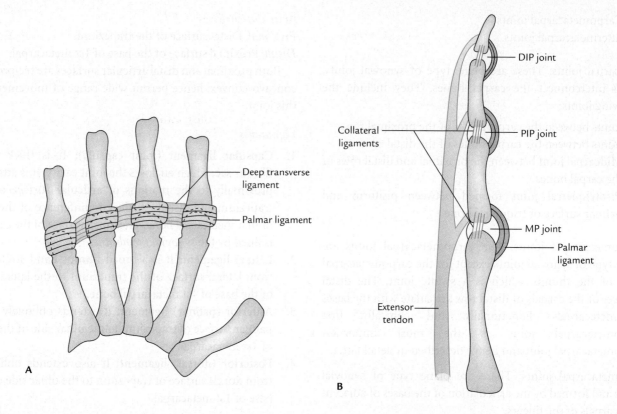

Fig. 12.5 Joints of the fingers: **A,** MP joints showing palmar and deep transverse ligaments; **B,** MP, PIP, and DIP joints showing palmar and collateral ligaments (DIP = distal interphalangeal, PIP = proximal interphalangeal, MP = metacarpophalangeal).

Metacarpophalangeal (MP) joints (Fig. 12.5A)

Type: They are synovial joints of ellipsoid/condylar variety.
Articular surfaces: They are formed by heads of metacarpals and bases of proximal phalanges.

Ligaments

1. **Palmar ligaments:** The palmar ligament is a fibrocartilaginous plate, which is more firmly attached to the phalanx than to the metacarpal. The palmar ligaments of second, third, fourth, and fifth MP joints are joined to each other by **deep transverse metacarpal ligament.**
2. **Medial and lateral collateral ligaments:** These are cord-like fibrous bands present on each side of the joint and extend from head of metacarpal to the base of phalanx.

Movements

- Flexion and extension
- Adduction and abduction
- Circumduction
- Limited rotation

Interphalangeal (IP) joints (Fig. 12.5B): Both proximal and distal interphalangeal (PIP and DIP) joints are synovial

joints of hinge variety. Their structure is similar to that of MP joints.

Movements

- Flexion and extension

MOVEMENTS OF THE HAND

To perform the various movements, the hand adopts a specific posture. Hence students must first understand the positions of hand at rest and during function.

POSITION OF THE HAND

Position of the hand at rest (Fig. 12.6)
It is the posture adopted by the hand when it is at rest (i.e., not performing any action).

The characteristic features of this position are:

1. Forearm is in semiprone position.
2. Wrist joint is slightly extended.
3. Fingers are partially flexed (index finger is not flexed as much as the other fingers).

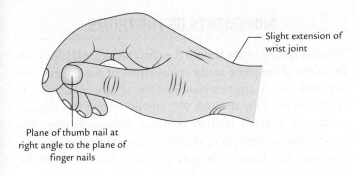

Slight extension of wrist joint

Plane of thumb nail at right angle to the plane of finger nails

Fig. 12.6 Position of the hand at rest.

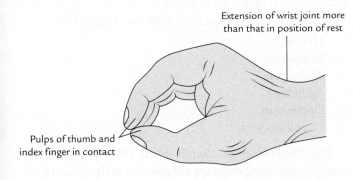

Extension of wrist joint more than that in position of rest

Pulps of thumb and index finger in contact

Fig. 12.7 Position of function of the hand.

4. Plane of thumb nail is at right angle to the plane of finger nails.

Position of hand during function (Fig. 12.7)
It is the posture adopted by hand when it is going to grasp an object between the thumb and index finger. The characteristic features of this position are:

1. Forearm is in semiprone position.
2. Wrist joint is slightly extended (more than that in position of rest).
3. All the fingers, including index finger, are partially flexed.
4. Thumb is rotated in such a way that the plane of thumb nail lies parallel with that of index finger and pulps of thumb and index finger are in contact.

N.B.
- Forearm bones are most stable when the forearm is in midprone position.
- When the wrist is partially extended: (a) flexor and extensor tendons of digits work to their best mechanical advantage and (b) flexors and extensors of carpus provide a stable base for movements of the digits.

CLASSIFICATION OF MOVEMENTS OF THE HAND

The movements of hand are classified into the following two types:

1. Prehensile.
2. Non-prehensile.

Non-prehensile movements: These are the movements in which objects are manipulated by pushing, tapping or lifting and involve movements of individual digits.

Prehensile movements (Fig. 12.8): These are of two types: (a) *precision grip* and (b) *power grip*. A third type called *hook grip* is used to suspend or pull the objects.

These movements are used for transmission of forces and not for skilled manipulation.

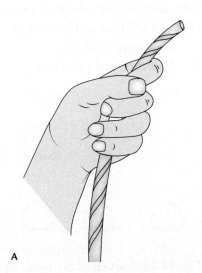

A

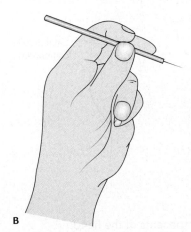

B

Fig. 12.8 Prehensile movements of the hand: **A**, power grip; **B**, precision grip.

FUNCTIONAL COMPONENTS OF THE HAND

The hand consists of the following three functional components (Fig. 12.9):

1. Central fixed component (central back bone).
2. Radial mobile component.
3. Ulnar mobile component.

The **central fixed component** is formed by the metacarpals of index and middle fingers.

The **mobile radial component** is formed by the thumb.

The **mobile ulnar component** is formed by the ring and little fingers.

N.B. The *mobile radial component* (thumb) comes into play in precision manipulations against the index finger:

- The thumb, index finger, and middle finger together form the so-called *radial digital tripod*.
- The mobile ulnar component is termed *ulnar hook*, which provides for stable power grip with palm or in 'hook grip'.
- The little finger is important for power grip whereas thumb is important for both power and precision grip.

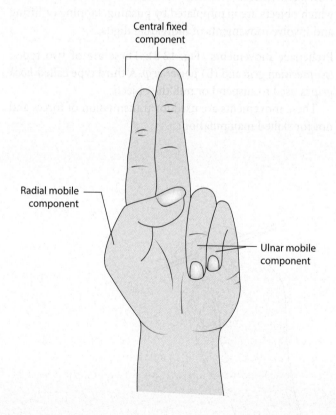

Fig. 12.9 Functional components of the hand.

MOVEMENTS OF THE THUMB

The metacarpal of the thumb (i.e., first metacarpal) does not lie in the same plane as the metacarpals of the fingers, but occupies a more anterior position (Fig. 12.10). In addition, it is rotated medially through 90°, and as a result its extensor surface is directed laterally and not backwards. For this reason, the movements of the thumb occur in planes at right angles to the planes of the corresponding movements of the fingers. The movements of thumb occur at carpometacarpal, metacarpophalangeal, and interphalangeal joints. The movements at the carpometacarpal joint of thumb are much freer than that of any other finger.

The various movements of thumb are (Fig. 12.11):

1. Flexion.
2. Extension.
3. Abduction.
4. Adduction.
5. Opposition.
6. Circumduction.

The movements of thumb, plane of movements, and muscles producing them are enumerated in the Table 12.3.

N.B. In addition to movements mentioned in Table 12.3, the following movements of thumb also take place:

- *Circumduction*, a combination of flexion, extension, abduction, and adduction.
- *Medial and lateral rotation*, which occurs along the long axis. *Medial rotation* is produced by opponens and flexors and *lateral rotation* by extensors.

MOVEMENTS OF THE FINGERS

The movements of fingers occur at metacarpophalangeal (MP) and proximal interphalangeal and distal interphalangeal (PIP and DIP) joints. The movements of fingers are:

1. Flexion and extension.
2. Abduction and adduction.

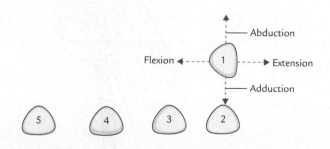

Fig. 12.10 Position of the metacarpals.

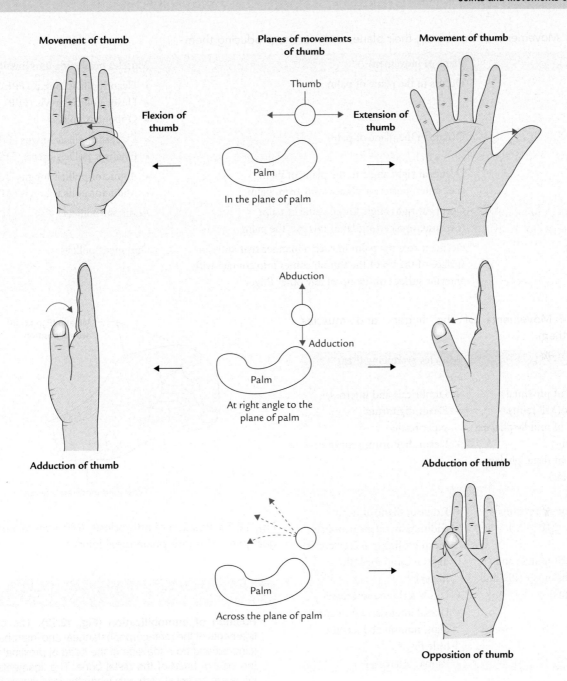

Fig. 12.11 Movements of the thumb.

The movements of finger are given in Table 12.4.

Flexion: It is a forward movement of fingers in the anteroposterior plane and occurs at MP, PIP, and DIP joints.

Extension: It is a backward movement of finger in the anteroposterior plane and occurs at MP, PIP, and DIP joints.

Abduction: It is a away movement of finger from the imaginary midline of the middle finger and occurs at MP joint.

Adduction: It is movement of fingers towards the imaginary midline of the middle finger and occurs at MP joint.

N.B. The movements of abduction and adduction fingers are possible only when fingers are in extended position because in this position the collateral ligaments of MP joints are slack. In flexed position of fingers the collateral ligaments of MP joint are taut.

The movements of fingers and muscles producing them are given in the Table 12.4.

Table 12.3 Movements of the thumb, their plane, and muscles producing them

Movement	Plane of movement	Muscles producing movement
Flexion	Occurs in the plane of palm	• Flexor pollicis longus (FPL) • Flexor pollicis brevis (FPB) • Opponens pollicis
Extension	Occurs in the plane of palm	• Extensor pollicis longus (EPL) • Extensor pollicis brevis (EPB)
Abduction	Occurs at right angle to the plane of palm (i.e., anteroposterior plane) away from palm	• Abductor pollicis longus (APL) • Abductor pollicis brevis (APB)
Adduction	Occurs at right angle to the plane of palm (i.e., anteroposterior plane) towards the palm	Adductor pollicis
Opposition	Occurs across the palm in such a manner that anterior surface of the tip of the thumb comes into contact with anterior surface of the tip of any other finger	Opponens pollicis

Table 12.4 Movements of the fingers and muscles producing them

Movement	Muscles producing them
Flexion • Flexion of proximal phalanx (MP joint) • Flexion of middle phalanx (PIP joint) • Flexion of distal phalanx (DIP joint)	• Lumbricals and interossei • Flexor digitorum superficialis • Flexor digitorum profundus
Extension • Extension of proximal phalanx (MP joint) • Flexion of middle and distal phalanges (PIP and DIP joints)	• Extensor digitorum (in addition by extensor indicis for index finger and extensor digiti minimi for little finger) • Lumbricals and interossei
Abduction	• Dorsal interossei (abductor digiti minimi abducts the little finger)
Adduction	• Palmar interossei

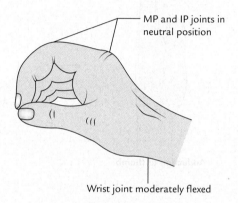

Fig. 12.13 Position of arthrodesis (MP = metacarpophalangeal joint, IP = interphalangeal joint).

Clinical correlation

• **Position of immobilization (Fig. 12.12):** The collateral ligaments of the metacarpophalangeal and interphalangeal joints extend from the side of the head of proximal bone to the side of base of the distal bone. The ligaments of MP joints are on full stretch only when the joint is fully flexed to 90°; on the other hand, ligaments of IP joint are stretched/taut only when the joint is fully extended. This knowledge is of vital importance when immobilizing the hand because contracture of the joints occurs within two weeks, if the joints are immobilized when the ligaments are lax/slack. Then the shortening of ligaments will cause irreversible joint contractures. Therefore, the position of immobilization of hand should be such that the MP joints are fully flexed and the interphalangeal joints are fully extended.

• **Position of arthrodesis* (Fig. 12.13):** The position of arthrodesis is one, in which wrist joint is moderately dorsiflexed (15–20°), and the MP and IP joint are set in neutral position.

***Arthrodesis** is a surgical procedure consisting of the obliteration of a joint space by doing bony fusion so that no movement can occur at the joint.

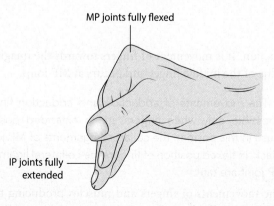

Fig. 12.12 Position of immobilization (MP = metacarpophalangeal joint, IP = interphalangeal joint).

Golden Facts to Remember

► Most important carpometacarpal joint	First carpometacarpal joint
► Position of forearm in which forearm bones are most stable	Midprone position
► All fingers are abducted by dorsal interossei *except*	Little finger, which is abducted by abductor digiti minimi
► Wrist complex consists of	Radio-carpal and midcarpal joints
► Palmar interossei are attached on all the metacarpals *except*	Third metacarpal (metacarpal of middle finger)

Clinical Case Study

An elderly man fell on the road with an outstretched right hand while trying to get into the moving bus. He developed localized pain and swelling on the dorsal aspect of his right wrist. He was taken to the nearby hospital, where on examination, the doctors observed a typical dinner fork deformity in the right hand. The X-ray of the region revealed a fracture of distal end of radius with posterior displacement of the distal fragment. A diagnosis of **Colles' fracture** was made.

Questions

1. What is Colles' fracture and how does it differ from Smith's fracture?
2. Which nerve is likely to be injured in Colles' fracture?
3. What is the position of styloid processes of radius and ulna before and after fracture?

Answers

1. It is the fracture of distal end of radius, about one inch proximal to the wrist joint with posterior displacement of the distal fragment. If the distal fragment is displaced anteriorly, it is called *Smith's fracture.*
2. Median nerve.
3. Before fracture (i.e., in normal state) the tip of styloid process of radius lies about 2 cm distal to that of ulna but after fracture, the tips of styloid processes of radius and ulna come to lie at the same level due to shortening of radius.

Major Nerves of the Upper Limb

The nerve supply to the upper limb is provided by the **brachial plexus** (described in detail in Chapter 5, page 70).

The five major nerves supplying the upper limb are:

1. Axillary nerve.
2. Musculocutaneous nerve.
3. Radial nerve.
4. Median nerve.
5. Ulnar nerve.

The study of five major nerves of the upper limb should be studied thoroughly and carefully because of their frequent involvement in various injuries and peripheral neuropathy.

AXILLARY NERVE (Fig. 13.1)

The axillary nerve (C5 and C6) arises from posterior cord of brachial plexus. It provides motor innervation to the deltoid and teres minor muscles and sensory innervation to the shoulder joint and to the skin over the lower lateral part of the shoulder. The branches of axillary nerve are shown in Figure 13.1 (for details see Chapter 5, page 70).

MUSCULOCUTANEOUS NERVE (Fig. 13.2)

The **musculocutaneous nerve** arises from lateral cord of the brachial plexus (C5, C6, and C7). It provides motor innervation to the muscles on the front of the arm and

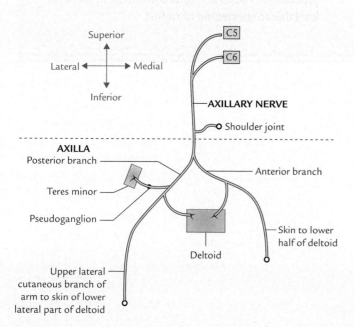

Fig. 13.1 Course and distribution of the axillary nerve.

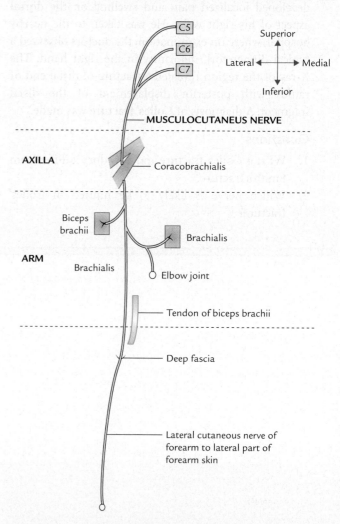

Fig. 13.2 Course and distribution of the musculocutaneous nerve.

sensory innervation to the skin of the lateral part of the forearm (for details see Chapter 8, page 96).

RADIAL NERVE (Fig. 13.3)

The radial nerve is a continuation of posterior cord of brachial plexus in the axilla. It is the *largest nerve of the brachial plexus*. It carries fibres from all the roots (C5, C6, C7, C8, and T1) of brachial plexus (but T1 fibres are not constant).

In the axilla, the radial nerve lies posterior to the third part of the axillary artery and anterior to the muscles forming the posterior wall of the axilla.

In the axilla, it gives off the following three branches:

1. *Posterior cutaneous nerve of arm* (which provides sensory innervation to skin on the back of the arm up to the elbow).
2. *Nerve to the long head of triceps.*
3. *Nerve to the medial head of triceps.*

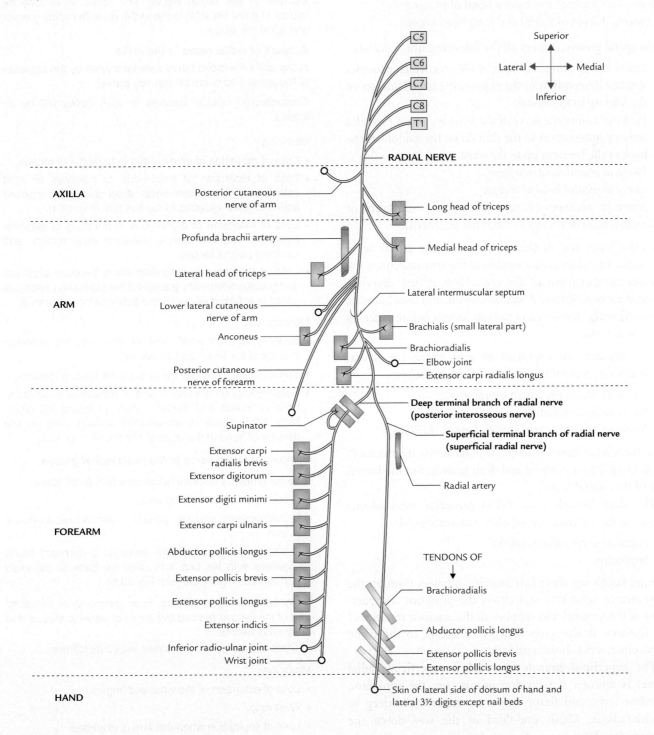

Fig. 13.3 Course and distribution of the radial nerve.

Radial nerve enters the arm at the lower border of the teres major. It passes between the long and medial heads of triceps to enter the lower triangular space, through which it reaches the spiral groove along with profunda brachii artery. The radial nerve in the spiral groove lies in direct contact with the humerus.

N.B. Boundaries of the Spiral Groove
Anteriorly: Middle one-third of the shaft of humerus.
Above: Origin of the lateral head of triceps.
Below: Origin of the medial head of triceps.
Posteriorly: Fibres of lateral and long head triceps.

In the spiral groove, it gives off the following five branches:

1. *Lower lateral cutaneous nerve of the arm,* which provides sensory innervation to the skin on the lateral surface of the arm up to the elbow.
2. *Posterior cutaneous nerve of the forearm,* which provides sensory innervation to the skin down the middle of the back of the forearm up to the wrist.
3. *Nerve to lateral head of triceps.*
4. *Nerve to medial head of triceps.*
5. *Nerve to anconeus* (it runs through the substance of medial head of triceps to reach the anconeus).

At the lower end of the spiral groove, the radial nerve pierces the lateral muscular septum of the arm and enters the anterior compartment of the arm. Here, it first descends between the brachialis and brachioradialis, and then between brachialis and extensor carpi radialis longus before entering the cubital fossa.

In the anterior compartment of arm above the lateral epicondyle, it gives off the following three branches:

1. Nerve to brachialis (small lateral part).
2. Nerve to brachioradialis.
3. Nerve to extensor carpi radialis longus (ECRL).

At the level of lateral epicondyle of humerus, it terminates by dividing into superficial and deep branches in the lateral part of the cubital fossa.

The **deep branch** (also called **posterior interosseous nerve**), in the cubital fossa supplies two muscles, viz.

1. Extensor carpi radialis brevis.
2. Supinator.

After supplying these two muscles, it passes through the substance of supinator and enters the posterior compartment of the forearm and supplies all the extensor muscles of the forearm. It also gives articular branches to the distal radio-ulnar, wrist, and carpal joints.

The **superficial branch** (also called **superficial radial nerve**) is sensory. It runs downwards over the supinator, pronator teres, and flexor digitorum superficialis deep to brachioradialis. About one-third of the way down the forearm (at about 7 cm above wrist), it passes posteriorly,

emerging from under the tendon of brachioradialis, proximal to the styloid process of radius and then passes over the tendons of anatomical snuff-box, where it terminates as cutaneous branches which provide sensory innervation to skin over the lateral part of the dorsum of hand and dorsal surfaces of lateral 3½ digits proximal to the nail beds.

Clinical correlation

Injuries of the radial nerve: The radial nerve may be injured at three sites: (a) in the axilla, (b) in the spiral groove, and (c) at the elbow.

A. Injury of radial nerve in the axilla

In the axilla the radial nerve may be injured by the pressure of the upper end of crutch (**crutch palsy**)

Characteristic clinical features in such cases will be as follows:

Motor loss

- Loss of extension of elbow—due to paralysis of triceps.
- Loss of extension of wrist—due to paralysis of wrist extensors. This causes **wrist drop** due to unopposed action of flexor muscles of the forearm (Fig. 13.4).
- Loss of extension of digits—due to paralysis of extensor digitorum, extensor indicis, extensor digiti minimi, and extensor pollicis longus.
- Loss of supination in extended elbow because supinator and brachioradialis are paralyzed but supination becomes possible in flexed elbow by the action of biceps brachii.

Sensory loss

- Sensory loss on small area of skin over the posterior surface of the lower part of the arm.
- Sensory loss along narrow strip on the back of forearm.
- Sensory loss on the lateral part of dorsum of hand at the base of thumb and dorsal surface of lateral 3½ digits. More often, there is an isolated sensory loss on the dorsum of hand at the base of the thumb (Fig. 13.5).

B. Injury of radial nerve in the radial/spiral groove

In radial groove, the radial nerve may be injured due to:

(a) midshaft fracture of humerus,
(b) inadvertently wrongly placed intramuscular injection, and
(c) direct pressure on radial nerve by a drunkard falling asleep with his one arm over the back of the chair (Saturday night paralysis; Fig. 13.6).

Injury to radial nerve occurs most commonly in the distal part of the groove beyond the origin of nerve to triceps and cutaneous nerves.

Clinical features in such cases will be as follows:

Motor loss

- Loss of extension of the wrist and fingers.
- Wrist drop.
- Loss of supination when the arm is extended.

- Sensory loss is restricted only to a variable small area over the dorsum of hand between the first and second metacarpals.

N.B. Extension of the elbow is possible but may be little weak because nerves to long and lateral heads of triceps arises in the axilla i.e., before the site of lesion.

C. Injury of radial nerve at elbow

Radial tunnel syndrome: It is an entrapment neuropathy of the deep branch of radial nerve at elbow. The compression of radial nerve at elbow may be caused by the following four structures:

(a) Fibrous bands, which can tether the radial nerve to the radio-humeral joint.
(b) Sharp tendinous margin of extensor carpi radialis brevis.
(c) Leash of vessels from the radial recurrent artery.
(d) Arcade of Frohse, a fibro-aponeurotic proximal edge of the superficial part of the supinator muscle.

Characteristic clinical features:

- Loss of extension of the wrist and fingers but no wrist drop.
- Pain over the extensor aspect of the forearm.

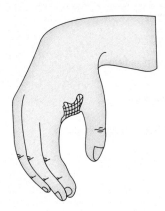

Fig. 13.4 Wrist drop resulting from radial nerve injury.

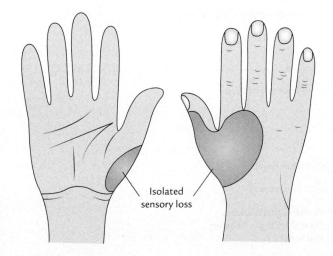

Isolated sensory loss

Fig. 13.5 Area of sensory loss in hand following radial nerve injury above the elbow.

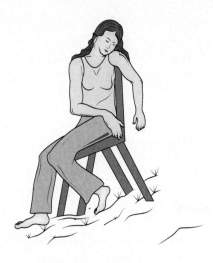

Fig. 13.6 Saturday night paralysis. Note drunk lady falling asleep with arm over the back of chair.

MEDIAN NERVE (Fig. 13.7)

The **median nerve** arises from brachial plexus in axilla by two roots: (a) lateral and (b) medial. The lateral root (C5, C6, and C7) arises from lateral cord of brachial plexus and medial root (C8 and T1) arises from medial cord of the brachial plexus. The medial root crosses in front of the third part of axillary artery to unite with lateral root in a Y-shaped manner either in front of or on the lateral side of the artery to form the median nerve. So the **root value of median nerve is C5, C6, C7, C8, and T1.**

In the axilla, the median nerve lies on the lateral side of the third part of the axillary artery. It enters the arm at the lower border of teres major.

In the arm, initially, median nerve lies lateral to brachial artery and then crosses in front of the artery from lateral to medial side at the level of midhumerus (i.e., level of insertion of coracobrachialis). After crossing, it runs downwards to enter cubital fossa.

In the cubital fossa, the median nerve lies medial to the brachial artery and tendon of biceps brachii. Here it is covered by bicipital aponeurosis, which separates it from the median cubital vein.

In the cubital fossa, it gives muscular branches from its medial side to supply all the superficial flexors of the forearm flexor carpi radialis, palmaris longus, and flexor digitorum superficialis) except flexor carpi ulnaris.

Median nerve leaves the cubital fossa by passing between the two heads of pronator teres. At this point, it gives off **anterior interosseous nerve.**

The anterior interosseous nerve is purely motor and supplies 2½ muscles:

1. Flexor pollicis longus.
2. Lateral half of the flexor digitorum profundus (FDP).
3. Pronator quadratus.

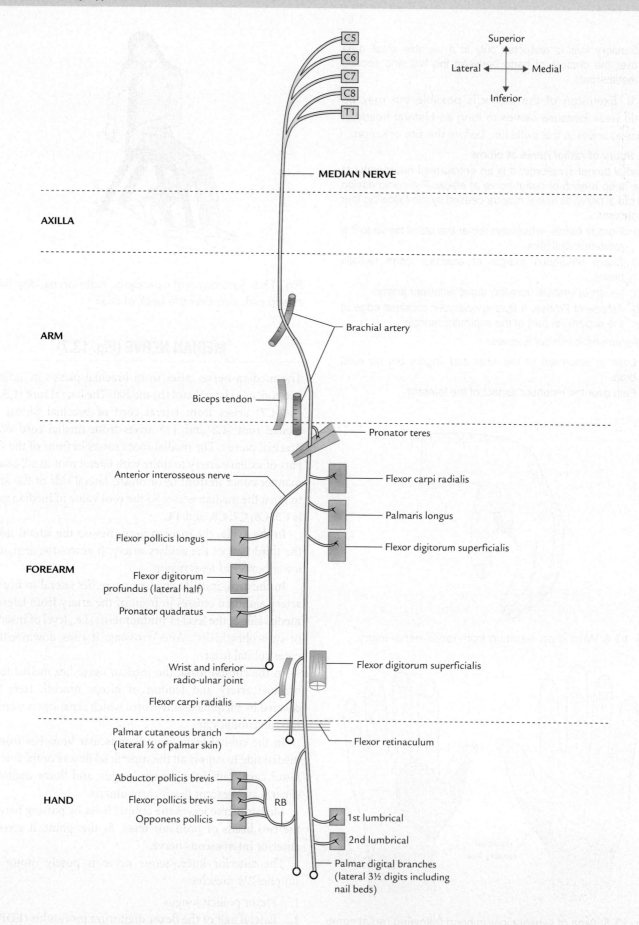

Fig. 13.7 Course and distribution of the median nerve (RB = recurrent branch).

In the forearm, the median nerve passes downwards behind the tendinous arch/bridge between the two heads of flexor digitorum superficialis and runs deep to the flexor digitorum superficialis. About 5 cm proximal to the flexor retinaculum, the median nerve emerges from the lateral side of the FDS and becomes superficial, lying lateral to the tendons of FDS and posterior to the tendon of palmaris longus.

In the midarm, the median nerve gives muscular branch to the radial head of flexor digitorum superficialis, which gives rise to tendon for index finger.

Before entering the carpal tunnel, it gives off its *palmar cutaneous branch,* which passes superficial to the flexor retinaculum to supply the skin over the thenar eminence and lateral part of the palm.

Median nerve enters the palm by passing through carpal tunnel where it lies deep to flexor retinaculum and superficial to the tendons of FDS, FDP, and FPL and their associated ulnar and radial bursae.

In the palm, the median nerve flattens at the distal border of the flexor retinaculum and divides into lateral and medial divisions. The lateral division gives a **recurrent branch,** which curls upwards to supply thenar muscles except the deep head of flexor pollicis brevis. It then divides into three palmar digital branches. The medial divisions give off two palmar digital nerves.

The five palmar digital nerves supply:

(a) sensory innervation to the skin of the palmar aspect of the lateral 3½ digits including nail beds and skin on the dorsal aspect of distal phalanges, and

(b) first and second lumbricals.

N.B.

- Median nerve is also termed **laborer's nerve** because the coarse movements of the hand required by laborers (e.g., digging the ground, lifting weight, etc.) are performed by long flexors of the forearm which are mostly supplied by the median nerve.

- It is also termed **'eye of the hand'** or *'peripheral eye'* because it provides sensory innervation to the pulp of the thumb and index finger which are used to see the thinness and texture of cloth and are also used for performing fine movements, e.g., buttoning a coat.

Clinical correlation

Injuries of the median nerve: The lesions of median nerve may occur at the following four sites: (a) at elbow, (b) at mid-forearm, (c) at wrist (distal forearm), and (d) in the carpal tunnel.

A. Injury of the median nerve at the elbow: At elbow the median nerve can be injured due to:

(a) supracondylar fracture of humerus,

(b) application of tight tourniquet during venipuncture, and

(c) entrapment of nerve between two heads of pronator teres or under the fibrous arch connecting the two heads of flexor digitorum superficialis.

Characteristic clinical features in such cases will be as follows:

- Forearm kept in supine position (loss of pronation), due to paralysis of pronator teres.
- Wrist flexion is weak—due to paralysis of all the flexors of forearm except medial half of FDP and flexor carpi ulnaris.
- Adduction of wrist—due to paralysis of FCR and unopposed action of FCU and medial half of FDP.
- No flexion is possible at the interphalangeal (IP) joints of index and middle fingers.
- *Benediction deformity of the hand* (Fig. 13.8A), i.e., when patient tries to make fist, the index and middle fingers remain straight, due to paralysis of both superficial and deep flexors of these fingers leading to loss of flexion at PIP and DIP joints. The ring and the little finger can be kept in flexed position due to intact nerve supply of medial half of the FDP.
- Loss of flexion of terminal phalanx of thumb, due to paralysis of FPL.
- *Ape-thumb deformity* (Fig. 13.8B), in which thenar eminence is flattened and thumb is laterally rotated and adducted, due to paralysis of muscles of thenar eminence and normal adductor pollicis, respectively.
- Loss of sensation in lateral half of the palm and lateral 3½ digits and also on the dorsal aspects of same digits (Fig. 13.9).

B. Injury of the median nerve at the mid-forearm: The injury of median nerve at mid-forearm results in *pointing index finger* due to paralysis of radial head of FDS muscle that continues as tendon of index finger; other signs and symptoms will be same as those which occur in lesion at distal forearm and wrist.

C. Injury of the median nerve at wrist (distal forearm): At wrist, median nerve and its palmar cutaneous branch may be injured just proximal to the flexor retinaculum by deep lacerated wounds (cut injury), e.g., suicidal cuts.

Characteristic clinical features in such a case will be as follows:

- *Ape-thumb deformity,* due to paralysis of muscles of thenar eminence.
- Loss of sensation on the lateral part of the palm (including that over the thenar eminence) and lateral 3½ digits including loss of sensation on the dorsal aspect of these digits (Fig. 13.9).

D. Injury in the carpal tunnel: The median nerve is injured in the carpal tunnel due to its compression and produces a clinical condition called **carpal tunnel syndrome.** The carpal tunnel is formed by anterior concavity of carpus and flexor retinaculum. The tunnel is tightly packed with nine long flexor tendons of fingers and thumb with their surrounding synovial sheaths and median nerve. The median nerve gets compressed in the tunnel due to its narrowing following a number of pathological conditions such as

(a) tenosynovitis of flexor tendons (idiopathic),

(b) myxedema (deficiency of thyroxine),

(c) retention of fluid in pregnancy,

(d) fracture dislocation of lunate bone, and

(e) osteoarthritis of the wrist.

Characteristic clinical features of the carpal tunnel syndrome are as follows:

- Feeling of burning pain or 'pins and needles' along the sensory distribution of median nerve (i.e., lateral 3½ digits) especially at night.
- There is no sensory loss over the thenar eminence because skin over thenar eminence is supplied by the palmar cutaneous branch of the median nerve, which passes superficial to flexor retinaculum.
- Weakness of thenar muscles.
- 'Ape-thumb deformity' may occur, if left untreated, due to paralysis of the thenar muscles.
- Positive **Tinel's sign** (Fig 13.10) and **Phalen's test** (Fig. 13.11).
- Reduced conduction velocity in the median nerve (<30 m/s) is diagnosis.

N.B. The signs and symptoms of the carpal tunnel syndrome are dramatically relieved by decompressing the tunnel by giving a longitudinal incision through flexor retinaculum.

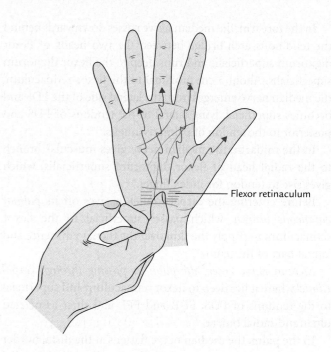

Fig. 13.10 Tinel's sign. Percussion over flexor retinaculum reproduces patient's symptoms.

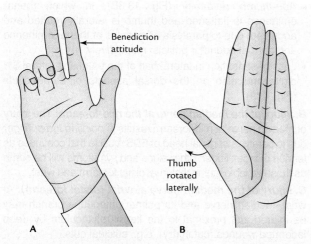

Fig. 13.8 Effects of the median nerve injury: **A,** benediction deformity of the hand (benediction attitude of hand); **B,** ape-thumb deformity.

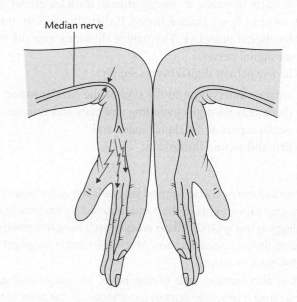

Fig. 13.11 Phalen's test. Flexion of both wrists against each other for one minute reproduces patient's symptoms.

ULNAR NERVE (Fig. 13.12)

The ulnar nerve arises in the axilla from the medial cord of brachial plexus (C8 and T1). It receives a contribution from the ventral ramus of C7. The C7 fibres in the ulnar nerve supply flexor carpi ulnaris.

In the axilla, the nerve lies medial to third part of axillary artery (between axillary artery and vein).

It enters the arm as part of main neurovascular bundle and runs distally along the medial side of the brachial

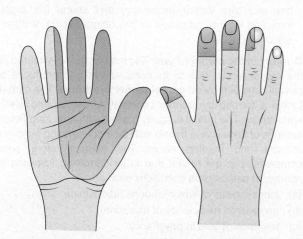

Fig. 13.9 Area of sensory loss in hand following injury of the median nerve.

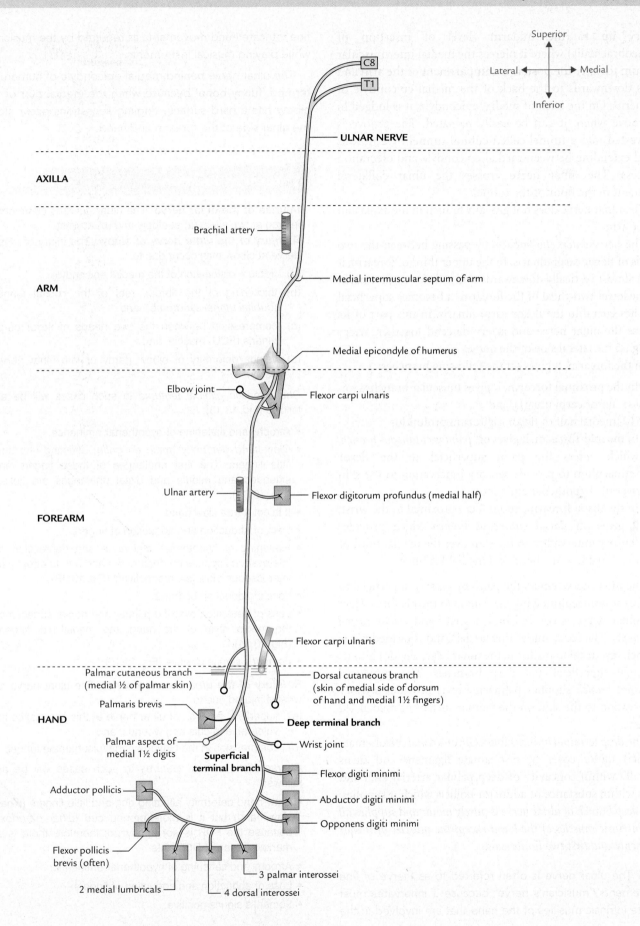

Fig. 13.12 Course and distribution of the ulnar nerve.

artery up to the midarm (level of insertion of coracobrachialis) where it pierces the medial intermuscular septum to enter the posterior compartment of the arm and runs downwards to the back of the medial epicondyle of humerus. On the back of medial epicondyle, it is lodged in a groove where it can be easily palpated. The groove is converted into a tunnel called **cubital tunnel** by a fibrous band extending between medial epicondyle and olecranon process. The ulnar nerve crosses the ulnar collateral ligament in the floor of the tunnel.

The ulnar nerve does not give any branch in the axilla and in the arm.

The *nerve enters the forearm* by passing between the two heads of flexor carpi ulnaris. In the upper third of forearm, it runs almost vertically downwards under flexor carpi ulnaris. In the lower two-third of the forearm, it becomes superficial and lies lateral to the flexor carpi ulnaris. In this part of its course the ulnar nerve and artery descend together, artery being on the lateral side of the nerve.

In the forearm, it gives off the following branches:

1. In the **proximal forearm,** it gives muscular branches to:
   (a) flexor carpi ulnaris, and
   (b) medial half of flexor digitorum profundus.
2. In the **mid-forearm**, it gives off *palmar cutaneous branch*, which enters the palm superficial to the flexor retinaculum to provide sensory innervation to the skin over the hypothenar eminence.
3. In the **distal forearm**, about 5 cm proximal to the wrist, it gives off *dorsal cutaneous branch* which provides sensory innervation to the skin over the medial third of the dorsum of the hand and medial 1½ finger.

The ulnar nerve enters the palm by passing superficial to the flexor retinaculum lying just lateral to the pisiform. Here the ulnar nerve is covered by a fascial band (*volar carpal ligament*). The space under this fascial band is termed **ulnar tunnel**. Just distal to pisiform, the ulnar nerve divides into its terminal superficial and deep branches. The *superficial terminal branch* supplies palmaris brevis provides sensory innervation to the skin on the palmar surface of medial 1½ fingers.

The *deep terminal branch* enters *Guyon's canal* (pisohamate tunnel) under cover of pisohamate ligament and turns laterally within concavity of deep palmar arterial arch and ends within substance of adductor pollicis which it supplies. The *deep branch of ulnar nerve is purely motor and supplies all the intrinsic muscles of the hand except the muscles of thenar eminence and first two lumbricals.*

N.B. The ulnar nerve is often referred to as '*nerve of fine movements*'/'**musician's nerve**' because it innervates most of the intrinsic muscles of the hand that are involved in the fine intricate hand movements as required by the musicians while playing musical instruments.

The ulnar nerve behind medial epicondyle of humerus is termed '**funny bone**' because when the medial part of the elbow hits a hard surface, tingling sensations occur along the ulnar side of the forearm and hand.

Clinical correlation

Injuries of the ulnar nerve: The ulnar nerve is commonly injured at two sites: (a) at elbow and (b) at wrist.

A. Injury of the ulnar nerve at elbow: The injury of ulnar nerve at elbow may occur due to:

(a) fracture dislocation of the medial epicondyle,

(b) thickening of the fibrous roof of the cubital tunnel (*cubital tunnel syndrome*), and

(c) compression between the two heads of flexor carpi ulnaris (FCU) muscle, and

(d) valgus deformity of elbow (tardy or late ulnar nerve palsy).

Characteristic clinical features in such cases will be as follows (Fig. 13.13):

- Atrophy and flattening of hypothenar eminence.
- *Claw-hand deformity* (*main en griffe*) affecting ring and little fingers. The first phalanges of these fingers are extended and middle and distal phalanges are flexed (Fig. 13.3A).
- It is not a true claw hand.
- Loss of abduction and adduction of fingers.
- Flattening of hypothenar eminence and depression of interosseous spaces on dorsum of hand due to atrophy of interosseous muscles, respectively (Fig. 13.3B).
- Loss of adduction of thumb.
- Loss of sensation over the palmar and dorsal surfaces of the medial third of the hand and medial 1½ fingers (Fig. 13.14).
- *Foment's sign* is positive (Fig. 13.15).*

B. Injury of the ulnar nerve at wrist: The ulnar nerve at wrist is injured due to

(a) superficial position of ulnar nerve at this site makes its vulnerable to cuts and wounds, and

(b) compression in the Guyon's canal/pisohamate tunnel.

Characteristic clinical features in such cases will be as follows:

- Claw-hand deformity affecting ring and little fingers (ulnar claw hand) but it is more pronounced (*ulnar paradox*) because the FDP is not paralyzed; therefore there is a marked flexion of DIP joints.
- Atrophy and flattening of hypothenar eminence.
- Loss of abduction and adduction of fingers.
- Foment's sign is positive.

N.B. Complete *claw hand* (Fig. 13.16): The combined lesions of the median and ulnar nerves at elbow cause a true/complete **claw-hand deformity**. The characteristic clinical features of a true claw hand are as follows:

- Hyperextension of the wrist and metacarpophalangeal (MP) joints.
- Flexion of interphalangeal (IP) joints.

---

*Foment's sign: The patient is asked to grasp the card between the thumb and index finger on the affected side and when the examining doctors pulls it, the flexion of distal phalanx of thumb occurs due to paralysis of adductor pollicis (i.e., Foment's sign is positive).

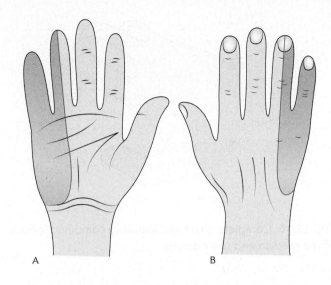

Fig. 13.14 Sensory loss in the hand following ulnar nerve injury: **A**, Palmar aspect; **B**, dorsal aspect.

The features of the three principal nerves (radial, median, and ulnar) of upper limb are summarized in Table 13.1.

AUTONOMOUS SENSORY AREAS OF THE HAND

An autonomous sensory area is that part of the dermatome that has no overlap from the adjacent nerves.

The autonomous sensory areas of the hand are used to test the integrity of nerves supplying the hand (e.g., ulnar, median, and radial). The autonomous sensory areas of the radial, median, and ulnar nerves are shown in Figure 13.17.

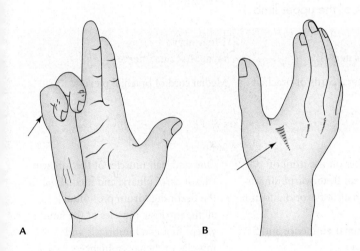

Fig. 13.13 Effects of the ulnar nerve injury: **A**, ulnar claw hand; **B**, hollowing of skin in the first web space on dorsal aspect of hand.

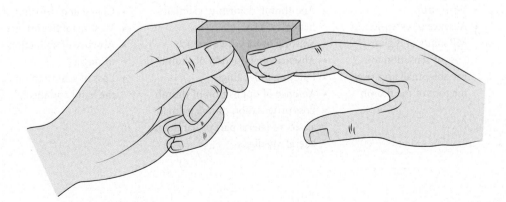

Fig. 13.15 Foment's sign to test the integrity of palmar interossei. The wrist should be dorsiflexed to rule out the action of long flexors of fingers.

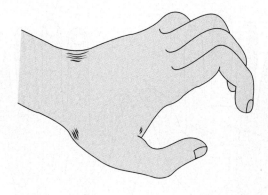

Fig. 13.16 Complete claw hand following combined lesions of the median and ulnar nerves.

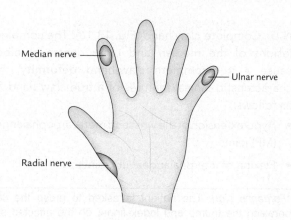

Fig. 13.17 Autonomous sensory areas of the radial, median, and ulnar nerves.

Table 13.1 Characteristics of radial, median, and ulnar nerves of the upper limb

Nerve	Radial nerve	Median nerve (syn. Laborer's nerve)	Ulnar nerve (syn. Musician's nerve)
Origin	Posterior cord of brachial plexus	Medial and lateral cords of brachial plexus	Medial cord of brachial plexus
Root value	C5–T1	C5–T1	C8–T1
Motor innervation	Supplies all the muscles on the back of arm and forearm	Supplies – all the muscles on the front of forearm except flexor carpi ulnaris and medial half of flexor digitorum profundus – muscle of thenar eminence and first two lumbricals	Supplies – One-and-half muscles of the forearm (flexor carpi ulnaris and medial half of the flexor digitorum profundus) – all the intrinsic muscles of the hand, except first two lumbricals and muscles of thenar eminence
Sensory innervation	• Posterior surface of the arm and forearm • Dorsal aspect of lateral 2/3rd of hand and lateral 3½ digits	Palmar aspect of lateral 2/3rd of hand, and lateral 3½ digits including their dorsal tips	Palmar aspect of medial 1/3rd of hand and medial 1½ fingers
Effects of lesion	• Wrist drop • Absence of extension of MP joints of digits • Loss of sensation to a variable small area over the root of the thumb	• Ape-thumb deformity (Simian's hand) • Wasting of thenar eminence • Absence of abduction of thumb • Pointing index finger • Absence of opposition of thumb • Loss of sensation on the palmar aspect of lateral part of hand and lateral 3½ digits	• Claw-hand deformity (*main en griffe*) • Wasting of hypothenar eminence • Absence of abduction and adduction of fingers • Loss of sensation on the ulnar side of the hand and medial 1½ digits

Table 13.2 Segmental innervation of the muscles of the upper limb

Segment	Muscles innervated
C5	• Deltoid • Supraspinatus, infraspinatus, and teres minor • Rhomboideus major and minor • Coracobrachialis, biceps brachii, and brachialis • Brachioradialis and supinator (*Abductors and lateral rotators of the shoulder; flexors and supinators of the forearm*)
C6	• Pectoralis major and minor • Subscapularis, latissimus dorsi, and teres major • Serratus anterior • Triceps • Pronator teres and pronator quadratus (*Adductors and medial rotators of the shoulder; extensors and pronators of the forearm*)
C7	Extensors and flexors of the wrist
C8	Long flexors and extensors of the fingers
T1	Small muscles of the hand

SEGMENTAL INNERVATION OF THE MUSCLES OF THE UPPER LIMB

The knowledge of these segmental values is of importance in the diagnosis of injuries to the nerves or to the spinal cord from which they arise. The segmental innervation of the muscles of the upper limb is given in Table 13.2. These are based on the clinical data observed by Kocher.

Golden Facts to Remember

➤ Largest nerve of the upper limb	Radial nerve
➤ Most serious disability of the median nerve lesion	Loss of ability to oppose the thumb to other fingers
➤ Largest nerve of brachial plexus	Radial nerve
➤ Most common site of the median nerve injury	Carpal tunnel
➤ Commonest peripheral neuropathy in the upper limb	Carpal tunnel syndrome (compression of median nerve in the carpal tunnel)
➤ Commonest cause of the carpal tunnel syndrome	Tenosynovitis of flexor tendons
➤ Commonest site of the ulnar nerve injury	At elbow, where it lies behind the medial epicondyle of the humerus
➤ Most reliable clinical test for the carpal tunnel syndrome	Cuff compression test (of Gilliatt and Wilson)
➤ Most common site of the radial nerve injury	Spiral groove
➤ Laborer's nerve	Median nerve
➤ Eye of the hand/peripheral eye	Median nerve in hand
➤ Musician's nerve	Ulnar nerve

Clinical Case Study

A 50-year-old female with history of rheumatoid arthritis complained of pain and 'pins and needles sensations' in lateral two-third of palm and palmar aspect of lateral 3½ digits of her right hand, which becomes severe at night and compels her to wake up at night. The examination revealed wasting of the thenar eminence, and hypoesthesia to light touch and pinprick over the palmar aspect of lateral 3½ digits. However, skin over the thenar eminence was not affected. The cuff compression test (of Gilliatt and Wilson) was positive.

Questions

1. Name the clinical condition on the basis of signs and symptoms.
2. Name the boundaries of carpal tunnel and enumerate its contents.
3. Compression of which nerve leads to the above condition?
4. Why does pain increase during night which makes the patient to wake up?
5. What is the most reliable clinical diagnostic test for the carpal tunnel syndrome? Give its brief account.

Answers

1. Carpal tunnel syndrome.
2. The carpal tunnel is bounded posteriorly by carpal bones and anteriorly by inelastic flexor retinaculum (transverse carpal ligament). It contains nine tendons of long flexors (e.g., tendons of FDS, FDP, and FPL) enclosed in synovial sheaths and median nerve.
3. Median nerve.
4. Due to accumulation of tissue fluid in the absence of the pump action of forearm muscles with arm at rest during night.
5. Cuff compression test (of Gilliatt and Wilson), when blood pressure (sphygmomanometer) cuff around the arm is inflated above the point of systolic blood pressure, the pain and paraesthesia is aggravated.

Introduction to Thorax and Thoracic Cage

The thorax is the upper part of trunk, which extends from root of the neck to the abdomen. In general usage, the term **chest** is used as a synonym for thorax. The cavity of trunk is divided by the diaphragm into an upper part called **thoracic cavity** and the lower part called the **abdominal cavity**. The thoracic cavity contains the principal organs of respiration– the lungs, which are separated from each other by bulky and movable median septum – the mediastinum. The principal structures in the mediastinum are **heart** and **great vessels**.

THORACIC CAGE

The thorax is supported by a skeletal framework called **thoracic cage**. It provides attachment to muscles of thorax, upper extremities, back, and diaphragm. It is osteocartilaginous and elastic in nature. It is primarily designed for increasing or decreasing the intrathoracic pressure so that air is sucked into lungs during inspiration and expelled from lungs during expiration—an essential mechanism of respiration.

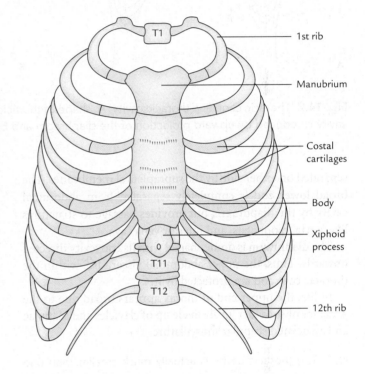

Fig. 14.1 Anterior aspect of thoracic cage.

FORMATION OF THORACIC CAGE (Fig. 14.1)

The **thoracic cage** is formed:
Anteriorly: by sternum (breast bone).
Posteriorly: by 12 thoracic vertebrae and intervening intervertebral discs.
Laterally: each side: by 12 pairs of ribs and associated 12 pairs of costal cartilages.

The **rib cage** is formed by sternum, costal cartilages, and ribs attached to the thoracic vertebrae.
The ribs articulate as follows:
1. **Posteriorly**—all the ribs articulate with the thoracic vertebrae.
2. **Anteriorly**—(a) the upper seven ribs (1st–7th) articulate with the side of sternum through their costal cartilages.

(b) The next three ribs (e.g., 8th, 9th, and 10th) articulate with each other through their costal cartilages.
(c) The lower two ribs (e.g., 11th and 12th) do not articulate and anterior ends of their costal cartilages are free.

N.B. The costal cartilages of 7th, 8th, 9th, and 10th ribs form a sloping costal margin.

SHAPE OF THORACIC CAGE (Fig. 14.2)

The thoracic cage resembles a truncated cone with its narrow end above and broad end below. The **narrow upper end** is continuous above with root of neck from which it is partly

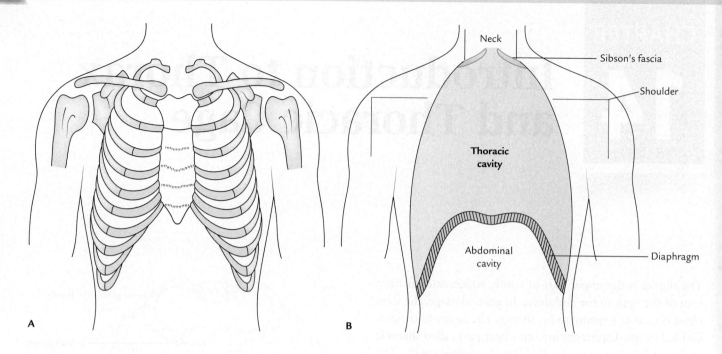

Fig. 14.2 Thoracic cage and thoracic cavity: **A,** shape of thoracic cage; **B,** schematic diagram to show how the size of thoracic cavity is reduced by upward projection of the diaphragm and by inward projection of the shoulder.

separated on either side by the suprapleural membranes. The **broad lower end** is completely separated from abdominal cavity by the diaphragm, but provides passage to structures like, aorta, esophagus, and inferior vena cava.

The **diaphragm** is dome shaped with its convexity directed upwards. Thus, the upper abdominal viscera lies within the thoracic cage and are protected by it.

In life, the upper end of thorax appears broad due to the presence of shoulder girdle made up of clavicles and scapulae and associated scapular musculature.

N.B. The thoracic cavity is actually much smaller than one assumes because the upper narrow part of thoracic cage appears broad (*vide supra*) and lower broad part of thoracic cage is encroached by the abdominal viscera due to dome-shaped diaphragm.

TRANSVERSE SECTION OF THORAX

In transverse section, the **adult thorax is kidney shaped** with transverse diameter more than the anteroposterior diameter (Fig. 14.3B, C). This is because the ribs are placed obliquely in adults.

In transverse section, the **thorax of infants below the age of two years is circular** with equal transverse and anteroposterior diameter (Fig. 14.3A). This is because the ribs are horizontally placed.

The transverse sections of thorax in adult and infant are compared in Table 14.1.

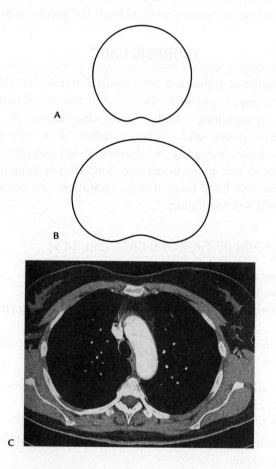

Fig. 14.3 The shape of thoracic cavity as seen in transverse section of thorax: **A,** in infant; **B,** in adult; **C,** transverse section of adult thorax in CT scan.

Table 14.1 Comparison of thoracic cavity as seen in transverse sections of the thorax in adult and infant

Thoracic cavity in adult	Thoracic cavity in infant
Kidney shaped	Circular
Ribs obliquely placed	Ribs horizontally placed
Transverse diameter can be increased by thoracic breathing (Hence respiration is thoraco-abdominal)	Transverse diameter cannot be increased by thoracic breathing (Hence respiration is purely abdominal)

Clinical correlation

The thorax up to 2 years after birth is circular in cross section. Therefore, the diameter of thorax cannot be increased within the circumference, the length of which remains constant. Therefore, in children up to the 2 years of age, the respiration is almost entirely abdominal.

Consequently, young **children are prone to suffer from pneumonia after abdominal operations**, because they resist breathing (being abdominal) due to pain. As a result the secretions in the lungs tend to accumulate, which may become infected and cause *pneumonia*.

SUPERIOR THORACIC APERTURE (THORACIC INLET)

The thoracic cavity communicates with the root of the neck through a narrow opening called *superior thoracic aperture* or *thoracic inlet*.

N.B. The superior thoracic aperture is called *thoracic outlet* by the clinicians because important arteries and T1 spinal nerves emerge from thorax through this aperture and enter the neck and upper limbs.

Anatomists refer to the superior thoracic aperture as **thoracic inlet** because air and food enter the thorax through trachea and esophagus, respectively.

Boundaries (Fig. 14.4)

Anteriorly: Superior border of manubrium sterni.

Posteriorly: Anterior border of the superior surface of the body of T1 vertebra.

Laterally (on each side): Medial border of first rib and its cartilage.

The upper end of anterior boundary lies 1.5 inches below the upper end of posterior boundary because first rib slopes downwards and forwards from its posterior end to anterior

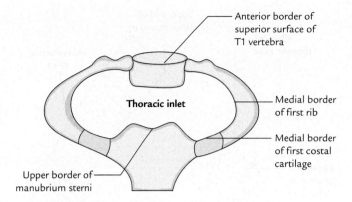

Fig. 14.4 Boundaries of the thoracic inlet.

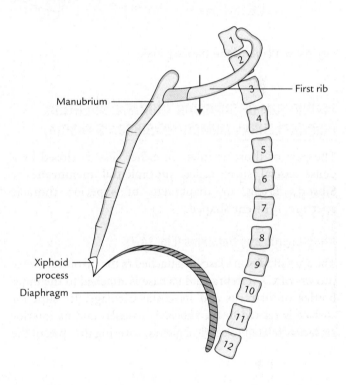

Fig. 14.5 Superior thoracic aperture; arrow (lateral view).

end (Fig. 14.5). Therefore, plane of thoracic inlet slopes (directed) downwards and forwards with an obliquity of about 45°. The upper border of manubrium sterni lies at the level of upper border of T3 vertebra (Fig. 14.6).

N.B. Due to downward and forward inclination of thoracic inlet, the apex of lung with the overlying pleura projects into the root of the lung.

Shape and Dimensions

Shape: Reniform/kidney shaped.
Dimensions: Transverse diameter: 4.5 inches.
Anteroposterior diameter: 2.5 inches.

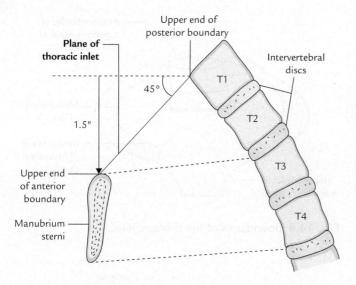

Fig. 14.6 Plane of the thoracic inlet.

DIAPHRAGM OF SUPERIOR THORACIC APERTURE (SUPRAPLEURAL MEMBRANE/SIBSON'S FASCIA)

The part of thoracic inlet, on either side, is closed by a dense fascial sheet called **suprapleural membrane** or **Sibson's fascia,** or diaphragm of superior thoracic aperture. It is **tent-shaped.**

Attachments and Relations (Fig. 14.7)

The apex of Sibson's fascia is attached to the tip of transverse process of C7 vertebra, and its base is attached to the inner border of first rib and its costal cartilage. Its superior surface is related to the subclavian vessels and its inferior surface is related to cervical pleura, covering the apex of the lung.

Functions

The functions of Sibson's fascia are as follows:

1. It protects the underlying cervical pleura, beneath which lies the apex of the lung.
2. It resists the intrathoracic pressure during respiration. As a result, the root of neck is not puffed up and down during respiration.

N.B. Morphologically, Sibson's fascia represents the spread out degenerated tendon of *scalenus minimus* (or *pleuralis*) *muscle.*

Structures Passing Through Thoracic Inlet (Fig. 14.8)

- Muscles
  1. Sternohyoid.
  2. Sternothyroid.
  3. Longus cervicis/longus colli.
- Arteries
  1. Right and left internal thoracic arteries.
  2. Brachiocephalic trunk/artery.
  3. Left common carotid artery.
  4. Left subclavian artery.
  5. Right and left superior intercostal arteries.
- Nerves
  1. Right and left vagus nerves.
  2. Left recurrent laryngeal nerve.
  3. Right and left phrenic nerves.
  4. Right and left first thoracic nerves.
  5. Right and left sympathetic chains.
- Veins
  1. Right and left brachiocephalic veins.
  2. Right and left 1st posterior intercostal veins.
  3. Inferior thyroid veins.

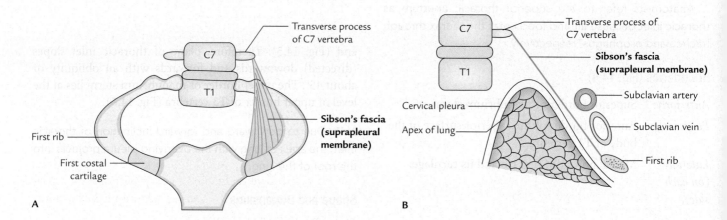

Fig. 14.7 Suprapleural membrane/Sibson's fascia: A, attachments; B, relations.

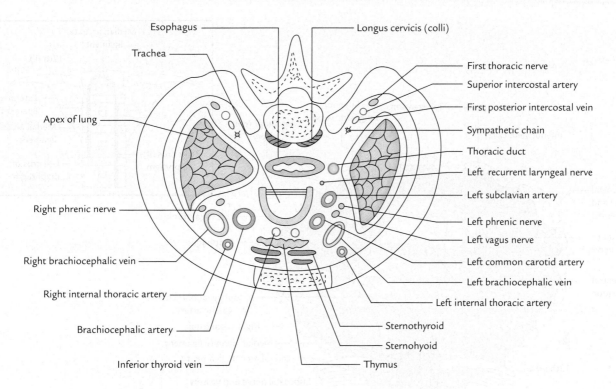

Esophagus — Longus cervicis (colli)
Trachea —
First thoracic nerve
Superior intercostal artery
First posterior intercostal vein
Apex of lung —
Sympathetic chain
Thoracic duct
Left recurrent laryngeal nerve
Left subclavian artery
Right phrenic nerve —
Left phrenic nerve
Left vagus nerve
Right brachiocephalic vein —
Left common carotid artery
Left brachiocephalic vein
Right internal thoracic artery —
Left internal thoracic artery
Brachiocephalic artery —
Sternothyroid
Sternohyoid
Inferior thyroid vein — Thymus

Fig. 14.8 Structures passing through the thoracic inlet.

- Lymphatics
  Thoracic duct.
- Others
  1. Anterior longitudinal ligament.
  2. Esophagus.
  3. Trachea.
  4. Right and left domes of cervical pleura.
  5. Apices of right and left lungs.

Clinical correlation

Thoracic inlet syndrome: The subclavian artery and lower trunk of the brachial plexus arch over the first rib, hence they may be stretched and pushed up by the presence of a congenitally hypertrophied scalenus anterior muscle or a cervical rib. This leads to thoracic inlet syndrome (also called *scalenus anterior syndrome* or *cervical rib syndrome*). It presents the following clinical features:

- Numbness, tingling, and pain along the medial side of forearm and hand, and wasting of small muscles of the hand due to the involvement of lower trunk of brachial plexus (T1).
- There may be ischemic symptoms in the upper limb such as pallor and coldness of the upper limb, and weak radial pulse due to compression of the subclavian artery.

INFERIOR THORACIC APERTURE (THORACIC OUTLET)

The inferior thoracic aperture is broad and surrounds the upper part of the abdominal cavity. The large musculoaponeurotic diaphragm attached to the margins of thoracic outlet separates the thoracic cavity from the abdominal cavity.

Boundaries

Anteriorly:	Xiphisternal joint.
Posteriorly:	Body of 12th thoracic vertebra.
Laterally (on each side):	Costal margin and 11th and 12th ribs.

DIAPHRAGM OF INFERIOR THORACIC APERTURE (Fig. 14.9)

The thoracic outlet is closed by a large dome-shaped flat muscle called **diaphragm**. Since it separates thoracic cavity from abdominal cavity, it is also termed **thoraco-abdominal diaphragm.**

The diaphragm is the **principal muscle of respiration**. It is dome shaped and consists of peripheral muscular part, and central fibrous part called **central tendon**.

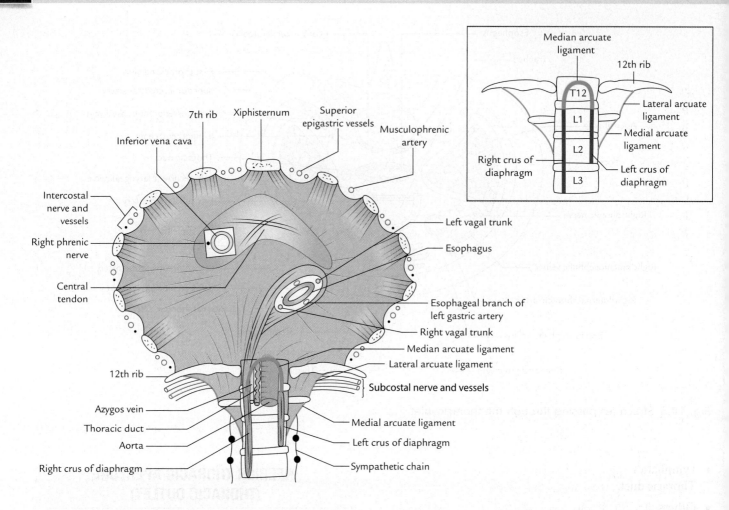

Fig. 14.9 Origin, insertion, and openings of the diaphragm. Figure in the inset shows details of vertebral origin of the diaphragm.

Origin

The origin of the diaphragm is divided into three parts, viz.

1. Sternal.
2. Costal.
3. Vertebral.

Sternal part: It consists of two fleshy slips, which arise from the posterior surface of the xiphoid process.

Costal part: On each side, it consists of six fleshy slips, which arise from the inner surface of lower six ribs near their costal cartilages.

Vertebral part: This part arises by means of (a) right and left crura of diaphragm and (b) five arcuate ligaments.

Crura

- *Right crus:* It is a vertical fleshy bundle, which arises from the right side of anterior aspects of the upper three lumbar vertebrae and intervening intervertebral discs.

- *Left crus:* It is vertical fleshy bundle, which arises from the left side of anterior aspects of upper two lumbar vertebrae and the intervening intervertebral discs.
  The medial margins of the crura are tendinous.

Arcuate ligaments

- **Median arcuate ligament** is an arched fibrous band stretching between the upper ends of two crura.
- **Medial arcuate ligament** is the thickened upper margin of the psoas sheath. It extends from the side of the body of L2 vertebra to the tip of the transverse process of L1 vertebra.
- **Lateral arcuate ligament** is the thickened upper margin of fascia covering the anterior surface of the quadratus lumborum. It extends from the tip of transverse process of L1 vertebra to the 12th rib.

N.B. The right crus is attached to more number of vertebrae because the right side diaphragm has to contract on the massive liver.

Insertion

From circumferential origin (*vide supra*), the muscle fibres converge towards the central tendon and insert into its margins.

The features of the central tendon are as follows:

1. It is trifoliate in shape, having (a) an anterior (central) leaflet, and (b and c) two tongue-shaped posterior leaflets. It resembles an equilateral triangle. The right posterior leaflet is short and stout, whereas the left posterior leaflet is thin and long.
2. It is inseparably fused with the fibrous pericardium.
3. It is located nearer to the sternum than to the vertebral column.

Surfaces and Relations

The **superior surface** of diaphragm projects on either side as **dome** or **cupola** into the thoracic cavity. Depressed area between the two domes is called **central tendon**. The superior surface is covered by endothoracic fascia and is related to the bases of right and left pleura on the sides and to the fibrous pericardium in the middle.

The **inferior surface** of diaphragm is lined by the diaphragmatic fascia and parietal peritoneum.

- *On the right side it is related to* (a) right lobe of the liver, (b) right kidney, and (c) right suprarenal gland.
- *On the left side it is related to* (a) left lobe of the liver, (b) fundus of stomach, (c) spleen, (d) left kidney, and (e) left suprarenal gland.

Openings of the Diaphragm

The openings of diaphragm are classified into two types: (a) major openings and (b) minor openings.

Major Openings

There are three named major openings, viz.

1. Vena caval opening.
2. Esophageal opening.
3. Aortic opening.

The location, shape, and vertebral levels of these openings are presented in Table 14.2.

The structure passing through three major opening of diaphragm are listed in Table 14.3.

N.B.

- Contraction of diaphragm enlarges the caval opening to enhance venous return.
- Contraction of diaphragm has a sphincteric effect on the esophageal opening (pinch-cock effect).

Table 14.2 Location, shape, and vertebral level of three major openings of the diaphragm

Opening	Location	Shape	Vertebral level
Vena caval opening	In the central tendon slightly to the right of median plane between the central and right posterior leaflets	Quadrangular or square	T8 (body)
Esophageal opening	Slightly to the left of median plane (The fibres of right crus split around the opening and act like pinch cock)	Oval or elliptical	T10 (body)
Aortic opening	In the midline behind the median arcuate ligament	Circular or round	T12 (lower border of the body)

Table 14.3 Structures passing through three major openings of the diaphragm

Opening	Structures passing through
Vena caval opening	- Inferior vena cava - Right phrenic nerve
Esophageal opening	- Esophagus - Right and left vagal trunks - Esophageal branches of left gastric artery
Aortic opening	From right to left these are: – Azygos vein – Thoracic duct – Aorta

- Contraction of diaphragm has no effect on the aortic opening because strictly it is outside the diaphragm.

Minor Openings

These are unnamed. Structures passing through these openings are as follows:

1. **Superior epigastric vessels** pass through the gap (*space of Larry*) between the muscular slips arising from xiphoid process and 7th costal cartilage.
2. **Musculophrenic artery** passes through the gap between the slips of origin from 7th to 8th ribs.

3. **Lower five intercostal nerves and vessels** (i.e., 7th–11th) pass through gaps between the adjoining costal slips.

4. **Subcostal nerves and vessels** pass deep to the lateral arcuate ligament.

5. **Sympathetic chain** passes deep to the medial arcuate ligament.

6. **Greater, lesser,** and **least splanchnic nerves** pass by piercing the crus of diaphragm on the corresponding side.

7. **Hemiazygos vein** pierces the left crus of the diaphragm.

Nerve Supply

The diaphragm is supplied by:

(a) right and left phrenic nerves, and

(b) lower five intercostal and subcostal nerves.

The **phrenic nerves** are both motor and sensory. The *right phrenic nerve* provides motor innervation to the right half of the diaphragm up to the right margin of esophageal opening, and *left phrenic nerve* provides motor innervation to the left half of the diaphragm up to the left margin of the esophageal opening.

The phrenic nerves provide sensory innervation to the central tendon of the diaphragm, and pleura and peritoneum related to it.

The **intercostal nerves** supply the peripheral parts of the diaphragm.

Arterial Supply

The diaphragm is supplied by the following arteries:

1. **Superior phrenic arteries** (also called *phrenic arteries*) from thoracic aorta.

2. **Inferior phrenic arteries,** from the abdominal aorta.

3. **Pericardiophrenic arteries,** from the internal thoracic arteries.

4. **Musculophrenic arteries,** the terminal branches of the internal thoracic arteries.

5. **Superior epigastric arteries,** the terminal branches of the internal thoracic arteries.

6. **Lower five intercostal** and **subcostal arteries** from the aorta.

Lymphatic Drainage

The lymph from diaphragm is drained into the following groups of lymph nodes:

1. **Anterior diaphragmatic lymph nodes,** situated behind the xiphoid process.

2. **Posterior diaphragmatic lymph nodes,** situated near the aortic orifice.

3. **Right lateral diaphragmatic nodes,** situated near the caval opening.

4. **Left lateral diaphragmatic nodes,** situated near the esophageal opening.

Actions of Diaphragm

The diaphragm acts to subserve the following functions:

1. **Muscle of inspiration:** The diaphragm is the main/principal muscle of respiration. When it contracts, it descends and increases the vertical diameter of the thoracic cavity (for details see page 223).

2. **Muscle of abdominal staining:** The contraction of diaphragm along with contraction of muscles of anterior abdominal wall raises the intra-abdominal pressure to evacuate the pelvic contents (voluntary expulsive efforts, e.g., micturition, defecation, vomiting, and parturition).

3. **Muscle of weight lifting:** By taking deep breath and closing the glottis, if possible to raise the intra-abdominal pressure to such an extent that it will help support the vertebral column and prevent its flexion. This assists the postvertebral muscles in lifting the heavy weights.

4. **Thoraco-muscular pump:** The descent of diaphragm decreases the intrathoracic pressure and at the same time increases the intra-abdominal pressure. This pressure change compresses the inferior vena cava, and consequently its blood is forced upward into the right atrium.

5. **Sphincter of esophagus:** The fibres of the right crus of diaphragm subserve a sphincteric control over the esophageal opening.

Clinical correlation

- **Diaphragmatic paralysis (paralysis of diaphragm):** The unilateral damage of phrenic nerve leads to *unilateral diaphragmatic paralysis.* The condition is diagnosed during fluoroscopy when an elevated hemidiaphragm is seen on the side of lesion, and showing paradoxical movements. The bilateral damage of phrenic nerves leads to complete diaphragmatic paralysis. It is a serious condition as it may cause respiratory failure.

- **Hiccups:** They occur due to involuntary spasmodic contractions of the diaphragm accompanied by the closure of the glottis. Hiccups normally occur after eating or drinking as a result of gastric irritation.

  The pathological causes of hiccups include diaphragmatic irritation, phrenic nerve irritation, hysteria, and uremia.

Development

The diaphragm develops in the region of neck from the following four structures (Fig. 14.10):

1. **Septum transversum**, ventrally.
2. **Pleuroperitoneal membranes** at the sides.
3. **Dorsal mesentery of esophagus**, dorsally.
4. **Body wall**, peripherally.

Most probably

- *Central tendon of diaphragm* develops from septum transversum.
- *Domes of diaphragm* develop from pleuroperitoneal membrane.
- *Part of diaphragm around the esophagus* develops from the dorsal mesentery of esophagus.

- Peripheral part of diaphragm, develops from the body wall.

For details of development, consult any textbook of Embryology.

N.B. The musculature of diaphragm develops from 3rd, 4th, and 5th cervical myotomes (C3, C4, C5), hence it receives its motor innervations from C3, C4, and C5 spinal segments (i.e., **phrenic nerve**). Later, when diaphragm descends from the neck to its definitive position (i.e., thoraco-abdominal junction), its nerve supply is dragged down. This explains the long course of the phrenic nerve.

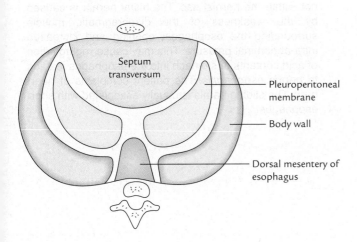

Fig. 14.10 Developmental components of the diaphragm.

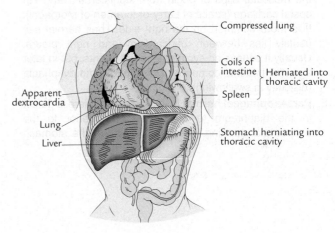

Fig. 14.11 Posterolateral hernia of diaphragm. (*Source:* Fig. 17.8, Page 190, *Textbook of Clinical Embryology*, Vishram Singh. Copyright Elsevier 2012, All rights reserved.)

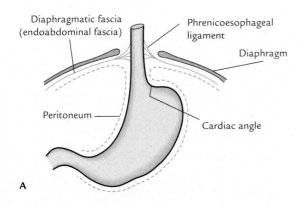
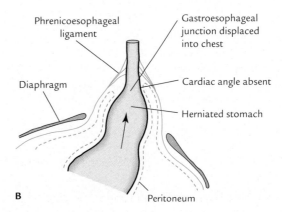

Fig. 14.12 Acquired hiatal (sliding) hernia: **A**, normal position of stomach; **B**, herniated stomach.

Clinical correlation

Diaphragmatic hernias

Congenital

The various types of congenital diaphragmatic hernias are as follows:

1. **Posterolateral hernia** (commonest congenital diaphragmatic hernia; Fig. 14.11): In this condition, there is herniation of abdominal contents into the thoracic cavity, which compress the lung and heart. The herniation occurs through the gap (pleuroperitoneal hiatus) between the costal and vertebral origins of the diaphragm called *foramen of Bochdalek*. The gap remains due to failure of closure of pleuroperitoneal canal. It occurs commonly on the left side (for details see *Clinical and Surgical Anatomy*, 2nd edition by Vishram Singh).

2. **Retrosternal hernia:** It occurs through the gap between the muscular slips of origin from xiphisternum and 7th costal cartilage (space of Larry or foramen of Morgagni). It is more common on the right side. Thus hernial sac usually lies between pericardium and right pleura. Usually it causes no symptoms in the infants, but in later age, the patients complain of discomfort and dysphagia (difficulty in swallowing).

3. **Paraesophageal hernia:** In this condition, there is defect in the diaphragm to the right and anterior to the esophageal opening. The anterior wall of the stomach rolls upwards in the hernial sac through this defect, until it becomes upside down in the thoracic cavity. An important feature of paraesophageal hernia is that the normal relationship of gastroesophageal junction in relation to diaphragm is not disturbed.

Acquired

The acquired diaphragmatic hernias may be either traumatic or hiatal (sliding).

1. **Traumatic hernia:** It may occur due to an open injury to the diaphragm by the penetrating wounds or closed injury to the diaphragm in road traffic accidents leading to sudden severe increase in the intra-abdominal pressure.

2. **Hiatal (sliding) hernia (Fig. 14.12):** This is the *commonest of all the internal hernias*. In sliding hernia, the gastroesophageal junction and cardiac end of stomach slides up into the thoracic cavity, but only anterolateral portion of the herniated stomach is covered by peritoneum, therefore the stomach itself is not within the hernial sac. The hiatal hernia is caused by the weakness of the diaphragmatic muscle surrounding the esophageal opening and increased intra-abdominal pressure. This may cause regurgitation of acid contents of stomach into the esophagus leading to *peptic esophagitis*. The patient complains of heart burn. The sliding hernia is usually associated with short esophagus.

Golden Facts to Remember

▶ Principal muscle of respiration/most important muscle of inspiration	Diaphragm
▶ Commonest congenital diaphragmatic hernia	Posterolateral hernia/herniation through foramen of Bochdalek
▶ Commonest of all the internal hernias	Acquired hiatal (sliding) hernia
▶ Superior thoracic aperture is called by clinicians as	Thoracic outlet
▶ Diaphragm receives its motor innervations from C3, C4, and C5 spinal segments (phrenic nerve) because	Musculature of diaphragm develops from 3rd, 4th, and 5th cervical myotomes in the region of the neck

Clinical Case Study

A male infant was brought to the hospital having markedly labored respiration and cyanosis. The heart sounds were displaced and there was an apparent dextrocardia. The left side of the chest was dull (flat) to percussion and had diminished breath sounds. The abdomen was characteristically scaphoid (i.e., boat shaped). The X-ray chest revealed the presence of bowel, spleen, and portions of the liver within thorax. A diagnosis of **congenital posterolateral (Bochdalek) hernia of diaphragm** was made.

Questions

1. Tell the congenital defect of diaphragm that leads to posterolateral hernia of Bochdalek.
2. Posterolateral (Bochdalek) hernia is common on which side—right or left?
3. What are the different types of congenital diaphragmatic hernia?
4. Which is the commonest congenital hernia of the diaphragm? Give its incidence.

Answers

1. Congenital gap between the vertebral and costal origins of the diaphragm due to failure of closure of pleuro-peritoneal canal.
2. It is three to five times more common on the left side.
3. (a) Posterolateral hernia, (b) retrosternal hernia, and (c) congenital paraesophageal or rolling hernia.
4. Posterolateral hernia of Bochdalek. Its incidence is 1:2000 births.

Bones and Joints of the Thorax

BONES OF THE THORAX

The bones of the thorax form the major part of the thoracic cage and provide support and protection to viscera (e.g., heart and lungs) present within the thoracic cavity. The thoracic cage is not static in nature, but dynamic as it keeps on moving at its various joints.

The bones of the thorax are:

1. Sternum.
2. Twelve pairs of ribs.
3. Twelve thoracic vertebrae.

STERNUM

The sternum (breast bone; Fig. 15.1A and B) is an elongated flat bone, which lies in the anterior median part of the chest wall. It is about 7 cm long.

PARTS

The sternum consists of the following three parts:

1. Upper part, the manubrium sterni/episternum.
2. Middle part, the body/mesosternum.
3. Lower part, the xiphoid process/metasternum.

The sternum resembles a dagger or a small sword in shape. Its three parts—manubrium, body, and xiphoid process represent the handle, blade, and point of the sword, respectively.

The upper part of sternum is broad and thick, whereas its lower part is thin and pointed. Its anterior surface is slightly rough and convex, while its posterior surface is smooth and slightly concave.

The manubrium and body of sternum lie at an angle of 163° to each other, which increases slightly during inspiration and decreases during expiration. The angle

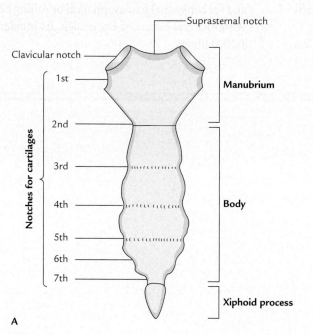

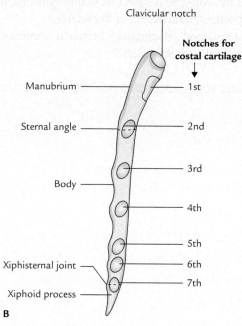

Fig. 15.1 Features of the sternum: **A**, anterior aspect; **B**, lateral aspect.

between long axis of manubrium and long axis of body of sternum is about 17°.

Anatomical Position

In anatomical position, the sternum as a whole is directed downwards and inclined slightly forward with its rough convex surface facing anteriorly. Its broad end is directed upwards and lower pointed end is directed downwards.

FEATURES AND ATTACHMENTS

Manubrium (Episternum; Figs. 15.1 and 15.2)

It is roughly quadrilateral in shape. It lies opposite to the third and fourth thoracic vertebrae. It is the thickest and strongest part of the sternum and presents the following features:

1. Two surfaces—anterior and posterior.
2. Four borders—superior, inferior, and lateral (right and left).

Anterior surface on each side provides attachment to the sternal head of sternocleidomastoid and pectoralis major muscles.

Posterior surface is smooth and forms anterior boundary of superior mediastinum.

- On each side, it provides attachment to two muscles:
  (a) *sternohyoid* at the level of clavicular notch, and
  (b) *sternothyroid* at the level of facet for 1st costal cartilage.

- Lower half is related to arch of aorta.
- Upper half is related to three branches of the arch of aorta, viz. brachiocephalic artery, left common carotid artery, left subclavian artery, and left brachiocephalic vein.

Upper border is thick, rounded, and concave. It presents a notch called *suprasternal notch* or *jugular notch*.
- It provides attachment to the interclavicular ligament.
- Clavicular notch on either side of suprasternal notch articulates with the clavicle to form *sternoclavicular joint*.

Lateral border presents two articular facets:
- Upper facet articulates with the 1st costal cartilage to form primary cartilaginous joint.
- Lower demifacet along with other demifacet in the body of sternum articulates with the 2nd costal cartilage.

Lower border articulates with the upper end of the body of sternum to form secondary cartilaginous joint called *manubriosternal joint*. The manubrium makes a slight angle with the body at this junction called **sternal angle** or **angle of Louis**. It is recognized by the presence of a transverse ridge on the anterior aspect of the sternum.

Body (Mesosternum; Figs 15.1 and 15.2)

The features of the body are as follows:

1. It is longer, narrower, and thinner than the manubrium.
2. It is broadest at its lower end.
3. Its **upper end** articulates with the manubrium at the sternal angle to form *manubriosternal joint*.

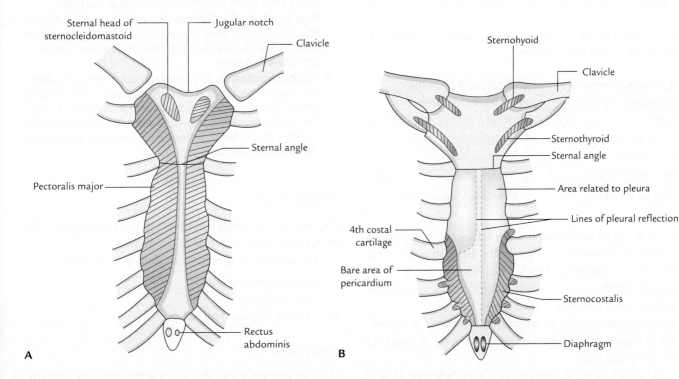

Fig. 15.2 Attachments on the sternum: **A**, anterior surface; **B**, posterior surface.

4. Its **lower end** articulates with the xiphoid process to form primary cartilaginous *xiphisternal joint.*
5. Its **anterior surface** presents three faint transverse ridges indicating the lines of fusion of four small segments called **sternebrae.** The anterior surface on each side gives origin to the pectoralis major muscle.
6. Its **posterior surface** is smooth and slightly concave.
   (a) Lower part of posterior surface gives origin to *sternocostalis muscle.*
   (b) On the right side of median plane, posterior surface is related to pleura, which separates it from the lung.
   (c) On the left side of median plane, upper half of the body is related to the pleura and lower half to the pericardium (*bare area of the pericardium*)
7. Its **lateral border** articulates with the 2nd–7th costal cartilages (to form synovial joints. Strictly speaking, 2nd costal cartilage articulates at the side of manubriosternal junction and 7th costal cartilage articulates at the xiphisternal junction).

Xiphoid Process (Metasternum; Figs 15.1 and 15.2)

1. It is the lowest and smallest part of the sternum.
2. It varies greatly in size and shape.
3. It may be bifid or perforated.
4. Its **anterior surface** provides insertion to the medial fibres of the rectus abdominis.
5. Its **posterior surface** gives origin to the sternal fibres of the diaphragm.
6. Its **tip** provides attachment to the upper end of linea alba.

Muscles attached on the posterior and anterior surfaces of sternum are summarized below:

Muscle attached on the anterior surface of the sternum	Muscles attached on the posterior surface of the sternum
• Sternal head of sternocleidomastoid	• Sternohyoid
	• Sternothyroid
• Pectoralis major	• Sternocostalis
• Rectus abdominis	• Diaphragm (sternal fibres)

N.B. Features of interest at the sternal angle: Sternal angle can be felt as a transverse ridge on the sternum about 5 cm below the suprasternal notch. *The sternal angle is an important surface bony landmark for many anatomical events accurate this level.* These are:
• Second costal cartilage articulates, on either side, with the sternum at this level, hence this level is *used for counting the ribs.*
• It lies at the level of intervertebral disc between T4 and T5 vertebrae.

• Horizontal plane passing through this level separates superior mediastinum from inferior mediastinum.
• Ascending aorta ends at this level.
• Arch of aorta begins and ends at this level.
• Descending aorta begins at this level.
• Trachea bifurcates into right and left principal bronchi at this level.
• Pulmonary trunk divides into right and left pulmonary arteries at this level.
• Upper border of heart lies at this level.
• Azygos vein arches over the root of right lung to end in the superior vena cava.

Clinical correlation

• **Sternal puncture:** Manubrium sterni is the preferred site for bone marrow aspiration because it is subcutaneous and readily accessible. The bone marrow sample is required for hematological examination. A thick needle is inserted into the upper part of manubrium to avoid injury to arch of aorta which lies behind the lower part. Sternal puncture is not advisable in children because in them the plates of compact bone of sternum are very thin and if needle passes through and through the manubrium it will damage the arch of aorta and its branches, leading to *fatal hemorrhage.*
• **Mid-sternotomy:** To gain access to the mediastinum for surgical operations on heart and great blood vessels, the sternum is often divided in the median plane called *mid-sternotomy.*
• **Funnel chest (pectus excavatum):** It is an abnormal shape of thoracic cage in which chest is compressed anteroposteriorly and sternum is pushed backward by the overgrowth of the ribs and may compress the heart.
• **Pigeon chest (pectus carinatum):** It is an abnormal shape of thoracic cage in which chest is compressed from side-to-side and sternum projects forward and downward like a keel of a boat.
• **Sternal fracture:** It is common in automobile accidents; e.g., when the driver's chest is hit against the steering wheel, the sternum is often fractured at the sternal angle. The backward displacement of fractured fragments may damage aorta, heart, or liver and cause severe bleeding which may prove fatal.

OSSIFICATION

The sternum develops from two vertical cartilaginous plates (**sternal plates**), which fuse in the midline.

The sternum ossifies from six double centres, viz.

1. One for manubrium.
2. Four for body.
3. One for xiphoid process.

Appearance

The centers appear in descending order for different parts of sternum as follows:

1. Manubrium: 5th month
2. Body
   (a) First sternebra: 6th month
   (b) Second sternebra: 7th month
   (c) Third sternebra: 8th month
   (d) Fourth sternebra: 9th month
   } of IUL*
3. Xiphoid process: 3rd year

Fusion

The fusion occurs as follows:

1. Fusion between sternal plates takes place from below upwards. It begins at puberty and completed by 25 years.
2. The xiphoid process fuses with the body at the age of 40 years.
3. Manubrium does not fuse with the body. As a result, the secondary cartilaginous manubriosternal joint usually persists throughout life. In about 10% individuals, fusion occurs in old age.

Clinical correlation

Sternal foramen and cleft sternum: The two sternal plates fuse in caudocranial direction. Sometimes sternebrae fail to fuse in the midline, as a result defect occurs in the body of sternum in the form of *sternal foramen* or *cleft sternum*. The cleft sternum is often associated with *ectopia cordis*.

RIBS

The ribs are flat, ribbon-like, elastic bony arches, which extend from thoracic vertebrae posteriorly to the lateral borders of the sternum anteriorly. Their anterior ends are connected to the costal cartilage. The ribs along with its costal cartilage constitute the **costa**. The ribs and their costal cartilages form greater part of the thoracic skeleton.

Number

Normally there are 12 pairs of ribs (but occurrence of accessory cervical or lumbar rib may increase them to 13 pairs or absence of 12th rib may reduce them to 11 pairs).

Arrangement and General Outline

1. The ribs are arranged one below the other and the gaps between the adjacent ribs are called *intercostals spaces.*
2. The length of ribs increases from 1st to 7th rib and then gradually decreases; hence, seventh rib is the longest rib.
3. The transverse diameter of thorax increases progressively from 1st to 8th rib, hence 8th rib has the greatest lateral projection.

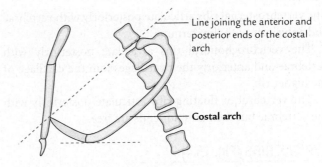

Line joining the anterior and posterior ends of the costal arch

Costal arch

Fig. 15.3 Costal arch (side view).

4. The ribs are arranged obliquely, i.e., their anterior ends lie at lower level than their posterior ends (Fig. 15.3).
5. The obliquity of ribs increases progressively from 1st to 9th rib, hence 9th rib is most obliquely placed.
6. The width of ribs gradually reduced from above downward.

The anterior ends of first seven ribs are connected to the sternum through their costal cartilages. The cartilages at the anterior ends of 8th, 9th, and 10th ribs are joined to the next higher cartilage. The anterior ends of 11th and 12th ribs are free and therefore called **floating ribs.**

N.B.

- The 10th rib usually have free anterior ends in Japanese.
- First rib slopes downwards along its entire extent.
- The middle of each costal arch (consisting of a rib and its costal cartilage) except the first rib lies at a lower level than a straight line joining the two ends of the costa (Fig. 15.3).

CLASSIFICATION

A. According to features

1. *Typical ribs:* 3rd–9th.
2. *Atypical ribs:* 1st, 2nd, 10th, 11th, and 12th.

The typical ribs have same general features, whereas the atypical ribs have special features and therefore can be differentiated from the remaining ribs.

B. According to relation with the sternum

1. *True ribs:* 1st–7th (i.e., upper 7 ribs).
2. *False ribs:* 8th–12th (i.e., lower 5 ribs).

True ribs articulate with the sternum anteriorly, whereas **false ribs** do not articulate with the sternum anteriorly.

C. According to articulation

1. Vertebrosternal ribs: 1st–7th.
2. Vertebrochondral ribs: 8th–10th.
3. Vertebral (floating) ribs: 11th and 12th.

*Intrauterine life.

The **vertebrosternal ribs** articulate posteriorly with vertebrae and anteriorly with the sternum.

The **vertebrochondral ribs** articulate posteriorly with vertebrae and anteriorly their cartilages join the cartilage of the higher rib.

The **vertebral** or **floating ribs** articulate posteriorly with the vertebrae but their anterior ends are free.

TYPICAL RIBS (Fig. 15.4)

Parts

Each rib has three parts: (a) anterior end, (b) posterior end, and (c) shaft.

The **anterior end** bears a concave depression.

The **posterior end** consists of head, neck, and tubercle.

The **shaft** is the longest part and extends between anterior and posterior ends. It is flattened and has inner and outer surfaces and upper and lower borders. It is curved with convexity directed outwards and bears a costal groove on its inner surface near the lower border. Five centimeters away from tubercle, it abruptly changes its direction, this is called **angle of the rib**.

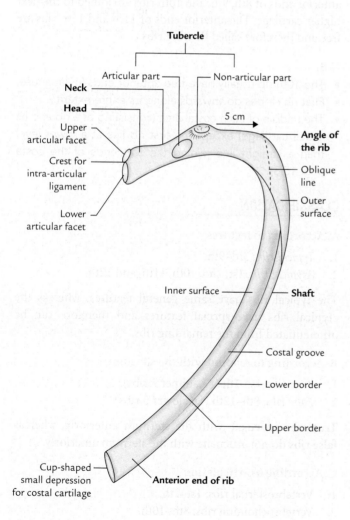

Fig. 15.4 Features of a typical rib.

Side Determination and Anatomical Position

The side of the rib can be determined by holding it in such a way that its posterior end having head, neck, and tubercle is directed posteriorly, its concavity faces medially and its sharp border is directed inferiorly.

In an **anatomical position**, the posterior end is higher and nearer the median plane than the anterior end.

Features and Attachments

Anterior (costal) end

It bears a small cup-shaped depression, which joins the corresponding costal cartilage to form a primary cartilaginous *costochondral joint*.

Posterior end

It presents head, neck, and tubercle.

Head

It has **two articular facets:** lower and upper.

1. The *lower larger facet* articulates with the body of numerically corresponding vertebra.
2. The *upper smaller facet* articulates with the next higher vertebra.

   The crest separating the two articular facets lies opposite the intervertebral disc.

Neck

1. It lies in front of the transverse process of the corresponding vertebra.
2. It has **two borders**—superior and inferior, and **two surfaces**—anterior and posterior.
3. The upper border is sharp crest like, whereas the lower border is rounded.
4. The posterior surface is rough and pierced by foramina.

Tubercle

1. It is situated on the outer surface of the rib at the junction of neck and shaft.
2. It is divided into **two parts**—medial *articular part* and lateral *non-articular part*. The articular part bears a small oval facet, which articulates with the transverse process of corresponding vertebra. The non-articular part is rough and provides attachment to ligaments.

Shaft

1. It is thin and flattened.
2. It presents **two surfaces**—outer and inner, **two borders**—upper and lower, and **two angles**—posterior and anterior.

Borders

Superior border

The superior border is thick and rounded, and presents outer and inner lips:

- The *outer lip* gives attachment to the external intercostal muscles.
- The *inner lip* gives attachment to the internal intercostal and intercostalis intimus muscles.

Lower border

The lower border is sharp and forms the lower border of the costal groove, and gives origin to the external intercostals muscle.

Surfaces

Outer surface

1. It is smooth and convex, and presents **two angles**—posterior and anterior.
   - The posterior angle (generally called only angle) is marked by an oblique ridge.
   - The anterior angle is marked by an indistinct oblique line.

Inner surface

It is smooth and concave. It presents a **costal groove** near its lower border. The costal groove becomes unrecognizable in the anterior part.

- The **costal groove** lodges intercostal nerve and vessels from above downwards, as follows (*Mnemonic:* VAN):
   1. Intercostal Vein.
   2. Intercostal Artery.
   3. Intercostal Nerve.
- The **internal intercostal** muscle is attached to the floor of the groove (intervening between intercostal nerves and vessels, and bone).

- The **intercostalis intimus** is attached to the upper border of the costal groove.

N.B. Three characteristic features of a typical rib:
- It is *curved* along its entire extent.
- It is *angulated*, i.e., presents two bends—one 5 cm in front of tubercle and one 2 cm behind the anterior end.
- It is *twisted*, so that the two ends of the rib cannot touch the same horizontal plane.
(*Mnemonic:* CAT – Curve, Angle, and Twist).

ATYPICAL RIBS

First Rib (Fig. 15.5)

Distinguishing Features

1. It is shortest, broadest, and most acutely curved.
2. Its shaft is flattened above downwards so that it has upper and lower surfaces, and outer and inner borders.
3. Its head is small, rounded, and bears a single circular articular facet to articulate with the side of first thoracic vertebra.
4. Its angle and tubercle coincide.
5. It has no costal groove on its inner surface.
6. Its neck is rounded and elongated. It is directed upwards, backwards and laterally.
7. Its anterior end is larger and thicker.

N.B. The shaft of the first rib slopes obliquely downwards and forwards to its sternal end. It is due to this obliquity that the pulmonary and pleural apices projects into the root of the neck.

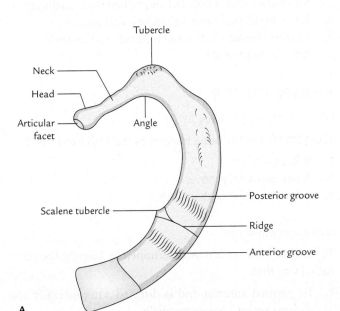

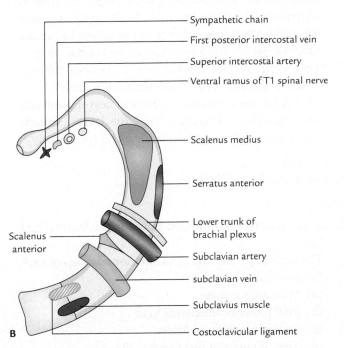

Fig. 15.5 First rib (left side) seen from above: **A**, general features; **B**, attachments and relations.

Side Determination

Side of the first rib can be determined by holding the rib in such a way that:

(a) its larger end is directed anteriorly and its smaller end is directed posteriorly,

(b) the surface of its shaft having two grooves separated by a ridge is directed superiorly, and

(c) its concave border is directed inwards and its convex border is directed outwards.

N.B. Trick for students for side determination of first rib: Keep the rib on the table top considering its position in your own body. Now note that the rib belongs to the side on which it's both ends touch the surface. If the rib is placed on the wrong side, then only its anterior end will be touching the surface.

Features and Attachments

Inner border

1. It presents a scalene tubercle about its middle. Tubercle and adjoining part of the upper surface provides attachment to the scalenus anterior muscle.

2. It provides attachment to the Sibson's fascia (suprapleural membrane).

Outer border

It provides origin to the first digitation of serratus anterior about its middle, just behind the groove for the subclavian artery.

Superior (upper) surface

1. It is crossed obliquely by two shallow grooves (anterior and posterior) separated by a slight ridge. The ridge is continuous with the scalene tubercle. The anterior groove lodges subclavian vein, while posterior groove lodges the subclavian artery and lower trunk of the brachial plexus.

2. The area behind posterior groove up to the costal tubercle provides attachment to the scalenus medius muscle.

3. The area in front anterior groove and near the anterior end provides attachment to **subclavius muscle** (anteriorly) and **costoclavicular ligament** (posteriorly).

Lower surface

It is related to the costal pleura.

Neck

1. It is elongated and directed upwards, backwards, and laterally.

2. The following structures form **anterior relations of neck** from medial to lateral side:

   (a) Sympathetic **chain**

   (b) First posterior intercostal **V**ein

   (c) Superior intercostal **A**rtery

   (d) Ventral ramus of first thoracic **N**erve.

Memory device: Chain pulling the VAN.

Second Rib (Fig. 15.6)

Distinguishing Features and Attachments

1. Its length is twice that of the second rib.

2. Its shaft is sharply/highly curved.

3. Its shaft is not twisted; hence both the ends of rib touch the table top when placed on it.

4. Near its middle, the outer convex surface of shaft presents a rough impression or prominent tubercle, which provides attachment to the serratus anterior muscle (lower part of first and whole of second digitation).

5. The outer surface of the shaft is directed outwards and upwards, while inner surface of the shaft is directed inwards and downwards.

6. Posterior part of internal surface presents a short costal groove.

7. The upper border and adjoining part of upper surface provide attachment to the scalenus posterior and serratus posterior superior muscles.

Tenth Rib

Distinguishing Features

It has single articular facet on its head, which articulates with the body of corresponding thoracic vertebra.

It is slightly shorter than the typical rib.

Eleventh Rib

Distinguishing Features

1. It has single large, articular facet on its head.

2. It has no neck and no tubercle.

3. Its anterior end is pointed and tipped with cartilage.

4. It has slight angle and a shallow costal groove.

5. Its inner surface is directed upwards and inwards.

6. It has a slight angle.

Twelfth Rib (Fig. 15.7)

Distinguishing Features

The 12th rib has the same features as the 11th except that:

1. It has no angle.

2. It has no costal groove.

3. It is much shorter than 11th.

Side Determination

The side of 12th rib can be determined by keeping the rib in such a way that:

1. Its pointed anterior end is directed anterolaterally and its broader end posteromedially.

2. Its slightly concave surface faces inwards and upwards.

3. Its sharper border is directed inferiorly.

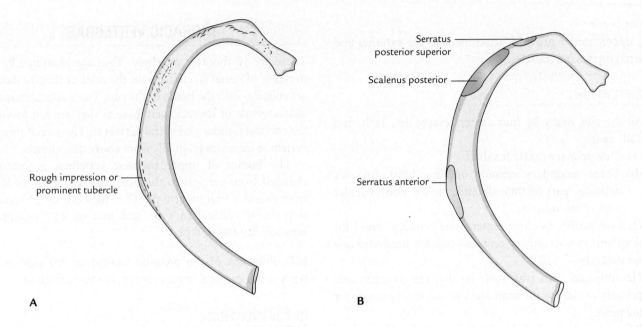

Fig. 15.6 Second rib (right): A, general features; B, attachments.

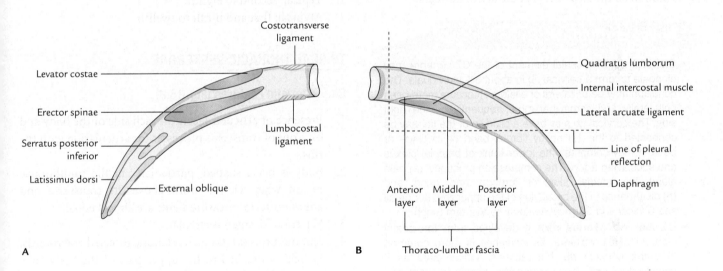

Fig. 15.7 Twelfth rib (right side) showing attachments: A, outer surface; B, inner surface.

Attachments

Outer surface

1. Near the tip, it provides attachment to the latissimus dorsi muscle above and external oblique muscle below.
2. Its medial half provides attachment to the erector spinae muscle.

Inner surface

1. An oblique line crossing the middle of this surface marks the line of *pleural reflection*.
2. Lower part of medial half provides attachment to the *quadratus lumborum muscle*.

3. Middle two-fourth near the upper border provides attachment to the *internal intercostal muscle*.
4. Upper part of lateral one-fourth near the tip provides attachment to the *diaphragm.*

Lower border

1. Close to head it provides attachment to the *lumbocostal ligament*, which stretches from transverse process of L1 vertebra.
2. *Lateral arcuate ligament* is attached to it just lateral to the quadratus lumborum.

Upper border

The upper border provides attachment to the external and internal intercostal muscles.

OSSIFICATION

- All the ribs ossify by four centers except 1st, 11th, and 12th ossify,
  - (a) One primary center for shaft.
  - (b) Three secondary centers: one for head, one for articular part of tubercle and one for non-articular part of the tubercle.
- First rib ossifies by three centers: one primary centre for shaft and two secondary centers—one for head and one for tubercle.
- Eleventh and 12th ribs ossify by two centers each: one primary center for the shaft and one secondary centre for the head.
- Primary centers of all the ribs appear at the 8th week of IUL.
- Secondary centers of all the ribs appear at puberty.
- Fusion in all the ribs occurs at the age of 20 years.

Clinical correlation

- **Cervical rib**: The costal element of the C7 vertebra may elongate to form a cervical rib in about 5% individuals. The condition may be unilateral or bilateral. It occurs more often unilaterally and somewhat more frequently on the right side. The cervical rib may have a blind tip or the tip may be connected to the 1st rib by fibrous band or cartilage or bone. It may compress the lower trunk of brachial plexus and subclavian artery. The compression produces: (a) pain along the medial side of forearm and hand and (b) disturbance in the circulation of the upper limb (for detail see *Clinical and Surgical Anatomy* by Vishram Singh.)
- **Lumbar rib (Gorilla rib)**: It develops from the costal element of L1 vertebra. Its incidence is more common than the cervical rib, but remains undiagnosed as it usually does not cause symptoms. It may be confused with the fracture of transverse process of L1 vertebra.
- **Fracture of rib**: Usually the middle ribs are involved in the fracture. The rib commonly fractures at its angle (posterior angle) as it is the weakest point.
- **Flail chest (stove-in-chest)**: When ribs are fractured at two sites (e.g., anteriorly as well as at an angle), the flail chest occurs. The flail segments of ribs are sucked in during inspiration and pushed out during expiration leading to a clinical condition called *paradoxical respiration*).

N.B.

- Fracture of ribs is rare in children as the ribs are elastic in them.
- First two ribs (1st and 2nd ribs) are protected by clavicle and last two ribs (11th and 12th) are mobile (floating), hence they are rarely injured.

THORACIC VERTEBRAE

There are 12 thoracic vertebrae. They are identified by the presence of costal facet/facets on the sides of their bodies for articulation with the heads of the ribs. These articulations are characteristic of thoracic vertebrae as they are not found in the cervical lumbar and sacral vertebrae. The size of thoracic vertebrae increases gradually from above downwards.

The bodies of upper thoracic vertebrae is gradually changed from cervical to thoracic type and those of lower from thoracic to lumbar type. Thus the body of T1 vertebra is typically cervical in type and that of T12 vertebra is typically lumbar in type.

N.B. Presence of the articular facet(s) on the side of the body is the *cardinal feature of the thoracic vertebrae*.

CLASSIFICATION

According to the features, the thoracic vertebrae are classified into two types:

1. Typical: second to eighth.
2. Atypical: first and ninth to twelfth.

TYPICAL THORACIC VERTEBRAE

Characteristic Features (Fig. 15.8)

1. Presence of articular facets on each side of the body and on front of transverse processes for articulation with the ribs.
2. Body is heart shaped, particularly in the midthoracic region when viewed from above. Its transverse and anteroposterior measurements are almost equal.
3. Vertebral foramen is circular.
4. Spinous process is long, slender, and directed downwards.
5. Pedicle is attached to the upper part of the body, thus making the inferior vertebral notch deeper.

Parts

The thoracic vertebra consists of two parts:

1. Body.
2. Vertebral arch.

The body and vertebral arch enclose a vertebral foramen in which lies the spinal cord surrounded by its meninges.

Body

1. It is heart shaped, when viewed from above.
2. Its anteroposterior and transverse dimensions are almost equal.
3. On each side, the bodies are two costal facets, superior, and inferior.

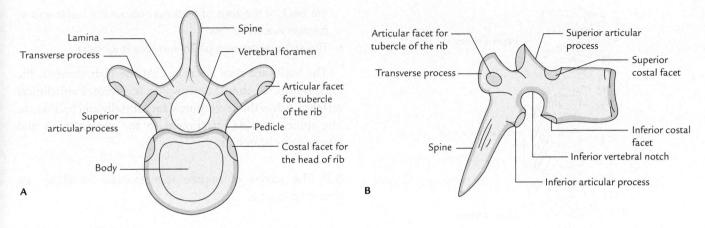

Fig. 15.8 Features of a typical thoracic vertebra: **A**, superior view; **B**, lateral view.

- *Superior facet* is larger and situated near the upper border of the body in front of the root of the pedicle.
- *Inferior facet* is smaller and situated near the lower border in front of the inferior vertebral notch.

Vertebral arch: It consists of a pair of pedicles anteriorly and two laminae, posteriorly:

- The *pedicles* (right and left) are short rounded bony bars, which project backwards and laterally from the posterior aspect of the body.
- The *laminae* (right and left)—each pedicle continues posteromedially as a vertical plate of bone. The laminae of two sides join with each other in the posterior midline.
- The *spinous process* arises in the midline where the two laminae meet posteriorly.
- *Two transverse processes*, one on either side arises from the junction of pedicle and lamina.
- *Two paired articular process*, two on each side spring from lamina, the superior articular process project rather more from pedicle than lamina, the inferior articular process springs from a lamina.

Features and Attachments
Body

1. The *upper larger costal facet* (actually demifacet) articulates with the head of the numerically corresponding rib.
2. The *lower smaller costal facet* (actually demifacet) articulates with the head of the next lower rib.
3. Anterior and posterior surfaces of body provide attachment to the anterior and posterior longitudinal ligaments, respectively. These ligaments are attached to both the upper end lower borders of the body.
4. Posterior surface of body is marked by vascular foramina for *basivertebral veins*, which are covered by the posterior longitudinal ligament.

Pedicles

1. They are attached nearer the superior border of body, as a result the *superior vertebral notch* is shallow and the *inferior vertebral notch* is deep.
2. The deep inferior vertebral notch together with small superior vertebral notch of next lower vertebra completes the intervertebral foramen, through which spinal nerve leaves the vertebral canal.

Laminae

1. They are short, broad, and thick; and overlap each other from above downwards.
2. Their margins give attachment to the ligamenta flava.

Superior Articular Processes
The articular facets on superior articular process are directed backwards and slightly laterally and articulate with the inferior articular facet of the next higher vertebra.

Inferior Articular Processes
The articular facet on inferior articular process is flat and faces forwards and little downwards and medially. It articulates with the superior articular facet of the next lower vertebra.

Transverse Processes
They are large club shaped and projects laterally and slightly backwards.

- The facet on the anterior aspect of the tip of transverse process articulates with the tubercle of the numerically corresponding rib.
- They provide attachments to the ligaments and muscles related to the rib cage and back.

Spine
The spines are directed downwards and backwards. The spinous processes of middle four vertebrae (i.e., from 5th to

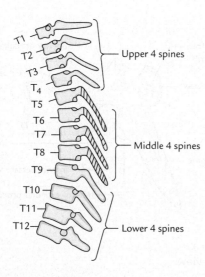

Fig. 15.9 Showing inclination of the spinous processes of thoracic vertebrae.

8th) are very long, vertical, and overlap each other. The spinous processes of upper four and lower four vertebrae are relatively short and less oblique in direction (Fig. 15.9).

N.B.

- The spinous process of T1 vertebra is most prominent and horizontal in its projection and can be palpated at

the back of the root of neck just below the lower end of median nuchal furrow.

- The spinous process of T8 vertebra is longest.

The backward slant decreases. At the 11th vertebra, the spine is directed almost downwards. It is termed **anticlinical vertebra**, below this level spine slants dorsally and backwards. The spines provide attachment to the supraspinous and interspinous ligaments.

N.B. The spines of middle four thoracic vertebrae are almost horizontal.

ATYPICAL THORACIC VERTEBRAE (Fig. 15.10)

First Thoracic Vertebra

Distinguishing Features

1. It resembles the 7th cervical vertebra.
2. The body is narrow anteroposteriorly. Its upper surface is concave from side to side with an upward projecting lip on either sides. The anterior border of inferior surface projects downwards.
3. The superior articular facet on the side of the body is circular and articulates with the whole of the facet on the head of the first rib.

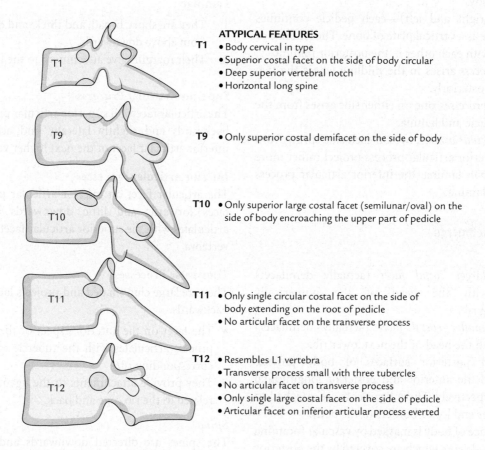

ATYPICAL FEATURES

T1
- Body cervical in type
- Superior costal facet on the side of body circular
- Deep superior vertebral notch
- Horizontal long spine

T9
- Only superior costal demifacet on the side of body

T10
- Only superior large costal facet (semilunar/oval) on the side of body encroaching the upper part of pedicle

T11
- Only single circular costal facet on the side of body extending on the root of pedicle
- No articular facet on the transverse process

T12
- Resembles L1 vertebra
- Transverse process small with three tubercles
- No articular facet on transverse process
- Only single large costal facet on the side of pedicle
- Articular facet on inferior articular process everted

Fig. 15.10 Features of atypical thoracic vertebrae.

4. The superior vertebral notches are deep (i.e., clearly seen) as in cervical vertebra.
5. The inferior articular facet is half (i.e., demifacet) articulates with the head of the 2nd rib.
6. The spinal process is nearly horizontal.

Ninth Thoracic Vertebra

Distinguishing Features

1. The lower costal facet on each side of body is absent
2. The body on each side possesses only superior costal facet (demifacet) for articulation with the 9th rib.

Tenth Thoracic Vertebra

Distinguishing Features

The body on each side possesses only single articular facet, which is semilunar or oval for articulation with the 10th rib. The costal facet encroaches on the upper part of the pedicle.

Eleventh Thoracic Vertebra

Distinguishing Features

1. Body on each side possesses single large circular costal facet for articulation with the head of the 11th rib. The costal facet extends onto the root of the pedicle.
2. Transverse processes are small and do not present costal facet on their tips (as 11th rib has no tubercle).

Twelfth Thoracic Vertebra

Distinguishing Features

1. It resembles the first lumbar vertebra.
2. Body on each side possesses a large single costal facet, which is more on the lower part of the pedicle than on the body.
3. Transverse process is small and presents three tubercles—superior, middle, and inferior. It has no articular facet (as 12th rib has no tubercle).

The three tubercles of the transverse process of 12th thoracic vertebra correspond with the following processes of the lumbar vertebra:

(a) Superior tubercle corresponds to the *mamillary process* of lumbar vertebra.
(b) Middle tubercle corresponds to the true *transverse process* of lumbar vertebra.
(c) Inferior tubercle corresponds to the *accessory process* of the lumbar vertebra.

The important distinguishing features of atypical thoracic vertebrae (i.e., 1st, 9th, 10th, 11th, and 12th) are enumerated in Table 15.1.

Table 15.1 Distinguishing features atypical thoracic vertebrae

Vertebra	Distinguishing features
T1	• Resembles 7th cervical vertebra • Superior costal facet is circular • Superior vertebral notch is deep and clearly seen
T9	• Presence of only superior demifacet
T10	• Presence of only single large complete costal facet
T11	• Presence of single large circular costal facet • Absence of articular facet on transverse process
T12	• Resembles 1st lumbar vertebra • Presence of single large circular facet extending onto the root of tubercle • Transverse process presents three tubercles: superior, inferior, and lateral

COSTAL CARTILAGES

The costal cartilages are made up of hyaline cartilage and are mainly responsible for providing elasticity and mobility of the chest wall.

First to 7th cartilages connect the respective ribs with the lateral border of the sternum and they increase in length from 1st to 7th.

Eighth to 10th cartilages at their anterior ends are connected with the lower border of the cartilage above and there is a gradual decrease in length from 8th to 10th.

Eleventh and 12th cartilages end in free pointed extremities.

JOINTS OF THE THORAX

The joints of thorax are as follows:

1. Costovertebral.
2. Costotransverse.
3. Costochondral.
4. Interchondral.
5. Manubriosternal.
6. Intervertebral.

COSTOVERTEBRAL JOINTS (Fig. 15.11)

These joints are formed by articulation of articular facets on the head of ribs and costal facets on the bodies of thoracic vertebrae.

The head of typical rib articulates with the body of numerically corresponding vertebra and also with the body of next higher vertebra.

Type

Synovial type of plane joint.

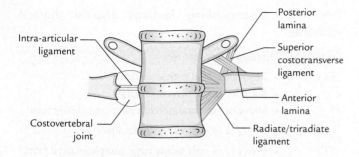

Fig. 15.11 Costovertebral joint.

Ligaments

1. **Capsular ligament (joint capsule):** It is the fibrous capsule that covers/encloses the joint and is attached to the articular margins.
2. **Radiate ligament/triradiate ligament:** It stretches from the anterior aspect of the head of rib and divides into three bands: upper, lower, and middle. The upper and lower bands are attached to the sides of upper and lower vertebrae. The middle band (also called *intra-articular ligament*) gets attached to the intervertebral disc.
3. **Intra-articular ligament:** It stretches from the crest between the two articular facets on the head of rib to the intervertebral disc and divides the joint cavity into two parts.

The 1st, 10th, 11th, and 12th ribs articulate with the bodies of numerically corresponding vertebrae.

N.B. Costovertebral joint of typical ribs have two joint cavities and those of atypical ribs have single joint cavity.

COSTOTRANSVERSE JOINTS (Fig. 15.12)

The tubercle articulates with the transverse process of the numerically corresponding vertebra to form a synovial joint. It is absent in 11th and 12th ribs.

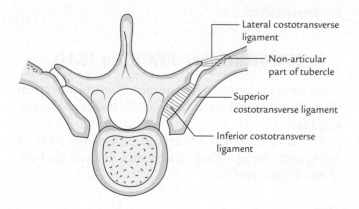

Fig. 15.12 Costotransverse joint.

Type

Plane type of synovial joint.

Ligaments

1. **Capsular ligament (joint capsule):** It is thin fibrous sac enclosing the joint.
2. **Superior costotransverse ligament:** It has two layers—anterior and posterior. The anterior layer stretches between the crest of rib and lower aspect of transverse process of vertebra above. The posterior layer stretches between the posterior aspects of the neck to the transverse process above.
3. **Inferior costotransverse ligament:** It extends from posterior aspect of the neck of rib to the transverse process of its own vertebra.
4. **Lateral transverse ligament:** It stretches between non-articular parts of tubercle to the tip of transverse process.

COSTOCHONDRAL JOINTS

The costochondral joints are primary cartilaginous joints between the anterior end of the rib and its cartilage. They permit no movements.

CHONDROSTERNAL JOINTS

These are joints between the medial ends of 1st–7th costal cartilages and lateral border of the sternum. They are often termed by clinicians as *sternocostal joints*.

First chondrosternal joint is primary cartilaginous joint (*synchondrosis*) and does not permit any movement.

N.B. The costal cartilage of 1st rib is united with manubrium sterni by a plate of fibrocartilage and hence it is not a typical primary cartilaginous joint (synchondrosis).

Second to seventh costal cartilages articulate with the sternum by synovial joints. Each joint has a single cavity, except the 2nd costosternal joint where the cavity is divided into two parts.

INTERCHONDRAL JOINTS

In interchondral joint, 7th–9th costal cartilages comes into contact with one another and articulate with each other by number of small synovial joints. At some sites, they are also united by ligaments. The union between the 9th and 10th costal cartilages is usually ligamentous.

MANUBRIOSTERNAL JOINT

The manubriosternal joint is formed between the lower end of the manubrium sterni and upper end of the body of sternum.

It is a secondary cartilaginous joint (**symphysis**) between manubrium and body of sternum. It permits slight sliding movements of body of sternum on the manubrium during respiration.

N.B. The *manubriosternal joint* is not a typical symphysis because as a rule bones taking part in the formation of a symphysis do not undergo bony union, but in many individuals after 30 years of age bony union does take place between the manubrium and the body of sternum.

INTERVERTEBRAL JOINTS

The intervertebral joints are formed

(a) between the bodies of the vertebrae, and
(b) between the articular processes of the vertebra.

JOINTS BETWEEN THE BODIES OF THE VERTEBRAE

These are secondary cartilaginous joint. The inferior and superior surfaces of the adjacent vertebral bodies are covered by thin plates of hyaline cartilages, which in turn are united by fibrocartilaginous intervertebral disc. The disc consists of an outer rim by fibrocartilage—*the annulus fibrosus* and a central core of gelatinous substance—the *nucleus pulposus.* These joints are held together by anterior and posterior longitudinal ligaments of the vertebral column (for details see *General Anatomy* by Vishram Singh).

JOINTS BETWEEN THE ARTICULAR PROCESSES

The joints between the superior and inferior articular processes of adjacent vertebrae are called **facet** (*zygapophysial)*

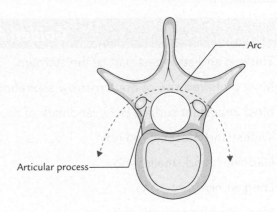

Fig. 15.13 The articular processes of thoracic vertebra are set on an arc.

joints. They are plane type of synovial joints and permit gliding movements. The zygapophysial joints of thoracic vertebrae are directed vertically. This limits flexion and extension, but facilitates rotation. The rotation is greatly facilitated because the articular process of thoracic vertebrae are set on an arc (Fig. 15.13). The ligaments are joint capsule, which encloses the articular surfaces. The accessory ligaments are: (a) ligaments flava between the laminae of adjacent vertebrae, (b) supraspinous, (c) infraspinous, and (d) intertransverse ligaments.

Movements

The movements of flexion and extension are best permitted in the cervical and the lumbar regions, while the rotatory movements are best seen in the thoracic region.

Golden Facts to Remember

► Thickest and strongest part of the sternum	Manubrium sterni
► Most preferred site of bone marrow aspiration	Manubrium sterni
► Most important surface bony landmark of thoracic cage	Sternal angle
► Widest and most curved rib	First
► Narrowest and smallest rib	Twelfth
► Longest rib	Seventh
► Most laterally projecting rib	Eighth
► Most oblique rib	Ninth
► Commonest accessory rib	Lumbar rib
► Gorilla rib	Lumbar rib
► Race in which anterior ends of 10th ribs are usually free	Japanese
► Smallest and most variable part of the sternum	Xiphoid process
► Thoracic vertebra with smallest body	T3
► Thoracic vertebra with longest spine	T8
► Anticlinical vertebra	T11

Clinical Case Study

A 25-year-old final year medical student told his Professor of Anatomy that he often feels pain in his right upper limb, and his radial pulse becomes feeble especially during exercise. He also told that sometimes he feels pain that radiates along the medial side of his forearm and hand. On examination, the professor noted a bony swelling in the root of the neck on the right side. X-ray neck revealed normal cervical spine. Chest X-ray, however, revealed the presence of cervical rib on the right side. The student was referred to an orthopedic surgeon who after physical examination and seeing reports advised the student to have his cervical rib removed, otherwise the vascular problem would worsen.

Questions

1. What is cervical rib?
2. Which structure is likely to be compressed by the cervical rib?
3. What complication could occur if the cervical rib is not removed?

Answers

1. The elongation of costal element of the transverse process of 7th cervical vertebra.
2. (a) Subclavian artery and (b) lower trunk of brachial plexus.
3. The cervical rib causes angulation of the subclavian artery over the first rib. Left untreated, a clot tends to form distal to the kinked vessel and portions of the clot (emboli) may enter the circulation of the upper limb, which may block one of the digital arteries in the hand and cause *gangrene* of finger tips. The prolonged compression of lower trunk brachial plexus (C8, T1) may cause wasting of the most of the small muscles of the hand.

Thoracic Wall and Mechanism of Respiration

The thoracic wall is formed posteriorly by the thoracic part of the vertebral column, anteriorly by the sternum and costal cartilages, and laterally by the ribs and the intercostal spaces. The floor of thorax is formed by the diaphragm and its roof is formed by suprapleural membranes. The diseases of thoracic viscera are the leading cause of death all over the world. Therefore, surface landmarks of the thorax are extremely important to the physicians in providing reference locations for performing inspection (visual observation), palpation (feeling with firm pressure), percussion (detecting densities through tapping), and auscultation (listening sounds with the stethoscope).

SURFACE LANDMARKS

BONY LANDMARKS

The bony landmarks of the thoracic wall are as follows (Fig. 16.1):

1. **Suprasternal notch (jugular notch):** It is felt just above the superior border of the manubrium sterni between the proximal medial ends of the two clavicles. It lies at the level of lower border of the body of T2 vertebra. The trachea can be palpated in this notch.
2. **Sternal angle (angle of Louis):** It is felt as a transverse ridge about 5 cm below the suprasternal notch. It marks the angle made between the manubrium and the body of the sternum (the angle between the long axis of manubrium and body of sternum is 163° posteriorly and 17° anteriorly). It lies at the level of intervertebral disc between the T4 and T5 vertebrae. The 2nd rib articulates on the either side with the sternum at this level. Hence it used as surface landmark for counting the ribs (for details see page 198).
3. **Xiphisternal joint:** It can be felt at the apex infrasternal/subcostal angle formed by the meeting of anterior end of subcostal margins. The xiphisternal joint lies at the level of the upper border of the body of T9 vertebra.

4. **Costal margin:** It forms the lower boundary of the thorax on each side and is formed by the cartilages of the 7th, 8th, 9th, and 10th ribs and the free ends of 11th and 12th ribs. The lowest point of costal margin is formed by the 10th rib and lies at the level of L3 vertebra.
5. **Subcostal angle:** It is situated at the inferior end of the sternum between the sternal attachments of the 7th costal cartilage.
6. **Thoracic vertebral spines:** The first prominent spine felt at the lower end of nuchal furrow (midline furrow on the back of neck) is the spine of C7 vertebra (**vertebra prominens**). All the thoracic spines are counted below this level. For reference, the 3rd thoracic spine lies at the level of root of spine of scapula and 7th thoracic spine lies at the level of inferior angle of the scapula.

SOFT TISSUE LANDMARKS

1. **Nipple:** In males, the nipple is usually located in the 4th intercostal space about 4 in (10 cm) from the midsternal line. In females, its position varies considerably.
2. **Apex beat of the heart:** It is lowermost and outermost thrust of cardiac pulsation, which is felt in the left 5th intercostal space 3.5 in (9 cm) from the midsternal line or just medial to the midclavicular line.

LINES OF ORIENTATION (Fig. 16.1)

The following imaginary lines are often used to describe surface locations on the anterior and posterior chest wall.

1. **Midsternal line:** It runs vertically downwards in the median plane on the anterior aspect of the sternum.
2. **Midclavicular line:** It runs vertically downwards from the midpoint of the clavicle to the midinguinal point. It crosses the tip of the 9th costal cartilage.
3. **Anterior axillary line:** It runs vertically downwards from the anterior axillary fold.

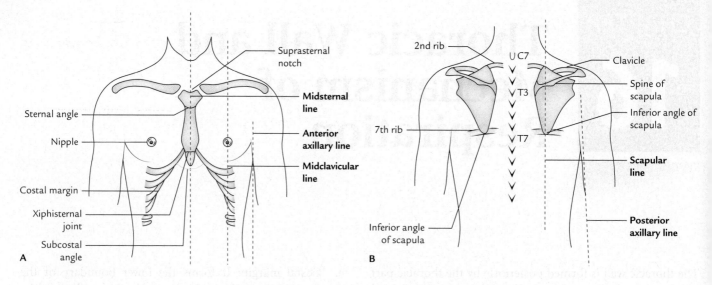

Fig. 16.1 Surface landmarks on the thoracic wall: **A**, anterior aspect; **B**, posterior aspect.

4. **Midaxillary line:** It runs vertically downwards from the point in the axilla located between the anterior and posterior axillary folds.
5. **Posterior axillary line:** It runs vertically downwards from the posterior axillary fold.
6. **Scapular line:** It runs vertically downwards on the posterior aspect of the chest passing through the inferior angle of the scapula with arms at the sides of the body.

COVERINGS OF THE THORACIC WALL

The thoracic wall is covered from superficial to deep by:

1. Skin.
2. Superficial fascia.
3. Deep fascia.
4. Muscles.

Skin: The skin covering thoracic wall is thin on its anterior aspect and thick on its back aspect. The distribution of hair is variable and depends on the age, sex, and race.

Cutaneous nerves: The cutaneous innervation on the front of thorax is provided by cutaneous branches of anterior primary rami of thoracic spinal nerves (T2–T6) in sequence from above downwards by the T2 at the level of 2nd rib to the T6 at the level of xiphoid process. The skin above the level of 2nd rib is supplied by the anterior primary ramus of C4 via supraclavicular nerves.

N.B.

*   The anterior rami of C5–T1 innervate the skin of the upper limb.
*   The cutaneous innervation on the back of thorax (on either side of midline for about 5 cm) is provided by posterior rami of thoracic spinal nerves.

Superficial fascia: The superficial fascia is more dense on the posterior aspect of the chest to sustain the pressure of the body when lying in the supine position. The superficial fascia on the front of the chest contains breast (mammary gland), which is rudimentary in males and well-developed in adult females. The breast is described in detail in Chapter 3.

Deep fascia: The deep fascia is thin and ill-defined (except in pectoral region) to allow free movement of the thoracic wall during breathing.

Muscles: The thoracic wall is liberally covered by the following extrinsic muscles:

1. **Muscles of upper limb:**
    (a) Pectoralis major and pectoralis minor muscles cover the front of thoracic wall.
    (b) Serratus anterior covers the side of thoracic wall.
2. **Muscles of abdomen:** Rectus abdominis and external oblique covers the lower part of the front of thoracic wall.
3. **Muscles of back:**
    (a) Trapezius and latissimus dorsi.
    (b) Levator scapulae, rhomboideus major and minor.
    (c) Serratus—posterior, superior, and inferior.
    (d) Erector spinae.

N.B.

*   The thoracic wall is more or less completely covered by extrinsic muscles except in the anterior and posterior median lines.
*   On the back, the thoracic wall is thinly covered by musculature in the region of triangle of auscultation (see page 62).

INTRINSIC MUSCLES (Figs 16.2–16.4)

The intrinsic muscles of the thoracic wall are arranged in three layers from superficial to deep. These are as follows (16.2A):

1. External intercostal muscle (superficial layer).
2. Internal intercostal muscle (intermediate layer).
3. Transversus thoracis muscle (deep layer).

The muscle layer is lined by the **endothoracic fascia**, which in turn is lined by the parietal pleura.

These three layers of muscles are comparable to the three layers of muscles in the abdominal wall.

The intercostal nerve and vessels form neurovascular bundle lie between the intermediate and deep layer (neurovascular plane).

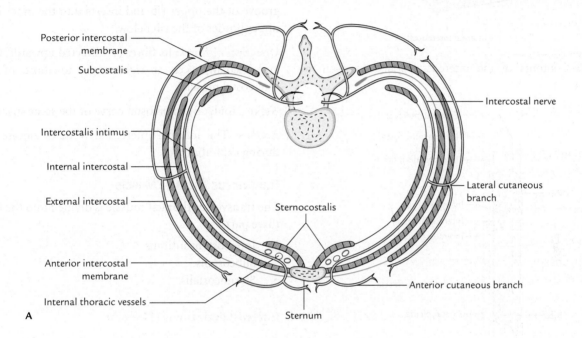

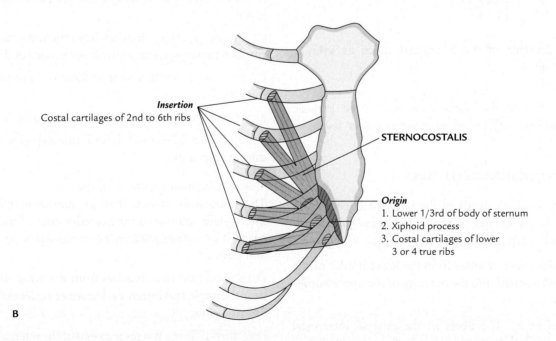

Fig. 16.2 Intrinsic muscles of the thoracic wall: A, layers of intrinsic muscles and course and branches of typical intercostal nerve; B, origin and insertion of sternocostalis muscle.

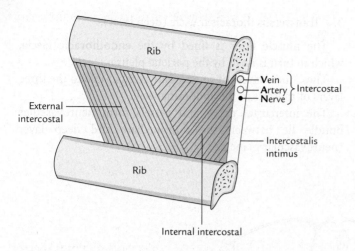

Fig. 16.3 Contents of the intercostal space as seen in dissection.

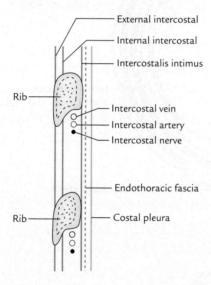

Fig. 16.4 Contents of the intercostal space as seen in vertical section.

N.B. In addition to the above-mentioned three intrinsic muscles there is another set of muscles called *levatores costarum*.

External Intercostal Muscle (11 Pairs)

Extent: Each muscle extends in the intercostal space from *tubercle of the rib* behind to the *costochondral junction* in front, where it is replaced by *anterior intercostal membrane*.

Origin and insertion: It arises from the lower border of the rib above and inserted into the outer lip of the upper border of rib below.

Direction of fibres: The fibres of the external intercostal muscle are directed downwards, forwards, and medially (*in the posterior part however, the fibres are directed downwards and laterally*).

Nerve supply: By intercostal nerve of the same space.

Actions: The external intercostal muscles elevate the ribs during inspiration.

Internal Intercostal Muscle (11 Pairs)

Extent: Each muscle extends in the intercostal space from the lateral border of sternum in front to the angle of rib behind, where it is replaced by the *posterior intercostal membrane*.

Origin and insertion: It arises from the floor of the costal groove of the upper rib and inserts into the inner lip of the upper border of the rib below.

Direction of fibres: Its fibres are directed upwards, forwards, and medially (i.e., at right angle to those of external intercostal muscle).

Nerve supply: By intercostal nerve of the same space.

Actions: The internal intercostal muscles elevate the ribs during expiration.

Transversus Thoracis Muscle

The transversus thoracis muscle is divided into the following three parts:

1. Intercostalis intimus.
2. Subcostalis.
3. Sternocostalis.

Intercostalis intimus (11 pairs)

Extent: It occupies the middle two-fourth of the intercostal space.

Origin and insertion: It arises from the inner surface of the rib above and inserts on to the inner surface of the rib below.

Direction of fibres: It is same as those of internal intercostal muscles.

Nerve supply: By intercostal nerve of the same space.

Actions: The intercostal intimi muscles elevate the ribs during expiration.

Subcostalis (total number variable)

The subcostalis muscle lies in the same plane as the intercostalis intimus in the posterior part of the intercostal space. It intervenes between the intercostal nerve and vessels, and pleura.

Origin and insertion: It arises from the inner surface of rib near the angle and inserts on the inner surface of the 2nd or 3rd rib below.

Direction of fibres: It is same as that of the internal intercostal muscle.

Nerve supply: By intercostal nerves.

Actions: Depressor of the ribs.

Sternocostalis (Fig. 16.2B)

The sternocostalis muscle one on either side is situated on the inner aspect of front of the chest wall (behind the sternum and costal cartilages) occupying the anterior part of the upper intercostal spaces, except the first space. The sternocostalis muscle intervenes between the anterior end of the intercostal nerves and the pleura.

Origin: It arises from (a) lower one-third of the posterior surface of the body of sternum, (b) posterior surface of the xiphoid process of the sternum, and (c) posterior surface of the costal cartilages of lower three or four ribs.

Insertion: The fibres diverge upwards and laterally as slips to be inserted into the lower border and inner surfaces of the costal cartilages of 2nd–6th ribs.

Nerve supply: By intercostal nerves.

Action: It draws down the costal cartilages in which it is inserted.

Levatores Costarum (12 Pairs)

These are a series of 12 small muscles placed on either side of the back of thorax, just lateral to the vertebral column.

Origin: It arises from the tip of transverse process from 7th to 11th thoracic vertebrae.

Insertion: Each muscle passes obliquely downwards and laterally to be inserted on to the upper edge and outer surface of the rib immediately below in the interval between the tubercle and angle.

Actions

1. Elevate and rotate the neck of rib in a forward direction.
2. Are rotators and lateral flexors of the vertebral column?

The origin insertion, extent, direction of fibres, nerve supply, and actions are given in Table 16.1.

INTERCOSTAL SPACES

The spaces between the two adjacent ribs (and their costal cartilages) are known as *intercostal spaces*. Thus there are 11 intercostal spaces on either side.

The 3rd–6th spaces are **typical intercostal spaces** because the blood and nerve supply of 3rd–6th intercostal spaces is confined only to thorax.

Table 16.1 Intrinsic muscles of the thoracic wall

Muscle	Origin	Insertion	Extent	Direction of fibres	Nerve supply	Actions
1. External intercostal	Lower border of rib above	Upper border (outer lip) of rib below	From costochondral junction to tubercle of rib (anteriorly it continues as *anterior intercostal membrane*)	Downwards, forwards, and medially	Intercostal nerve of the same space	Elevates the rib during inspiration
2. Internal intercostal	Floor of the costal groove of the rib above	Upper border (inner lip) of rib below	From lateral border of sternum to the angle of rib (posteriorly it continues as *posterior intercostal membrane*)	Upwards, forwards and medially	Intercostal nerve of same space	Elevates the rib during expiration
3. Transversus thoracis						
(a) Intercostalis intimus	Inner surface of rib above	Inner surface of rib below	Confined to the middle 2/4th of the intercostal space	Upwards, forwards and medially	Intercostal nerve of same space	Elevates the rib during expiration
(b) Subcostalis	Inner surface of rib near angle	Inner surface of 2nd or 3rd ribs below	Confined to posterior parts of lower spaces only	Upwards, forwards and medially	Intercostal nerves	Depressor of ribs
(c) Sternocostalis	– Lower 1/3rd of the posterior surface of the body of sternum – Posterior surface of xiphoid process – Posterior surface of costal cartilages of lower 3 or 4 ribs near sternum	Costal cartilages 2nd to 6th ribs	Inner surface of front wall of chest	Upwards and laterally	Intercostal nerves	Draws 2nd to 6th cartilages downwards

CONTENTS OF A TYPICAL INTERCOSTAL SPACE

Each space contains the following structures (Fig. 16.4):

1. Three intercostal muscles, viz.
   (a) External intercostal.
   (b) Internal intercostal.
   (c) Innermost intercostal (intercostalis intimus).
2. Intercostal nerves.
3. Intercostal arteries.
4. Intercostal veins.
5. Intercostal lymph vessels and lymph nodes.

N.B. *Plane of neurovascular bundle in the intercostal space:* The neurovascular bundle consisting of intercostal nerve and vessels lies between the internal intercostal and innermost intercostal muscles, i.e., between the intermediate and deepest layers of muscles.

They are arranged in the following order from above downwards:

1. Intercostal Vein.
2. Intercostal Artery.
3. Intercostal Nerve.

(*Mnemonic:* VAN)

INTERCOSTAL MUSCLES

Intercostal muscles are a group of muscles that are present in the intercostal space and help form and move the chest wall.

The following muscles constitute intercostal muscles:

1. External intercostal muscle.
2. Internal intercostal muscle.
3. Innermost intercostal muscle (intercostalis intimi).

N.B. Strictly speaking, the intercostalis intimi is not present in the intercostal space as it lies on the deeper aspects of the ribs.

Nerve supply: By intercostal nerves.

Actions

The actions of intercostal muscles are as follows:

1. They act as strong supports for the rib preventing their separation.
2. They act as elevators of the ribs during respiration. External intercostal muscles act during inspiration, while others act during expiration.

The intercostal muscles are described in detail on page 213–214.

INTERCOSTAL NERVES

The 12 pairs of thoracic spinal nerves supply the thoracic wall. As soon as they leave, the intervertebral foramina they divide into anterior and posterior rami (Fig. 16.5).

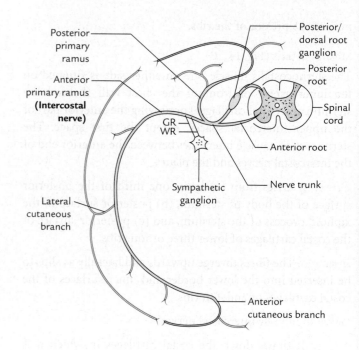

Fig. 16.5 Typical thoracic spinal nerve (GR = grey rami communicantes, WR = white rami communicantes).

The anterior primary rami of upper 11 thoracic spinal nerves (T1–T11) are called **intercostal nerves** as they course through the intercostal spaces. The anterior primary ramus of the 12th thoracic spinal nerve runs in the abdominal wall below the 12th rib, hence it is called **subcostal nerve.**

N.B. Unique features: The intercostal nerves are anterior primary rami of thoracic spinal nerves. They are segmental in character unlike the anterior primary rami from other regions of spinal cord which form nerve plexuses viz. cervical, brachial, lumbar and sacral.

Classification

The intercostal nerves are classified into the following two groups:

1. Typical intercostal nerves (3rd, 4th, 5th, and 6th).
2. Atypical intercostal nerves (1st, 2nd, 7th, 8th, 9th, 10th, and 11th).

The **typical intercostal nerves** are those which remain confined to their own intercostal spaces.

The **atypical spinal nerves** extend beyond the thoracic wall and partly or entirely supply the other regions.

TYPICAL INTERCOSTAL NERVE

Course and Relations

The typical intercostal nerve after its origin turns laterally behind the sympathetic trunk, and then enters the **intercostal space** between the parietal pleura and posterior intercostal membrane. It then enters the **costal groove** of the corresponding rib to course laterally and forwards.

In costal groove it comes into relation with corresponding intercostal vessels and forms **neurovascular bundle** of the intercostal space.

In the intercostal space, vein, artery and nerve lie in that order from above downwards.

Near the sternal end of the intercostal space, the intercostal nerve crosses in front of the internal thoracic artery. Then it pierces internal intercostal muscle, anterior intercostal membrane, and pectoralis major muscle to terminate as **anterior cutaneous nerve.**

N.B.

- In the posterior part of intercostal space, the intercostal nerve lies between the pleura and posterior intercostal membrane.
- In the remaining greater part of intercostal space, it lies between the internal intercostal and intercostalis intimus muscles.

Branches

1. **Rami communicantes:** Each nerve communicates with the corresponding thoracic ganglion by white and grey rami communicantes.
2. **Muscular branches:** These are small tender branches from the nerve, which supply intercostal muscles and serratus posterior and superior.
3. **Collateral branch:** It arises in the posterior part of the intercostal space near the angle of the rib and runs in the lower part of the space along the upper border of the rib below in the same neurovascular plane. It supplies intercostal muscles, parietal pleura, and periosteum of the rib.
4. **Lateral cutaneous branch:** It arises in the posterior part of the intercostal space near the angle of the rib and accompanies the main nerve for some distance, then pierces the muscles of the lateral thoracic wall along the midaxillary line. It divides into anterior and posterior branches to supply the skin on the lateral thoracic wall.
5. **Anterior cutaneous branch:** It is the terminal branch of the nerve, which emerges on the side of the sternum. It divides into medial and lateral branches and supplies the skin on the front of the thoracic wall.

ATYPICAL INTERCOSTAL NERVES

The atypical intercostal nerves are as follows:

1. **First intercostal nerve:** The greater part of this nerve joins the ventral ramus C8 spinal nerve to form lower trunk of the brachial plexus. The remaining part of the nerve is very small and it lacks both lateral and anterior cutaneous branches.
2. **Second intercostal nerve:** Its lateral cutaneous branch is called **intercostobrachial nerve.** It courses across the axilla and joins the medial cutaneous branch of the arm. The intercostobrachial nerve supplies the skin of the floor of the axilla and upper part of the medial side of the arm. *In coronary arterial disease, the cardiac pain is referred along this nerve to the medial side of the arm.*
3. **Seventh to eleventh intercostal nerves:** These nerves leave the corresponding intercostal spaces to enter into the abdominal wall; hence they are called **thoraco-abdominal nerves.** These nerves supply intercostal muscles of the corresponding intercostal spaces. In addition they supply:
   (a) muscles of anterior abdominal wall, e.g., external oblique, internal oblique, transverse abdominis, and rectus abdominis muscles, and
   (b) skin and parietal peritoneum covering the outer and inner surfaces of the abdominal wall, respectively.

Clinical correlation

- **Root pain/girdle pain:** Irritation of intercostal nerves caused by the diseases of thoracic vertebrae produces severe pain which is referred around the trunk along the cutaneous distribution of the affected nerve. It is termed *root pain* or *girdle pain*.
- **Sites of eruption of cold abscess on the body wall:** Pus from the tuberculous thoracic vertebra/vertebrae (Pott's disease) tends to track along the neurovascular plane of the space and may point at three sites of emergence of cutaneous branches of the thoracic spinal nerve, viz. (a) just lateral to the sternum, (b) in the midaxillary line, and (c) lateral to the erector spinae muscle (Fig. 16.6).
- **Herpes zoster:** In herpes zoster (shingles) involving the thoracic spinal ganglia, the cutaneous vesicles appear in the dermatomal area of distribution of intercostal nerve. It is an extremely painful condition.
- **Intercostal nerve block** is given to produce local anesthesia in one or more intercostal spaces by injecting the anesthetic agent around the nerve trunk near its origin, i.e., just lateral to the vertebra.
- **Thoracotomy:** The conventional thoracotomy (postero-lateral) is performed along the 6th rib. The neurovascular bundle is protected from injury by lifting the periosteum of the rib.
- Considering the position of neurovascular bundle in the intercostal space, it is safe to insert the needle, a little above the upper border of the rib below.

INTERCOSTAL ARTERIES

The thoracic wall has rich blood supply. It is provided by the posterior and anterior intercostal arteries.

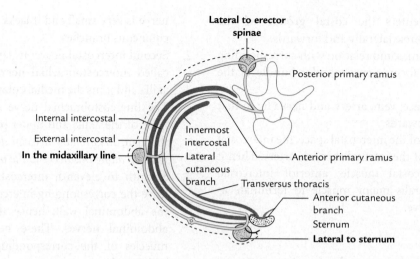

Fig. 16.6 Sites of eruption of tuberculous cold abscess on the body wall. (*Source*: Fig. 3.1, Page 104, *Clinical and Surgical Anatomy*, 2e, Vishram Singh. Copyright Elsevier 2007 All rights reserved.)

Each intercostal space contains one posterior and two anterior intercostal arteries (upper and lower).

POSTERIOR INTERCOSTAL ARTERIES (Fig. 16.7)

There are 11 pairs of intercostal arteries, one in each space. They supply the greater part of the intercostal spaces.

Origin

1. The 1st and 2nd posterior intercostal arteries are the branches of superior intercostal artery—a branch of the costocervical trunk.
2. The 3rd–11th posterior intercostal arteries arise directly from the descending thoracic aorta (Fig. 16.7A).

Course and Relations

In front of the vertebral column (Fig. 16.7B)

- The right posterior intercostal arteries are longer than the left because the descending aorta lies on the left side of the front of the vertebral column. They pass behind the esophagus, thoracic duct, azygos vein, and sympathetic chain but in front of the anterior aspect of vertebral body.
- The left posterior intercostal arteries are smaller and pass behind the hemiazygos vein and sympathetic chain, but in front of the side of the vertebral body

In the intercostal space

In the intercostal space, the posterior intercostal artery lies between the intercostal vein above and the intercostal nerve below. The neurovascular bundle in the intercostal space lies between the internal intercostal and intercostalis intimus muscles.

Termination

Each posterior intercostal artery ends at the level of costochondral junction by anastomosing with the upper anterior intercostal artery of the space.

Branches

1. **Dorsal branch:** It supplies the spinal cord, vertebra and muscles, and skin of the back.
2. **Collateral branch:** It arises near the angle of the rib and runs forwards along the upper border of the rib below and ends by anastomosing with the lower anterior intercostal artery.
3. **Muscular branches:** They supply intercostal, pectoral, and serratus anterior muscles.
4. **Lateral cutaneous branch:** It closely follows the lateral cutaneous branch of the intercostal nerve.
5. **Mammary branches (external mammary arteries):** They arise from posterior intercostals arteries of the 2nd, 3rd, and 4th intercostal spaces and supply the breast mammary gland.
6. **Right bronchial artery:** It arises from right 3rd posterior intercostal artery.

Clinical correlation

- **Paracentesis thoracis:** During *paracentesis thoracis* (aspiration of fluid from pleural cavity), the needle should never be inserted medial to the angle of the rib to avoid injury to the posterior intercostal artery, as it crosses the space obliquely from below upwards (for details see page 216).
- **Coarctation of aorta:** In *coarctation of aorta* (narrowing of arch of aorta), the posterior intercostal arteries are markedly enlarged and cause notching of the ribs, particularly in their posterior parts.

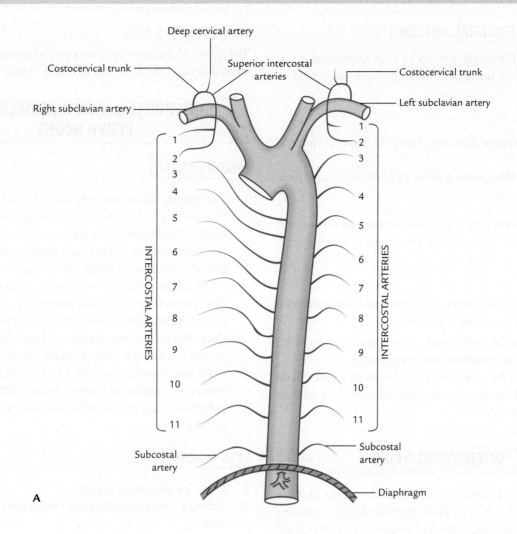

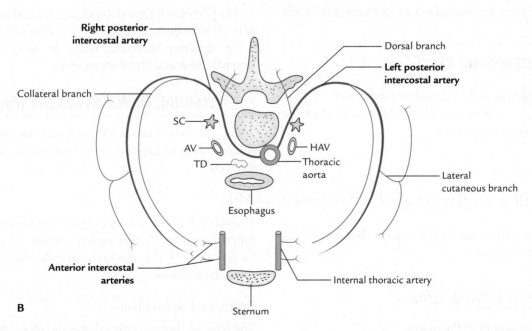

Fig. 16.7 Posterior intercostal arteries: A, origin; B, course and relations (SC = sympathetic chain, AV = azygos vein, TD = thoracic duct, HAV = hemiazygos vein).

ANTERIOR INTERCOSTAL ARTERIES

There are two intercostal arteries in each intercostal space. They are present in the upper nine intercostal spaces only.

Origin

1. In 1st–6th spaces they arise from the internal thoracic artery.
2. In 7th and 9th spaces, they arise from musculophrenic artery.

N.B. The 10th and 11th intercostal spaces do not extend forward enough to have anterior intercostal arteries.

Termination

The anterior intercostal arteries are short and end at the level of costochondral junction as follows:

1. Upper anterior intercostal artery anastomoses with corresponding posterior intercostal artery.
2. Lower anterior intercostal artery anastomoses with collateral branch of the corresponding posterior intercostal artery.

INTERCOSTAL VEINS

The number of intercostal vein corresponds to the number of intercostal arteries, i.e., each intercostal space contains two anterior intercostal veins and one posterior intercostal vein. Their tributaries correspond to the branches of the arteries.

ANTERIOR INTERCOSTAL VEINS

1. They are present only in the upper nine spaces.
2. Each space contains two veins and accompanies the anterior intercostal arteries.

Termination

1. In upper six spaces, they end in the internal thoracic vein.
2. In seventh, eighth, and ninth spaces, they end in the musculophrenic vein.

POSTERIOR INTERCOSTAL VEINS

1. They are present in all the spaces.
2. Each space contains only one posterior intercostal vein.
3. Each vein accompanies the posterior intercostal artery.
4. Its tributaries correspond to the branches of posterior intercostal artery.

Termination (Fig. 16.8)

The mode of drainage (termination) of posterior intercostal veins differs on the right and left sides (Table 16.2).

INTERCOSTAL LYMPH VESSELS AND LYMPH NODES

LYMPH VESSELS

1. The lymph vessels from the anterior parts of the spaces drain into anterior intercostal/internal mammary lymph nodes. The efferent from these nodes unite with those of tracheobronchial and brachiocephalic nodes to form the bronchomediastinal trunk, which drains into subclavian trunk on the right side and thoracic duct on the left side.
2. The lymph vessels from the posterior parts of the spaces drain into posterior intercostal nodes. The efferent from the posterior intercostal nodes of lower four spaces unite to form a slender lymph trunk, which descends and drain into the *cysterna chyli*. The efferent from posterior intercostal nodes of upper spaces drain into right lymphatic duct on the right side and thoracic duct on the left side.

LYMPH NODES

1. Posterior intercostal nodes.
2. Anterior intercostal/internal mammary (parasternal) nodes.

The posterior intercostal nodes are located in the posterior part of the intercostal spaces on the necks of the ribs.

The anterior intercostal nodes lie along the course of internal thoracic (mammary) artery.

INTERNAL THORACIC ARTERY (Fig. 16.9)

There are two internal thoracic arteries, right and left, situated deep to anterior chest wall, one on either side of sternum.

Origin

The internal thoracic artery arises from the first part of the subclavian artery (lower surface), about 2.5 cm above the medial end of the clavicle, opposite the origin of the thyrocervical trunk.

Course and Termination

The internal thoracic artery descends behind the medial end of the clavicle and upper six coastal cartilages, about 1 cm away from the lateral margin of the sternum. It ends in the 6th intercostal space by dividing into *superior epigastric* and *musculophrenic arteries*.

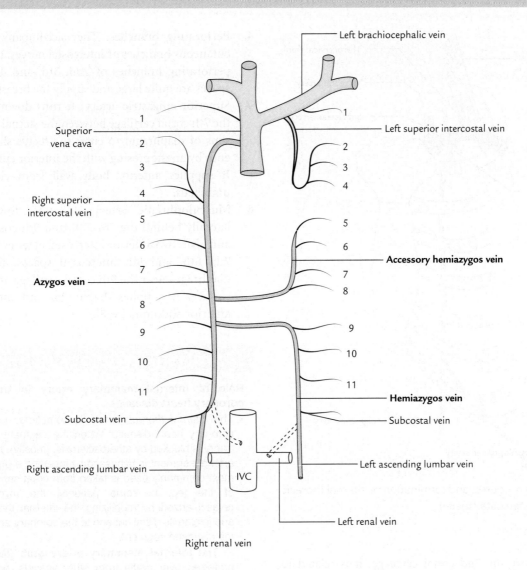

Fig. 16.8 Drainage of posterior intercostal veins. Note that posterior intercostal veins are numbered 1–11 from above downwards.

Table 16.2 Mode of termination of right and left posterior intercostal veins

Right posterior intercostal veins	Left posterior intercostal veins
1st (highest) drains into the right brachiocephalic vein	1st (highest) drains into left brachiocephalic vein
2nd, 3rd, and 4th join to form *right superior intercostal vein*, which in turn drains into the azygos vein	2nd, 3rd, and 4th join to form *left superior intercostal vein*, which in turn drains into left brachiocephalic vein
5th–11th drain into the azygos vein	• 5th–8th drain into accessory azygos vein • 9th–11th drain into hemiazygos vein
Subcostal vein drains into the azygos vein	Subcostal vein drains into the hemiazygos vein

Relations

Anteriorly: From above downwards, it is related to:

- Medial end of the clavicle.
- Internal jugular vein.
- Brachiocephalic vein.

- Phrenic nerve.
- Pectoralis major.
- Upper six costal cartilages.
- External intercostal membranes.
- Internal intercostal muscles.
- Upper six intercostal nerves.

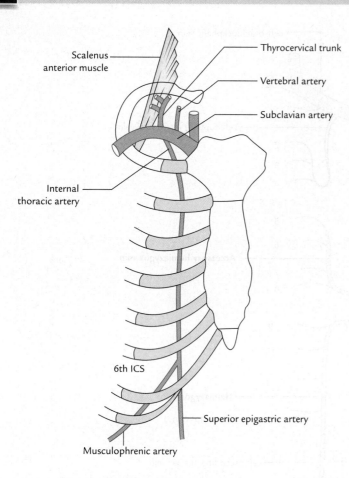

Fig. 16.9 Origin, course, and termination of internal thoracic artery (ICS = intercostal space).

Posteriorly:

- Above the 2nd costal cartilage, it is related to endothoracic fascia and pleura.
- Below the 2nd costal cartilage, it is related to sternocostalis muscle, which intervenes between the artery and the endothoracic fascia and pleura.

N.B. The internal mammary artery is accompanied by two venae comitantes, which unite at the level of 3rd costal cartilage to form the *internal thoracic (mammary) vein*, which runs upwards along the medial side of the artery to terminate into the brachiocephalic vein at the root of the neck.

Branches

1. **Pericardiophrenic artery:** It arises in the root of the neck above the 1st costal cartilage, and descends along with phrenic nerve to the diaphragm. It supplies pericardium and pleura.
2. **Mediastinal branches:** They are small inconstant twigs, which supply connective tissue, thymus, and front of the pericardium.
3. **Anterior intercostal arteries:** They are two for each of the upper six intercostal spaces.

4. **Perforating branches:** They accompany the anterior cutaneous branches of intercostal nerves. In females, the perforating branches of 2nd, 3rd, and 4th intercostal spaces are quite large and supply the breast.
5. **Superior epigastric artery:** It runs downwards behind the 7th costal cartilage between the sternal and 1st costal slips of diaphragm to enter the rectus sheath where it ends by anastomosing with the inferior epigastric artery. It supplies anterior body wall from clavicle to the umbilicus.
6. **Musculophrenic artery:** It runs downwards and laterally behind the 7th, 8th, and 9th costal cartilages, and gives two anterior intercostal arteries to each of the 7th, 8th, and 9th intercostal spaces. It pierces the diaphragm near the 9th costal cartilage, to reach under surface. It supplies diaphragm and muscles of the anterior abdominal wall.

Clinical correlation

Role of internal mammary artery in treatment of coronary heart diseases:

- The *internal thoracic artery* is sometimes used to treat coronary heart disease. When the segment of coronary artery is blocked by atherosclerosis, (mostly), the diseased arterial segment is bypassed by inserting a graft. The graft most commonly used is taken from great saphenous vein of the leg. In some patients, the myocardium is revascularized by mobilizing the internal thoracic artery and joining its distal cut end to the coronary artery distal to the diseased segment.

  The **internal mammary artery graft (IMA graft)** is preferred over grafts from other vessels, because IMA graft lasts long. Recently it has been found that internal mammary arteries are less prone to develop atherosclerosis because of their histological peculiarity. The walls of these arteries contain only elastic tissue and the cells of their endothelial lining secrete some chemicals, which prevents atherosclerosis. The left internal mammary artery is preferred over right internal mammary artery, because it is easier to access it.
- Earlier the *internal thoracic artery* was used to be ligated in the 3rd intercostal space in order to reinforce the blood supply to the heart by diverting blood from this artery to its *pericardiophrenic branch*. This procedure is now obsolete.

MECHANISM OF RESPIRATION

The respiration consists of two alternate phases of (a) inspiration and (b) expiration, which are associated with alternate increase and decrease in the volume of thoracic cavity, respectively. During inspiration, the air is taken in (*inhaled*) and during expiration, the air is taken out (*exhaled*).

Rate of Respiration

The average rate of respiration is 18 per minute in normal resting state of an adult. It is faster in children and slower in the elderly.

INSPIRATION

During inspiration the volume of thoracic cavity increases, which creates a negative intrathoracic pressure, consequently air is sucked into the lungs.

An increase in the capacity of thoracic cavity occurs vertically, anteroposteriorly, and transversely (i.e., side to side).

Vertical Diameter

Theoretically, the vertical diameter of the thoracic cavity can increase, if the roof of the thoracic cavity is raised or its floor lowered or both. The roof of thoracic cavity is formed by **tough suprapleural membrane**, which is fixed, hence cannot move up and down. However, the floor of thoracic cavity is formed by the freely movable diaphragm. Thus when the diaphragm contracts, its central tendon descends, and its domes are flattened. As a result, there is an increase in the vertical diameter of the thoracic cavity (Fig. 16.10).

Anteroposterior Diameter

An increase in anteroposterior diameter of the thoracic cavity occurs when sternum moves forwards and upwards.

Each rib acts a lever, the fulcrum of which lies just lateral to the tubercle of the rib. Thus two arms of lever are greatly disproportional, e.g., posterior arm is very short and anterior arm is very long. Thus slight movement at the vertebral end of the rib is greatly magnified at the anterior end of the rib (Fig. 16.11).

Since anterior ends of the ribs are at a lower level than their posterior ends, during elevation of the ribs, when their anterior ends move upwards and forwards, they carry with them the sternum. (This movement occurs mostly in vertebrosternal ribs.) Consequently, the anteroposterior diameter of the thoracic cavity is increased. This movement

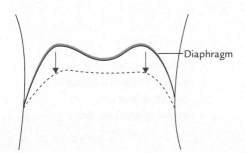

Fig. 16.10 Increase in vertical diameter of the thoracic cavity due to descent of diaphragm.

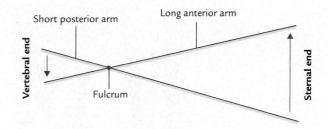

Fig. 16.11 Increase in anteroposterior diameter of thoracic cavity because the ribs act as levers with fulcrum just lateral to the tubercle.

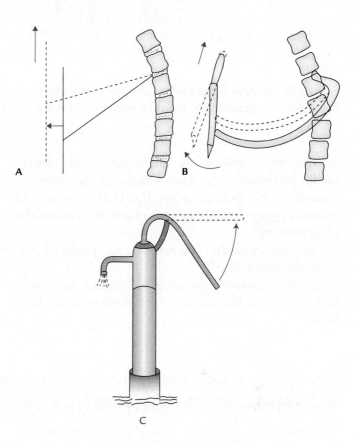

Fig. 16.12 Increase in anteroposterior diameter of the thoracic cavity due to movements of sternum: A, idealized representation; B, actual movement of sternum; C, real life pump.

is termed **pump-handle movement** because sternum moves up and down like a handle of pump during respiration (Fig. 16.12).

Transverse Diameter

The middle of the shaft of the ribs lies at the lower level than the plane passing through its two ends (anterior and posterior; Fig. 15.3). This arrangement resembles a **bucket handle**. Therefore, during elevation of the ribs, the shafts of

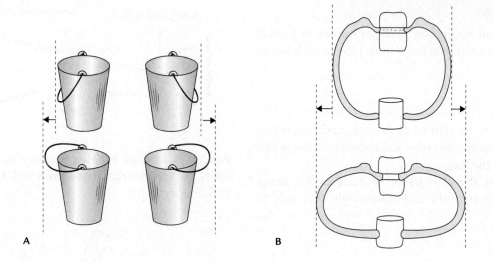

Fig. 16.13 Increase in transverse diameter of the thoracic cavity due to bucket-handle movements of vertebrochondral rib: A, idealized representation; B, actual movements of the ribs.

the ribs move outwards like the bucket handle—**bucket handle movement**. This causes increase in the transverse diameter of the thoracic cavity (Fig. 16.13). The axis of movement passes from the tubercle of this rib to the middle of the sternum.

The bucket-handle movement is produced by vertebrochondral ribs.

The main factors responsible for increase in various diameters of the thoracic cavity are summarized in Table 16.3.

Table 16.3 Factors responsible for the increase in various diameters of the thoracic cavity during inspiration

Diameter	Factors responsible for increase
Vertical	Descent (contraction) of the diaphragm
Anteroposterior	**Pump-handle movement** of the sternum (brought about by the elevation of vertebrosternal ribs)
Transverse	**Bucket-handle movement** of the vertebrochondral ribs

Table 16.4 Muscles acting during different types of respiration

Type of respiration	Inspiration (elevation of ribs)	Expiration (depression of ribs)
Quiet respiration	• External intercostal muscles • Diaphragm	• Passive • No muscles
Deep respiration	• External intercostal muscles • Scalene muscles • Sternocleidomastoid • Levatores costarum • Serratus posterior superior • Diaphragm	• Passive • No muscles
Forced respiration	• All the muscles involved in deep inspiration (*vide supra*) • Levator scapulae • Trapezius • Rhomboids • Pectoral muscles • Serratus anterior	• Quadratus lumborum • Internal intercostal muscles • Transverse thoracis • Serratus posterior inferior

EXPIRATION

The expiration is the passive process brought about by

(a) elastic recoil of the alveoli of the lungs,
(b) relaxation of the intercostal muscles and the diaphragm, and
(c) increase in the tone of the muscles of anterior abdominal wall.

TYPES OF RESPIRATION (BREATHING)

The respiration is classified into the following three types:

1. Quiet respiration.
2. Deep respiration.
3. Forced respiration.

In **quiet respiration**, the movements are normal as described above.

In **deep respiration**, movements described for quiet respiration are increased. The 1st rib is elevated by scalene and sternocleidomastoid muscles.

In **forced respiration**, all movements are exaggerated. The scapula is fixed and elevated by trapezius, levator scapulae, rhomboideus major, and rhomboideus minor muscles, so that pectoral muscles and serratus anterior can raise the ribs.

The muscles acting during different types of respiration (i.e., respiratory muscles) are enumerated in Table 16.4.

Clinical correlation

Posture of patient during asthmatic attack: During asthmatic attack (characterized by breathlessness/difficulty in breathing), the patient is most comfortable on sitting up, leaning forwards and fixing the arms on the bed/table. This is because in the sitting position, the diaphragm is at its lowest level, allowing maximum ventilation. Fixation of arms fixes the scapulae, so that the pectoral muscles and serratus anterior may act on the ribs which they elevate.

Golden Facts to Remember

▶ Anterior primary rami of all the thoracic spinal nerves are intercostal nerves *except*	Anterior primary ramus of T12 spinal nerve which is *subcostal nerve*
▶ Main movement to increase the anteroposterior diameter of the thoracic cavity	*Pump-handle movement* of sternum brought about by the elevation of vertebrosternal ribs (2nd–6th ribs)
▶ Main movement to increase the transverse diameter of the thoracic cavity	*Bucket-handle movement* of vertebrochondral ribs
▶ Main factor responsible for increase of vertical diameter of the thoracic cavity	Contraction of the diaphragm
▶ Position of body in which diaphragm lies at the highest level	Supine position
▶ Position of body in which diaphragm lies at the lowest level	Sitting position
▶ Principal muscle of respiration	Diaphragm
▶ Muscle of weight lifting	Diaphragm

Clinical Case Study

A 55-year-old patient came to the hospital with complaints of weakness, loss of weight, and pain on the back of chest. On examination, tenderness was noted on percussion, in the region of thoracic spine. Small bulges were also seen on the surface of the chest at three sites: (a) lateral to the sternum, (b) in the midaxillary line, and (c) lateral to the erector spinae muscle. The X-ray of thoracic spine revealed *collapse of vertebral bodies* of T5 and T6 vertebrae and a *perispinal soft tissue shadow.* He was diagnosed as a case of **Pott's disease.**

Questions

1. What is Pott's disease?
2. What is the cause of perispinal soft tissue shadow?
3. Mention the anatomical basis of small bulges noted on the surface of the chest wall (*vide supra*).

Answers

1. Tuberculosis of spine (i.e., vertebrae).
2. Perispinal abscess.
3. The pus from the region of tubercular spine (**cold abscess**) tracks around the thoracic wall along the plane of neurovascular bundle and points on the surface of the chest at the sites of exit of cutaneous branches of the intercostal nerve, i.e., (a) lateral to the erect spinae muscle, (b) in the midaxillary line, and (c) just lateral to the sternum.

CHAPTER 17

Pleural Cavities

The thoracic cavity is divided into three compartments (Fig. 17.1): right and left lateral compartments and middle compartment. Each lateral compartment is occupied by a

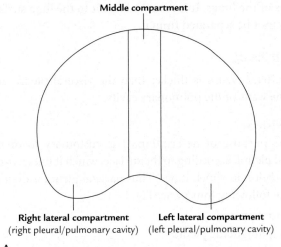

Middle compartment

Right lateral compartment
(right pleural/pulmonary cavity)

Left lateral compartment
(left pleural/pulmonary cavity)

A

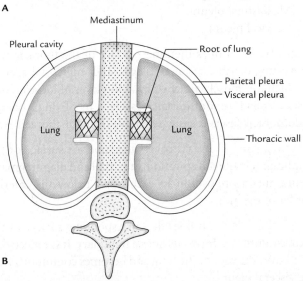

Mediastinum

Pleural cavity

Root of lung

Parietal pleura
Visceral pleura

Lung   Lung

Thoracic wall

B

Fig. 17.1 Compartment of the thoracic cavity: **A**, empty compartments; **B**, lateral compartments occupied by lung enclosed in the serous sac (pleural sac).

lung enclosed in the serous sac called **pleural cavity**. The middle compartment contains, essentially, all the thoracic structures except lungs, such as heart with its pericardium, great blood vessels that leave or enter the heart, structures that traverse the thorax to enter the abdomen in passing from the neck to the abdomen or from abdomen to neck such as esophagus, vagus nerves, phrenic nerves, and thoracic duct.

The mass of tissues and organs occupying the middle compartment form a mobile septum—**mediastinum** that completely separates the two pleural cavities.

PLEURAL CAVITIES (Fig. 17.2)

Each lung is invested by and enclosed in a serous sac which consists of two continuous serous membranes—the **visceral pleura** and **parietal pleura**. The visceral pleura invests all the surfaces of the lung forming its shiny outer surface, whereas the parietal pleura lines the pulmonary cavity (i.e., thoracic wall and mediastinum).

The space between the visceral and parietal pleura is called **pleural cavity**.

A little description of development of lung makes it is easier to understand the relationship of the lung and pleura.

During early embryonic life, each lateral compartment of the thoracic cavity is occupied by a closed serous sac, which is invaginated from the medial side by the developing lung and as a result of this invagination, it converted into a double-layered sac. The outer layer is called **parietal pleura** and the inner layer is called **visceral pleura**. The visceral pleura is continuous with parietal pleura at the root of the lung. The parietal and visceral layers are separated from each other by a slit-like potential space called **pleural cavity**. The pleural cavity is normally filled with a thin film of tissue fluid, which lubricates the adjoining surfaces of the pleura and allows them to move on each other without friction.

The two layers become continuous with each other by means of a **cuff of pleura**, which surrounds the root of the lung consisting of structures entering and leaving the lung at the hilum of the lung, such as principal bronchi and

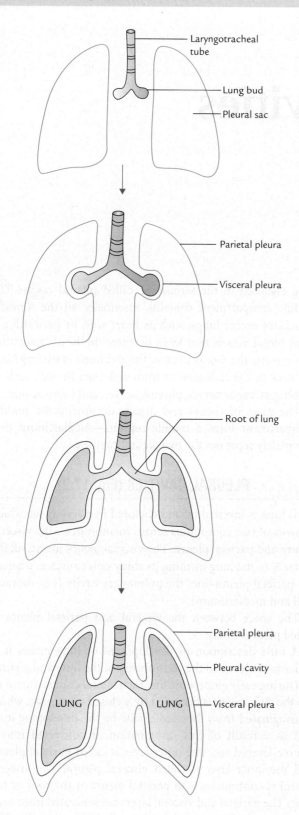

Fig. 17.2 Invagination of developing lungs into the closed serous sacs.

pulmonary vessels. To allow the movement of principal bronchi and pulmonary vessels during respiration, the cuff of pleura hangs down as loose triangular fold called **pulmonary ligament**. The pulmonary ligament extends from

root of the lung as far down as the diaphragm between the lung and the mediastinum.

PLEURA

The pleura-like peritoneum is a serous membrane lined by flattened epithelium (mesothelium). The lining epithelium secretes a watery lubricant—the **serous fluid.**

LAYERS OF THE PLEURA

The pleura consist of two layers: (a) visceral pleura and (b) parietal pleura. The moistened space between the two layers is called *pleural cavity (vide supra).*

Visceral Pleura (Pulmonary Pleura)

The visceral pleura completely covers the surface of the lung except at the hilum and along the attachment of the pulmonary ligament. It also extends into the depths of the fissures of the lungs. It is firmly adherent to the lung surface and cannot be separated from it.

Parietal Pleura

The parietal pleura is thicker than the visceral pleura and lines the walls of the pulmonary cavity.

Subdivisions

For the purpose of description, it is customary to divide parietal pleura, according to the surface, which it lines, covers or the region in which it lies. Thus parietal pleura is divided into the following four parts (Fig. 17.3):

1. Costal pleura.
2. Diaphragmatic pleura.
3. Mediastinal pleura.
4. Cervical pleura.

Costal pleura: It lines the inner surface of the thoracic wall (consisting of ribs, costal cartilages, and intercostal spaces) to which it is loosely attached by a thin layer of loose areolar tissue called **endothoracic fascia.** In living beings, endothoracic fascia is easily separable from the thoracic wall.

Diaphragmatic pleura: It covers the superior surface of the diaphragm. In quiet respiration, the costal and diaphragmatic pleura are in opposition to each other below the inferior border of the lung.

Mediastinal pleura: It lines the corresponding surface of the mediastinum and forms its lateral boundary. It is reflected as a cuff over the root of the lung and becomes continuous with the visceral pleura.

Cervical pleura: It is the dome of parietal pleura, which extends into the root of the neck about 1 inch (2.5 cm) above the medial end of clavicle and 2 inches (5 cm) above the 1st

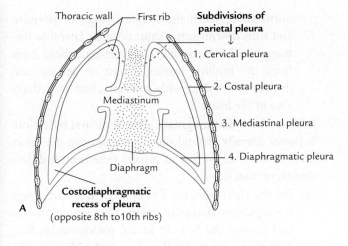

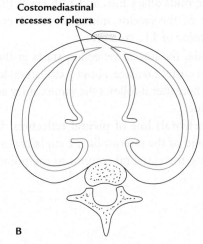

Fig. 17.3 Reflection of the pleura as seen in: **A**, vertical section of the thoracic cavity; **B**, transverse section of the thoracic cavity.

costal cartilage. It is called **cupola** and covers the apex of the lung. Therefore, utmost caution should be taken while penetrating this area with anesthetic needle. It is covered by the **suprapleural membrane**.

Relations of cervical pleura: The relations of cervical pleura are as follows:

Arteriorly: Subclavian artery and scalenus anterior muscle.

Posteriorly: Neck of 1st rib and structures passing in front of it (see page 201).

Laterally: Scalenus medius muscle.

Medially: Great vessels of the neck.

PULMONARY LIGAMENT (Fig. 17.4)

The pleura surround the root of the lung similar to the cuff (sleeve) of the jacket around the wrist (Fig. 17.4A). It extends down as a fold called **pulmonary ligament**. The pulmonary ligament extends from the root of the lung as far down as the diaphragm between the lung and the mediastinum. The fold is filled with loose areolar tissue and contain few lymphatics.

Functions

The functions of pulmonary ligaments are as follows:

1. It provides a *dead space* into which the pulmonary veins can expand during increased venous return as during exercise.

2. It allows the descent of the root of the lung with the descent of diaphragm during inspiration. As a result, the apex of lung comes down from the tough suprapleural membrane leaving an empty space below the membrane. Now the apex of lung can expand into this empty space.

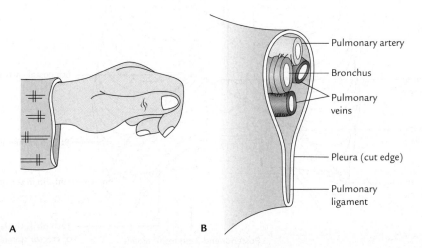

Fig. 17.4 Root of lung and pulmonary ligament: **A**, cuff (sleeve) of jacket simulating pulmonary ligament; **B**, structures forming the root of lung.

SURFACE MARKINGS OF THE PLEURA (Fig. 17.5)

The knowledge of reflexion of parietal pleura on the surface of the chest wall is of great importance while carrying out various medical and surgical procedures.

The reflection of parietal pleura can be marked on the surface by the following lines:

1. **Cervical pleura:** It is marked by a curved line (with convexity directed upwards) drawn from sternoclavicular joint to the junction of medial third and middle third of the clavicle. The summit of dome of pleura lies 1 inch (2.5) above the medial one-third of the clavicle.

2. **Anterior (costomediastinal) line of pleural reflection:** It differs on the two sides:

   (a) **On the right side**, it extends downwards and medially from the right sternoclavicular joint to the midpoint of the sternal angle, and then descends vertically up to the midpoint of the xiphisternal joint.

   (b) **On the left side**, it extends downwards and medially from the left sternoclavicular joint to the midpoint of the sternal angle, then descends vertically only up to the level of the 4th costal cartilage. It then arches

outwards to reach the sternal margin of sternum and runs downwards a short distance lateral to this margin to reach the 6th costal cartilage, about 3 cm from the midline leaving a part of pericardium directly in contact with anterior chest wall (**bare area of the heart**).

3. **Inferior (costodiaphragmatic) line of pleural reflection:** It passes laterally around the chest wall from the lower limit of the anterior line of pleural reflection. It differs slightly on two sides:

   (a) **On the right side,** the line of reflection starts from the xiphisternal joint or behind the xiphoid process and crosses the 8th rib in the midclavicular line, 10th rib in the midaxillary line, and 12th rib at the lateral border of the erector spinae muscle, 2 cm lateral to the spine of T12 vertebra.

   (b) **On the left side,** the line of reflection starts at the level of the 6th costal cartilage, about 2 cm lateral to the midline. Thereafter it follows the same course as on the right side.

4. **Posterior (costovertebral) line of pleural reflection:** It ascends from the end of the inferior line, 2 cm lateral to the T12 spine along the vertebral column to the point,

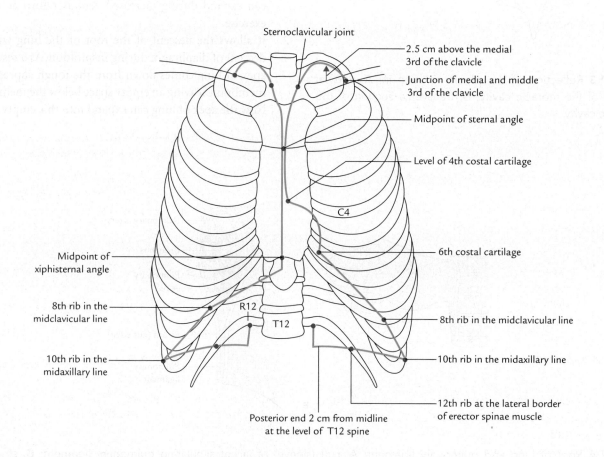

Fig. 17.5 Schematic diagram showing lines of pleural reflection.

2 cm lateral to the spine of C7 vertebra. The costal pleura becomes mediastinal pleura along this line.

N.B. The inferior margin of the lung passes more horizontally than the inferior margin of the pleura. Consequently, it crosses the 6th rib in the midclavicular line, 8th rib in the midaxillary line, and 10th rib at the lateral border of the erector spine.

The ribs crossed by inferior margin of the lung and pleura in *midclavicular line, midaxillary line,* and *lateral to erector spine* are compared below:

Inferior margin of lung: 6th rib, 8th rib, and 10th rib
Inferior margin of pleura: 8th rib, 10th rib, and 12th rib

RECESSES OF THE PLEURA (Fig. 17.3)

Normally the space between the parietal and visceral pleura is only a potential space and is filled with thin film of serous fluid. However in areas of pleural reflection on to the diaphragm and mediastinum, the space between the parietal and visceral pleura is greatly expanded. These expanded regions of pleural cavity are called **pleural recesses.** They are essential for lung expansion during deep inspiration. Thus *pleural recesses serve as reserve spaces of pleural cavity for the lungs to expand during deep inspiration.* The recesses of pleura are as follows:

1. Costodiaphragmatic recesses (right and left).
2. Costomediastinal recesses (right and left).

N.B. In addition to the above recesses of pleura, there are three more small recesses, viz.

- *Right and left retroesophageal recesses*
  These are formed by the reflection of mediastinal pleura behind the esophagus. Each recess is thought to be occupied by a part of the lung, and contributes to the retrocardiac space seen in the radiographs of the chest.
- *Infracardiac recess*
  It is a small recess of right pleural sac which sometimes extends beneath the inferior vena cava.

Costodiaphragmatic recess (Fig. 17.3A): It is located inferiorly between the costal and diaphragmatic pleurae. Vertically it measures about 5 cm and lies opposite the 8th–10th ribs along the midaxillary line. The costodiaphragmatic recesses are the most dependent parts of the pleural cavities, hence the fluid of pleural effusion first collect at these sites.

Costomediastinal recess (Fig. 17.3B): It is located anteriorly between the costal and mediastinal pleurae and lies between sternum and costal cartilages. The right costomediastinal recess is possibly occupied by the anterior margin of the right lung even during quiet breathing. The left costomediastinal recess is large due to the presence of cardiac

notch in the left lung. Its location can be confirmed clinically by percussion (tapping) of the chest wall. As one moves during tapping from the area of underlying lung tissue to the area of left costomediastinal recess unoccupied by lung tissue, a change in tone, from resonant to dull, is noticed. This is called the area of **superficial cardiac dullness.**

Clinical correlation

- **Radiological appearance of pleural effusion:** When a small quantity of fluid collects in the costodiaphragmatic recess (pleural effusion) the costodiaphragmatic angle is obliterated (widening of the angle). It is seen as radiopaque shadow with a fluid line in X-ray chest. This may be the first indication of pleural effusion. Therefore recesses of pleura are examined routinely in the chest radiographs.

  The costodiaphragmatic recess can be entered through the 9th and 10th intercostal spaces without penetrating the lung in patient with quiet breathing because it lies opposite 8th–10th ribs.
- **Sites of extension of pleura beyond the thoracic cage:** There are five sites, where pleura extends beyond the thoracic cage.

  These sites are as follows:
  1. On either side in the root of the neck (as domes of pleura).
  2. In the right xiphisternal angle.
  3. On either side in the costovertebral angle.

  The pleura can be punctured inadvertently at these sites during surgical procedures.

NERVE SUPPLY OF THE PLEURA

The **parietal pleura** develops from somatopleuric layer of the lateral plate of mesoderm, hence it is supplied by the somatic nerves and is sensitive to pain:

- Costal and peripheral part of the diaphragmatic pleura is supplied by the *intercostal nerves.*
- Mediastinal and central part of the diaphragmatic pleura is supplied by the *phrenic nerve.*

The **visceral pleura** develops from splanchnopleuric layer of the lateral plate of mesoderm, hence it is supplied by the autonomic (sympathetic) nerves (T2–T5) and is insensitive to pain.

Clinical correlation

Referred pain of pleura: The pain from central diaphragmatic pleura and mediastinal pleura is referred to the neck or shoulder through phrenic nerves (C3, C4, and C5) because skin at these sites has same segmental supply through the supraclavicular nerves (C3, C4, and C5).

BLOOD SUPPLY AND LYMPHATIC DRAINAGE OF THE PLEURA

Blood supply of parietal pleura is same as that of the thoracic wall and blood supply of the visceral (pulmonary) pleura is same as that of the lung.

Table 17.1 enumerates the differences between parietal and visceral pleura.

Clinical correlation

- **Pleurisy or pleuritis:** It is the inflammation of the parietal pleura. Clinically it presents as pain, which is aggravated by respiratory movements and radiates to thoracic and abdominal walls. It is commonly caused by *pulmonary tuberculosis.* The pleural surface becomes rough due to accumulation of inflammatory exudate. Due to roughening of the pleural surfaces friction occurs between the two layers of pleura during respiratory movements. Thus *pleural rub* can be heard with stethoscope on the surface of the chest wall during inspiration and expiration.
- The collection of serous fluid, air, blood, and pus in the pleural cavity is termed *hydrothorax* (pleural effusion) pneumothorax, hemothorax, and pyothorax (empyema), respectively.
- **Pleural effusion** (Fig. 17.6): Normally the pleural cavity contains only 5–10 ml of clear fluid, which lubricates the pleural surfaces to allow their smooth movements without friction. The excessive accumulation of fluid in the pleural cavity is called *pleural effusion.* It usually occurs due to inflammation of pleura. The pleural effusion leads to decreased expansion of lung on the side of effusion. Clinically it can be detected with decreased breath sounds and dullness on percussion on the site of effusion.
- **Thoracocentesis/pleural tab:** It is a procedure by which an excess fluid is aspirated from the pleural cavity. It is performed with the patient in sitting position. Usually the needle is inserted in the 6th intercostal space in the midaxillary line. The needle is inserted into the lower part of the intercostal space along the upper border of the rib to avoid injury to the intercostal nerve and vessels. The needle passes in succession through skin, superficial fascia, serratus anterior, intercostal muscles, endothoracic fascia, and parietal pleura to reach the pleural cavity.
- **Pneumothorax (Fig. 17.7):** Accumulation of air in the pleural cavity is called *pneumothorax.*
  - *Spontaneous pneumothorax:* As the name indicates, in this condition, air enters pleural cavity suddenly due the rupture of emphysematous bullae of the lung.
  - *Open pneumothorax:* This condition occurs due to stab wounds on the thoracic wall piercing the pleurae, leading to the communication of air in the pleural cavity with the outside (atmospheric) air. Consequently, each time when patient inspires, the air is sucked into the pleural cavity. Sometimes the clothing and the layers of thoracic wall combine to form a valve so that air enters through the wound during inspiration, but cannot exit through it. In these circumstances, air pressure builds up continuously in the pleural cavity on the wounded side which pushes the mediastinum to the opposite

Table 17.1 Differences between the parietal and visceral pleurae

Parietal pleura	Visceral pleura
Lines the thoracic wall and mediastinum	Lines the surface of the lung
Develops from the somatopleuric mesoderm	Develops from the splanchnopleuric mesoderm
Innervated by the somatic nerves	Innervated by the autonomic nerves
Sensitive to pain	Insensitive to pain
Blood supply and lymphatic drainage is same as that of thoracic wall	Blood supply and lymphatic drainage is same as that of the lung

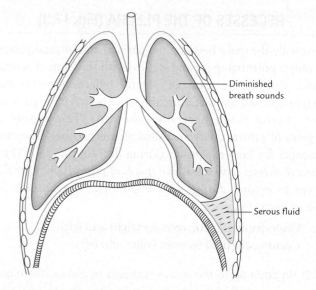

Fig. 17.6 Pleural effusion.

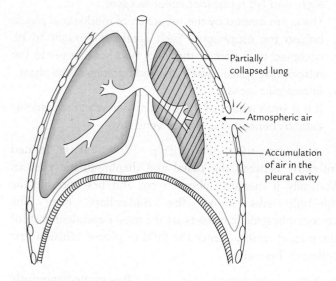

Fig. 17.7 Pneumothorax.

(healthy) side. This is called *tension pneumothorax.* The tension pneumothorax is characterized by (a) collapse of lung on the affected side, and (b) compression of lung on the healthy side.

Golden Facts to Remember

- Most dependent part of the pleural cavity — Costodiaphragmatic recess

- Most preferred site for the pleural aspiration — Midaxillary line in the 6th intercostal space

- Nerve providing sensory innervation to the parietal pleura overlying the right dome of diaphragm — Right phrenic nerve

- Area of superficial cardiac dullness — Area on the front of chest left to sternum between 4th and 6th costal cartilages

Clinical Case Study

A 30-year-old female visited the hospital and complained that she had been feeling severe pain on the right side of her chest for past two weeks and has little difficulty in breathing. She also told that pain often radiated to the anterior abdominal wall. On auscultation the doctor noticed the absence of breath sounds over the inferior lobe of her right lung. The X-ray chest PA view revealed blunting of right costodiaphragmatic angle and line of fluid level. She was diagnosed as a case of **pleural effusion**.

Questions

1. What is (a) pleural cavity and (b) pleural effusion?
2. Enumerate the recesses of pleura.
3. What is the anatomical basis of radiation of pain to the anterior abdominal wall?
4. Mention the (a) cause of pleural effusion and (b) site where pleural fluid collects first.

Answers

1. (a) Potential space between parietal and visceral layers of the pleura.
   (b) Accumulation of serous fluid in the pleural cavity.
2. Right and left costomediastinal recesses and right and left costodiaphragmatic recesses.
3. The peripheral part of diaphragmatic pleura and costal pleura are supplied by intercostal nerves. The lower five intercostal nerves also supply the muscle of anterior abdominal wall. Hence pain is often referred to the anterior abdominal wall.
4. (a) Inflammation of pleura (i.e., pleuritis).
   (b) Costodiaphragmatic recess being the most dependent.

Lungs (Pulmones)

LUNGS (PULMONES)

The **lungs** or **pulmones** are the principal organs of respiration. The two lungs (right and left) are situated in the thoracic cavity, one on either side of the mediastinum enclosed in the pleural sac. The main function of lungs is to oxygenate the blood, i.e., exchange of O_2 and CO_2 between inspired air and blood. Each lung is large conical/pyramidal shaped with its base resting on the diaphragm and its apex extending into the root of the neck. The right lung is larger and heavier than the left lung. The right lung weighs about 700 g and left lung 650 g. The right lung has three lobes and the left lung has two lobes. The lobes are separated by deep prominent fissures on the surface of the lung and are supplied by two lobar bronchi (Fig. 18.1).

The lungs are attached to the trachea and heart by principal bronchi and pulmonary vessels, respectively.

In newborn baby and people living in clean environment, the lungs are rosy pink in color, but in people living in polluted areas or those who are smokers, have the lungs are brown or black in color, and mottled in appearance due to inhaled carbon particles.

In the adults, the lungs are spongy in texture and crepitate on touch due to the presence of air in their alveoli. They float in water. In fetus and stillborn children, the lungs are solid and do not crepitate on touch due to the absence of air in their alveoli. They sink in water.

EXTERNAL FEATURES

Each lung presents the following features (Figs 18.1 and 18.2):

1. Apex.
2. Base.

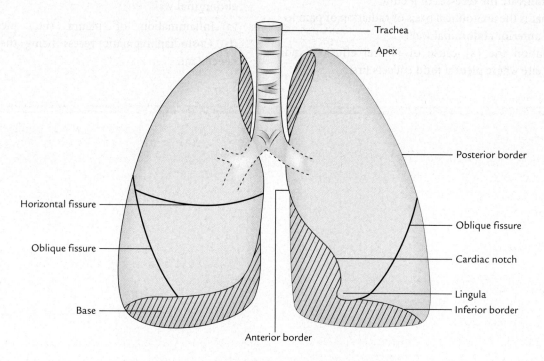

Fig. 18.1 Trachea and lungs as seen from the front.

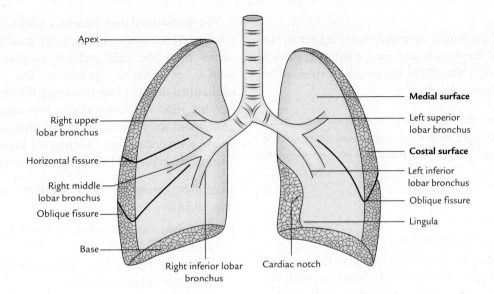

Apex

Right upper lobar bronchus

Horizontal fissure

Right middle lobar bronchus

Oblique fissure

Base

Right inferior lobar bronchus

Medial surface

Left superior lobar bronchus

Costal surface

Left inferior lobar bronchus

Oblique fissure

Lingula

Cardiac notch

Fig. 18.2 Lobes of the lung with lobar bronchi.

3. Three borders (anterior, posterior, and inferior).
4. Two surfaces (costal and medial).

Anatomical position and side determination

The side of lung can be determined by holding the lung in such a way that:

(a) its conical end (*apex*) is directed upwards and its broader end (*base*) is directed downwards,

(b) its convex surface (*costal surface*) is directed outwards and its flat medial surface presenting hilum is directed inwards,

(c) its thin margin (*anterior margin*) should face forwards and its rounded border (*posterior border*) should face backwards.

N.B. The side should not be determined by number of fissures and lobes as they are variable.

The external features are discussed in detail in the following text.

APEX

The apex is rounded/blunt superior end of the lung. It extends into the root of the neck about 3 cm superior to the anterior end of the 1st rib and 2.5 cm above the medial one-third of the clavicle. It is covered by cervical pleura and suprapleural membrane.

Relations

Anterior: (a) Subclavian artery, (b) internal thoracic artery, and (c) scalenus anterior.

Posterior: Neck of 1st rib and structures in front of it, e.g., (a) ventral ramus of first thoracic nerve, (b) first posterior intercostal artery, (c) first posterior intercostal vein, and (d) sympathetic chain.

N.B.
• All the structures related to the apex are separated from it by suprapleural membrane.
• Apex is grooved by subclavian artery on the medial side and on the front.

Clinical correlation

Pancoast syndrome: It occurs due to involvement of structures related to the posterior aspect of the apex of lung by the cancer of the lung apex.

Clinical features
• Pain along the medial side of forearm and hand, and wasting of small muscles of the hand due to involvement of ventral ramus of T1.
• *Horner's syndrome*, due to involvement of sympathetic chain.
• Erosion of first rib.

N.B. Cancer of lung apex may spread to involve neighboring structures, such as subclavian or brachiocephalic vein, subclavian artery, phrenic nerve causing following signs and symptoms.
• Venous engorgement and edema in neck, face, and arm due involvement of subclavian and brachiocephalic veins.
• Diminished brachial and/or radial pulse due to compression on subclavian artery.
• Paralysis of hemidiaphragm due to infiltration of phrenic nerve.

BASE

The base is lower semilunar concave surface, which rests on the dome of the diaphragm, hence it is also sometimes called *diaphragmatic surface*.

Relations

On the right side, the lung is separated from the liver by the right dome of the diaphragm, and on the left side, the left lung is separated from the spleen and fundus of stomach by the left dome of the diaphragm.

N.B. The base of the right lung is deeper (i.e., more concave) because right dome of diaphragm rises to the more superior level due to the presence of liver underneath it.

BORDERS

The borders of the lungs are as follows:

1. **Anterior border:** It is thin and shorter than the posterior border. The anterior border of right lung is vertical. The anterior border of left lung presents a wide **cardiac notch**, which is occupied by the heart and pericardium. In this region, the heart and pericardium is uncovered by the lung. Hence this region is responsible for an **area of superficial cardiac dullness**. Below the cardiac notch, it presents a tongue-shaped projection called **lingula**.
2. **Posterior border:** It is thick and rounded. It extends from spine of C7 vertebra to the spine of T10 vertebra.
3. **Inferior border:** It is semilunar in shape and separates the costal and medial surfaces.

SURFACES

The surfaces of the lungs are costal and medial.

Costal Surface

It is large, smooth, and convex. It is covered by the costal pleura and endothoracic fascia.

Relations

It is related to the lateral thoracic wall. (In embalmed and hardened lung, the costal surface presents impressions of the ribs.)

The number of ribs related to this surface is as follows:

- Upper 6 ribs in midclavicular line.
- Upper 8 ribs in midaxillary line.
- Upper 10 ribs in scapular line.

Medial Surface

It is divided into two parts (a) small posterior **vertebral part**, and (b) large anterior **mediastinal part**.

Relations

The **vertebral part** is related to the vertebral column, posterior intercostal vessels, and greater and lesser splanchnic nerves.

The **mediastinal part** presents a hilum, and it is related to mediastinal structures such as heart, great blood vessels, and nerves. Since the right and left surfaces of mediastinum consists of different structures. The relations of the mediastinal surface of the two lungs differ because structures forming right and left surfaces of mediastinum differ. To understand the relations of the mediastinal surfaces of the lungs, the students are advised to know the structures forming the right and left surfaces of the mediastinum.

Structures forming right surface of mediastinum (Fig. 19.3A):

1. The right mediastinal surface mainly consists of right atrium.
2. Above the right atrium are present superior vena cava and right brachiocephalic vein.
3. Behind these structures are present the trachea and esophagus.
4. The azygos vein, a large venous channel, runs upwards along the side of vertebral column and arches over the root of the right lung to terminate into the superior vena cava.
5. Three neural structures, viz. (a) right phrenic nerve, (b) right vagus nerve, and (c) right sympathetic chain.

   - The **phrenic nerve** runs to diaphragm passing superficial to three venous structures from above downwards—(i) superior vena cava, (ii) right atrium, and (iii) inferior vena cava. This course is in front of the root of the lung.

The **vagus nerve** lies against the right side of the trachea and travels behind the lung root. Here it breaks up into branches to take part in the formation of posterior pulmonary plexus and esophageal plexus.

The **sympathetic trunk** runs in the paravertebral gutter. The splanchnic nerves leave its lower half, run medially, and pierce the crura of diaphragm to reach the abdomen.

Structures forming left surface of the mediastinum (Fig. 19.3B):

1. The left ventricle and aorta are the main structures forming the left surface of the mediastinum.
2. Aorta ascends at first, arches over the left lung root, and then descends behind the lung root.
3. Three greet vessels (brachiocephalic trunk, left common carotid artery, and left subclavian vein) arise from the aortic arch and ascend up to reach the root of the neck.
4. The esophagus as it descends through thorax shifts to the left behind the heart and gently crosses the line of the descending aorta.
5. Three neural structures, viz. (a) left phrenic nerve, (b) left vagus nerve, and (c) left sympathetic chain.

Table 18.1 Relations of the mediastinal surfaces of the right and left lungs

Mediastinal surface of the right lung	Mediastinal surface of the left lung
Right atrium	Left ventricle
Superior and inferior vena cavae	Ascending aorta
Azygos vein	Arch of aorta and descending thoracic aorta
Right brachiocephalic vein	Left subclavian and left common carotid arteries
Esophagus and trachea	Esophagus and thoracic duct
Three neural structures	Four neural structures
• Right phrenic nerve	• Left phrenic vein
• Right vagus nerve	• Left vagus nerve
• Right sympathetic chain	• Left recurrent pharyngeal nerve
	• Left sympathetic chain

- The **left phrenic nerve** crosses the aortic (left) side, passes in front of the lung root, and runs down superficial to left ventricle to reach the diaphragm.
- The **left vagus nerve** is held away from the trachea by the aortic arch. Here it gives recurrent laryngeal branch, which hooks under the aortic arch, ascends up into the tracheoesophageal groove. Below the aortic arch, the vagus nerve runs behind the lung root and breaks up into posterior pulmonary and esophageal branches.
- The position of **sympathetic trunk** and **splanchnic nerves** is similar to those of the right side.

The relations of mediastinal surfaces of right and left lungs are given in Table 18.1 and shown in Figures 18.3 and 18.4.

The impressions produced by mediastinal structures on the medial surfaces of lungs are shown in Figures 18.5 and 18.6.

LOBES AND FISSURES (Figs 18.1 and 18.2)

The **right lung is divided into three lobes**: superior, middle, and inferior by two fissures—(a) an oblique fissure and (b) a horizontal fissure.

The **left lung is divided into two lobes**: (a) superior and (b) inferior by an oblique fissure.

1. **Oblique fissure:** A long oblique fissure runs obliquely downwards and forwards crossing the posterior border about 6 cm (2 inches) below the apex and inferior border about 7.5 cm (3 inches) lateral to the midline. It separates the superior and middle lobes from the inferior lobe.

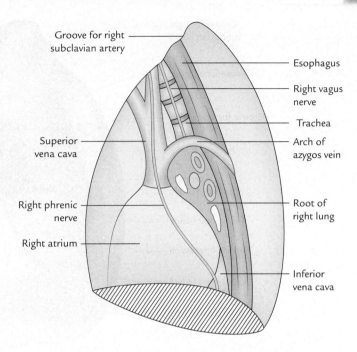

Fig. 18.3 Structures related to the mediastinal surface of the right lung.

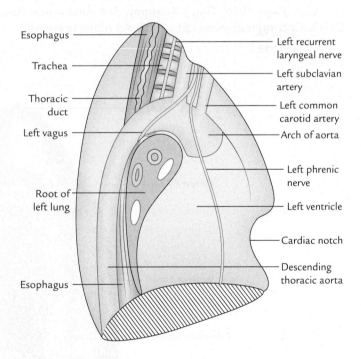

Fig. 18.4 Structures related to the mediastinal surface of the left lung and producing impression on this surface.

2. **Horizontal fissure:** A short horizontal fissure is present only in the right lung. It starts from oblique fissure at the midaxillary line and runs horizontally forward to the anterior border of the lung. It separates the superior and middle lobes.

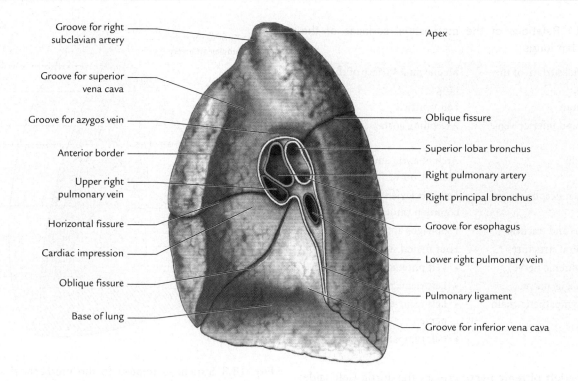

Fig. 18.5 The impressions produced by mediastinal structures on the medial surface of the right lung. (*Source:* Fig. 63.6, Page 1066, *Gray's Anatomy: The Anatomical Basis of Clinical Practice,* 39th ed., Susan Standring (Editor-in-Chief). *Copyright* Elsevier Ltd., 2005, All rights reserved.)

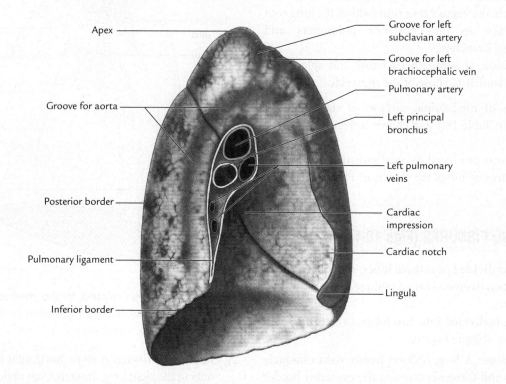

Fig. 18.6 The impressions produced by mediastinal structures on the medial surface of the left lung. (*Source:* Fig. 63.7, Page 1067, *Gray's Anatomy: The Anatomical Basis of Clinical Practice,* 39th ed., Susan Standring (Editor-in-Chief). Elsevier Ltd, 2005, All rights reserved.)

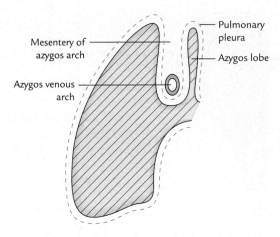

Fig. 18.7 Formation of azygos lobe of the lung.

The **oblique fissure** in left lung runs obliquely downwards and forwards crossing the posterior border about 6 cm below the apex and inferior border almost at its apex. It separates the superior lobe from the inferior lobe.

N.B.

- The *oblique fissure* acts as a plane of cleavage so that during inspiration, the upper part of lung expands forwards and laterally, whereas the lower part of the lung expands downwards and backwards.
- In X-ray chest PA view, the horizontal fissure is visible in 60% of the cases. The oblique fissure is usually visible in X-ray chest lateral view.
- Oblique fissure of left lung is more vertical than the oblique fissure of the right lung.

Clinical correlation

- **Identification of the completeness of the fissure:** It is important before performing lobectomy (i.e., removal of the lobe of the lung because individuals with incomplete fissures are more prone to develop postoperative air leakage than those with complete fissures).
- **Accessory lobes and fissures**
  - Lobe of azygos vein (Fig. 18.7): Sometimes the medial part of the superior lobe is partially separated by a fissure of variable length, which contains the terminal part of the azygos vein, enclosed in the free margin of a mesentery derived from the mediastinal pleura. This is termed *lobe of azygos vein*. It varies in size and sometimes includes the apex of the lung.
  - A left horizontal fissure is a normal variant found in 10% of the individuals.

ROOT OF THE LUNG

The root of lung is a short broad pedicle connecting the medial surface of the lung with the mediastinum. It consists of structures entering and leaving the lung at hilum.

The **hilum** is the area on the mediastinal surface of the lung through which structures enter or leave the lung.

The root of lung is surrounded by a tubular sheath derived from the mediastinal pleura.

COMPONENTS

The root of lung consists of the following structures:

1. Principal bronchus in the left lung, and eparterial and hyparterial bronchi in the right lung.
2. Pulmonary artery.
3. Pulmonary veins (two in number).
4. Bronchial arteries (one on the right side and two on the left side).
5. Bronchial veins.
6. Lymphatics of the lung.
7. Anterior and posterior pulmonary plexuses of the nerves.

N.B. The root of lung lies opposite the bodies of T5, T6, and T7 vertebrae.

ARRANGEMENT OF STRUCTURES IN THE ROOT OF THE LUNG AT THE HILUM (Fig. 18.8)

The arrangement of structures in the roots of the lungs is as follows:

1. **From before backwards (it is more or less similar on two sides):**
   (a) Pulmonary vein (superior)
   (b) Pulmonary artery
   (c) Bronchus (left principal bronchus on the left side, and eparterial, and hyparterial bronchus on the right side).

   Mnemonic: VAB (Vein, Artery, and Bronchus).

2. **From above downwards (it differs on two sides):**

Right side	Left side
• Eparterial bronchus	Pulmonary artery
• Pulmonary artery	Left principal bronchus
• Hyparterial bronchus	Inferior pulmonary vein
• Inferior pulmonary vein	

N.B. The difference in the arrangement of structures from above downwards on the two sides is because right principal bronchus before entering the lung at hilum divides into two lobar bronchi, the upper lobar bronchus passes above the pulmonary artery (**eparterial bronchus**) and lower lobar bronchus passes below the pulmonary artery (**hyparterial bronchus**).

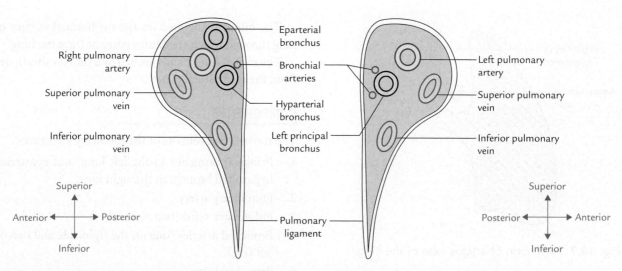

Fig. 18.8 Arrangement of structures in the roots of right and left lungs.

RELATIONS OF THE ROOT OF THE LUNG

Anterior:
- Phrenic nerve.
- Anterior pulmonary plexus.
- Superior vena cava (on right side only).

Posterior:
- Vagus nerve.
- Posterior pulmonary plexus.
- Descending thoracic aorta (on left side only).

Superior:
- Arch of azygos vein (on right side only).
- Arch of aorta (on left side only).

Inferior:
- Pulmonary ligament.

Clinical correlation

Hilar shadow in chest radiograph: In X-ray chest posteroanterior (PA) view, the root of each lung casts a radiopaque shadow called **hilar shadow** in the medial one-third of the lung field. The shadow is in fact cast by pulmonary vessels when seen end on. The enlargements of bronchopulmonary lymph nodes (hilar lymph nodes) increase the density of the hilar shadows.

The differences between the right and left lungs are given in Table 18.2.

SURFACE MARKINGS (Fig. 18.9)

1. **Margins:** The lung margins approximately coincide with those of the pleura (see page 241), except at the following points:
   (a) *Lower border:* The lower border of each lung is two-rib spaces higher than the lower border of the pleura. Thus, it lies along the line, which cuts
      (i) 6th rib in the midclavicular line,
      (ii) 8th rib in the midaxillary line, and
      (iii) 10th rib at the lateral border of erector spinae and ends 2 cm lateral to the spine of T10 vertebra.
   (b) *Anterior border:* The anterior border of the left lung has a distinct notch (the cardiac notch), which passes laterally behind the 4th and 5th intercostal spaces.
   (c) *Posterior border:* Its lower end ends at the level of spine of T10 vertebra.

2. **Fissures**
   (a) The *oblique fissure* is marked by a line drawn obliquely downwards and outwards from 1 inch (2.5 cm) lateral to the T5 spine to the 6th costal cartilage about 1½ inches (4 cm) from the midline. *In clinical practice, ask the patients to abduct the shoulder to its full extent; the line of **oblique fissure** in*

Table 18.2 Differences between the right and left lungs

	Right lung	Left lung
Size and shape	Larger, shorter, and broader	Smaller, longer, and narrower
Weight	700 g	650 g
Lobes	Three (upper, middle, and lower)	Two lobes (upper and lower)
Fissure	Two (horizontal and oblique)	One (oblique)
Anterior border	Straight	Not straight (presents a cardiac notch)
Hilum	Two bronchi (eparterial and hyparterial)	One bronchus (left principal bronchus)

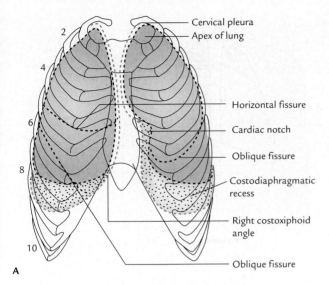

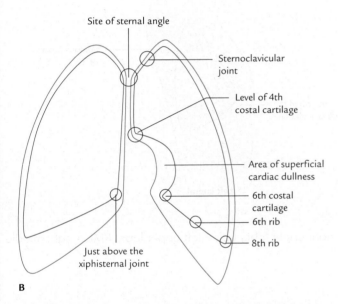

Fig. 18.9 Surface markings of the lung and pleura on the front: **A**, shows the relationship of lungs and pleurae in the thoracic case; **B**, shows outlines of lung and pleura. Note outline of lung are shown by blue line and pleura by red line.

this position corresponds to the medial border of the rotated scapula.

(b) The *transverse fissure* is marked by a line drawn horizontally along the 4th costal cartilage, and meets the oblique fissure where the latter crosses the 5th rib.

Clinical correlation

Auscultation of lungs: Visualization of lungs from the surface for listening lung sounds (Fig. 18.10): During auscultation of lung sounds, it is of utmost importance for the clinicians to visualize the lungs from the surface as follows:

- *Anteriorly:* The right side of chest primarily presents upper and middle lobes separated by the horizontal fissure at about the 5th rib in the midaxillary line to 4th rib at the sternum. The left side of chest primarily presents upper lobe, which is separated from the lower lobe by oblique fissure extending from the 5th rib in the midaxillary line to the 6th rib at the midclavicular line.
- *Posteriorly:* Except for apices, posterior aspect of chest on either side primarily presents lower lobe extending from spinous process of T3–T10 or T12 vertebrae.
- *Right lateral:* The lung lies deep to the area extending from axilla to the level of the 7th or 8th rib. The upper lobe is demarcated at the level of the 5th rib in the midaxillary line and 6th rib in the midclavicular line.
- *Left lateral:* The lung lies deep to the area extending from axilla to the 7th or 8th rib. The upper lobe is demarcated at the level of the 5th rib in the midaxillary line and 6th rib in the midclavicular line.

N.B. *Key points to remember during auscultation of lungs:*
- The superior lobe of the right lung is audible above the 4th rib.
- The middle lobe of the right lung is audible between the 4th and the 6th rib.
- The lower lobes of both lungs are audible below the 6th rib on the front.
- The inferior lobes of the right and left lungs are best examined on the back, especially in the region of the triangle of auscultation.

INTERNAL STRUCTURE

The lung is mainly made up of **intrapulmonary bronchial tree**, which is concerned with the conduction of air to-and-fro from the lung, and **pulmonary units**, which are concerned with the gaseous exchange within the lung (for detailed structure see textbooks on Histology).

BRONCHIAL TREE (Fig. 18.11)

The bronchial tree consists of principal bronchus, lobar bronchi, terminal bronchioles, and respiratory bronchioles.

Principal Bronchi (Figs 18.12 and 18.13)

The trachea divides outside the lungs, at the level of the lower border of T4 vertebra, into two primary (principal) bronchi—right and left for right and left lung, respectively:

1. **Right principal bronchus** is shorter, wider, and more vertical. It is about 1 inch (2.5 cm) long and lies more or less in line with the trachea.
2. **Left principal bronchus** is narrower, longer, and more horizontal than the right. It is about 2 inches (5 cm) long and does not lie in line with the trachea.

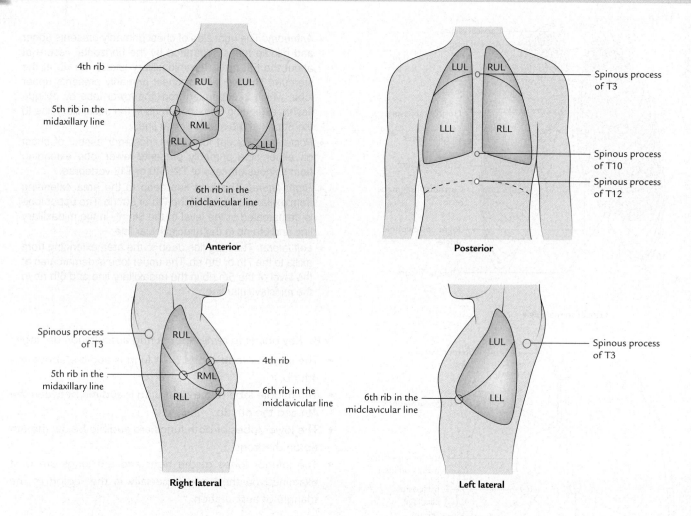

Fig. 18.10 Surface projection of different lobes of lungs (RUL = right upper lobe, LUL = left upper lobe, RML = right middle lobe, RLL = right lower lobe, LLL = left lower lobe).

The long axis of right principal bronchus deviates about 25° from the long axis of the trachea, whereas long axis of the left principal deviates about 45° from the long axis of the trachea.

The left principal bronchus passes to the left below the arch of aorta and in front of the esophagus.

Clinical correlation

- **Aspiration of foreign body into the right principal bronchus:** The inhaled foreign bodies usually enter in the right principal bronchus because it is shorter, wider and in line with the trachea. Since the inhaled foreign particles tend to enter in the right principal bronchus, hence in the right lung. As a result, lung abscess occurs more commonly in the right lung.
- **Bronchoscopy** (Fig. 18.14): It is a procedure, in which a flexible, fibre-optic bronchoscope is introduced in the trachea to visualize the interior of the trachea and bronchi. The **carina**, a keel-like median ridge at the bifurcation of the trachea is an important landmark visible through the bronchoscope. The widening and distortion of the angle between the principal bronchi (distorting the position of

carina) seen in bronchoscopy is serious prognostic sign, since it usually indicates carcinomatous involvement of tracheobronchial lymph nodes. The carina of trachea is also a very sensitive area for cough reflex.

- **Bronchiogenic carcinoma**: It is the commonest cancer in the males especially in chronic cigarette smokers. It usually arises from epithelial lining of the bronchi and forms well-circumscribed grey white mass in the lung. A presence of circular shadow (popularly called *coin-shadow*) in plane X-ray chest (PA view) may be the only finding in an otherwise asymptomatic patient.

The bronchiogenic carcinoma may spread (metastasis) to brain by both arterial and venous routes as under:

– *Arterial root*

  Lung capillaries → pulmonary vein → left atrium → left ventricle → aorta → internal carotid and vertebral arteries → brain

– *Venous route*

  Bronchial veins → azygos vein → external vertebral venous plexus → internal vertebral venous plexus → cranial dural venous sinuses → brain.

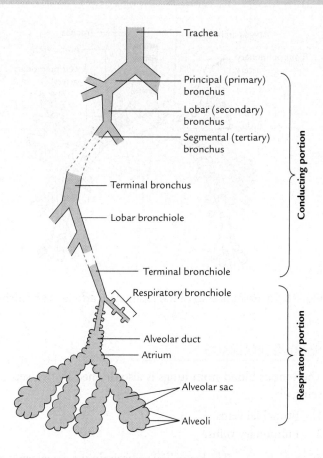

Fig. 18.11 Bronchial tree.

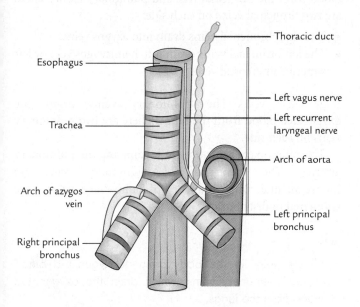

Fig. 18.12 Relation of principal bronchi.

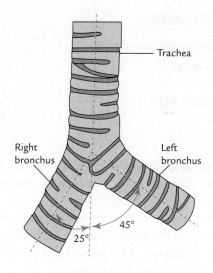

Fig. 18.13 Trachea and principal bronchi.

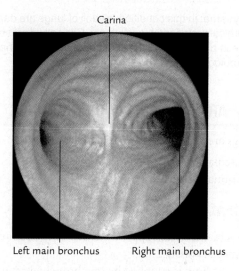

Fig. 18.14 Lower end of trachea and its main branches as seen on bronchoscopy. (*Source:* Fig. 3.48A, Page 151, *Gray's Anatomy for Students*, Richard L Drake, Wayne Vogl, Adam WM Mitchell. Copyright Elsevier Inc. 2005, All rights reserved.)

LOBAR BRONCHI

On entering the lung, the right principal bronchus divides (gives off) three lobar bronchi, one for each lobe of the right lung. The left principal bronchus on entering the lung divides into two lobar bronchi, one for each lobe of the left lung.

TERTIARY (SEGMENTAL) BRONCHI

Each lobar bronchus divides into segmental (tertiary) bronchi, one for each bronchopulmonary segment.

The segmental bronchi divide repeatedly to form very small bronchi called **terminal bronchioles**. The terminal bronchioles give off *respiratory bronchioles,* which lack cartilage in their walls.

Each **respiratory bronchiole** aerates a small portion of lung called **pulmonary units**, which is concerned with gaseous exchange within the lung.

PULMONARY UNITS

Each pulmonary unit consists of

(a) alveolar ducts,
(b) atria,
(c) air saccules, and
(d) alveoli.

N.B.

- The respiratory bronchiole represents the transitional zone/part between the conducting and respiratory portions of the respiratory system.
- The alveoli are specialized sac-like structures which form greater part of the lungs. They are the main sites for the gaseous exchange of oxygen and carbon dioxide between the inspired air and blood.

Clinical correlation

Emphysema: In this condition, alveoli of lungs are damaged by chemicals released by pollutants. Clinically it presents as shortness of breath and the chest appears barrel shaped in chest radiograph.

ARTERIAL SUPPLY OF THE LUNGS

The lungs are supplied by two sets of arteries, viz.

1. Bronchial arteries.
2. Pulmonary arteries.

BRONCHIAL ARTERIES

The bronchial arteries supply nutrition to the bronchial tree and pulmonary tissue.

The right lung is supplied by one bronchial artery, which arises from the right third posterior intercostal artery or from upper left bronchial artery. The left lung is supplied by two bronchial arteries, which arise from descending thoracic aorta.

PULMONARY ARTERIES

The pulmonary arteries supply deoxygenated blood to the lungs. There is one pulmonary artery for each lung. They are the branches of the pulmonary trunk.

The right and left pulmonary arteries lie anterior to the principal (primary) bronchi as they enter the hilum of their respective lungs. The right pulmonary artery is crossed superiorly by the arch of the azygos vein; whereas the left pulmonary artery lies inferior to the arch of aorta, at the level of T5 vertebra. The pulmonary arteries divide into lobar branches in the hilum and subsequently divide into terminal/segmental branches. The segmental branches, branch successively corresponding with the segmental branches of the bronchial tree (Fig. 18.15).

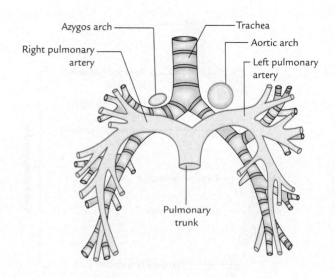

Fig. 18.15 Relationship of the pulmonary arteries to bronchi.

VENOUS DRAINAGE

The venous blood from lungs is also drained by two sets of veins, viz.

1. Bronchial veins.
2. Pulmonary veins.

Bronchial veins: The bronchial veins drain the deoxygenated blood from the bronchial tree and pulmonary tissue. There are two bronchial veins on each side:

- The right bronchial veins drain into azygos veins.
- The left bronchial veins drain into hemiazygos vein or left superior intercostal vein.

Pulmonary veins: The pulmonary veins drain the oxygenated blood from the lungs. There are two pulmonary veins on each side.

The pulmonary veins do not accompany the pulmonary arteries. The tributaries of pulmonary veins are intersegmental, while branches of pulmonary arteries are segmental in distribution.

N.B.

- All the veins in the body drain deoxygenated blood except pulmonary veins, which drain the oxygenated blood from the lungs.
- All the arteries of the body supply oxygenated blood except pulmonary arteries, which supply deoxygenated blood to the lungs.
- The bronchial arteries provide nutrition to the bronchial tree, as far as the respiratory bronchioles, i.e., non-respiratory portions of the lungs.
- The respiratory portions of the lungs are nourished by pulmonary capillary beds and atmospheric air in the alveoli.

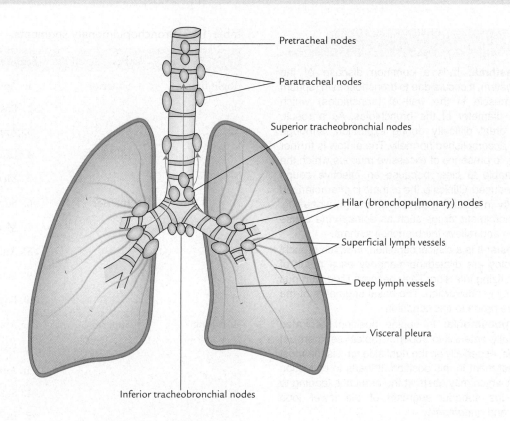

Pretracheal nodes

Paratracheal nodes

Superior tracheobronchial nodes

Hilar (bronchopulmonary) nodes

Superficial lymph vessels

Deep lymph vessels

Visceral pleura

Inferior tracheobronchial nodes

Fig. 18.16 Lymphatic drainage of the lungs.

LYMPHATIC DRAINAGE

The lymphatic drainage of the lung is clinically important because lung cancer spreads by lymphatic path.

The lymph from the lung is drained by two sets of lymph vessels (Fig. 18.16):

1. Superficial vessels.
2. Deep vessels.

Superficial lymph vessels: These vessels drain the peripheral lung tissue lying beneath the visceral pleura. They form the **superficial (subpleural) plexus** beneath the visceral pleura. The vessels from plexus pass around the borders and margins of the fissures of lung to reach the hilum where they drain into the **bronchopulmonary (hilar) lymph nodes**.

Deep lymph vessels: These vessels drain the bronchial tree, pulmonary vessels, and connective tissue septa and form **deep plexus**. The vessels from deep plexus run along the bronchi and pulmonary vessels towards the hilum of the lung passing through **pulmonary lymph nodes** located within the lung substance, and finally drain into **bronchopulmonary (hilar) lymph nodes**.

Thus both superficial and deep lymphatic plexuses drain into bronchopulmonary (hilar) lymph nodes. From hilar lymph nodes, the lymph is drained into the superior and inferior *tracheobronchial lymph nodes* located superior and inferior to the bifurcation of the trachea, respectively. These nodes in turn drain into pre- and paratracheal lymph nodes, and right and left bronchomediastinal lymph trunk, which finally drain into right lymphatic duct and thoracic duct on the right and left sides respectively.

N.B. All the lymph from the lung is drained into *tracheobronchial lymph nodes* (located at the hilum), which in turn drain into *bronchomediastinal lymph nodes*.

NERVE SUPPLY

The lung is supplied by both parasympathetic and sympathetic nerve fibres:

The **parasympathetic fibres** are derived from the vagus nerve and **sympathetic fibres** are derived from T2 to T5 spinal segments. Both provide motor supply to the bronchial muscles and secretomotor supply to the mucous glands of the bronchial tree.

The **parasympathetic fibres** cause bronchoconstriction/ bronchospasm, vasodilatation, and increased mucous secretion. The **sympathetic fibres** cause bronchodilatation, vasoconstriction, and decreased mucous secretion.

The afferent impulse arising from the bronchial mucous membrane and stretch receptors in the alveolar walls pass to the central nervous system through both sympathetic and parasympathetic fibres.

- **Bronchial asthma:** It is a common disease of the respiratory system. It occurs due to bronchospasm (spasm of smooth muscle in the wall of bronchioles) which reduces the diameter of the bronchioles. As a result, patient has great difficulty during expiration, although inspiration is accomplished normally. The airflow is further impeded due to presence of excessive mucous which the patient is unable to clear because an effective cough cannot be produced. Clinically the asthma is characterized by (a) difficulty in breathing (dyspnea) and (b) wheezing. The sympathomimetic drugs such as epinephrine cause vasodilatation and relieve the bronchial asthma.

- **Bronchiectasis:** It is a clinical condition, in which bronchi and bronchioles are dilated permanently as a result of chronic necrotizing infection. They become filled with pus leading to airway obstruction. The basal segments of the lower lobe are prone to this condition.

- **Aspiration pneumonia:** In supine position, aspirated material usually enters into superior (apical segment) of the lower lobe, especially on the right side for it is the most dependent segment in this position. It leads to collection of secretions which may obstruct the bronchus leading to collapse of the superior segment of the lower lobe (*atelectasis*) and *pneumonia*.

Table 18.3 Bronchopulmonary segments

	Lobes	Segments
Right lung	• Superior	1. Apical
		2. Posterior
		3. Anterior
	• Middle	4. Lateral
		5. Medial
	• Inferior	6. Superior (apical)
		7. Medial basal
		8. Anterior basal
		9. Lateral basal
		10. Posterior basal
Left lung	• Superior	1. Apical
		2. Posterior
		3. Anterior
		4. Superior lingular
		5. Inferior lingular
	• Inferior	6. Superior (apical)
		7. Medial basal
		8. Anterior basal
		9. Lateral basal
		10. Posterior basal

BRONCHOPULMONARY SEGMENTS

The bronchopulmonary segments are well-defined, wedge-shaped sectors of the lung, which are aerated by tertiary (segmental) bronchi (Fig. 18.17).

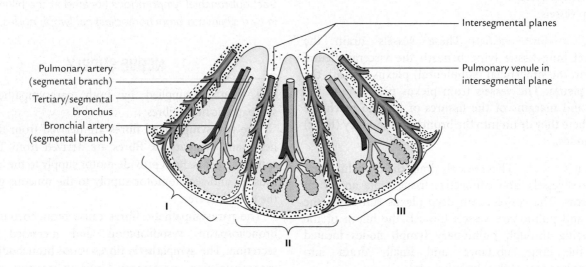

Intersegmental planes

Pulmonary venule in intersegmental plane

Pulmonary artery (segmental branch)

Tertiary/segmental bronchus

Bronchial artery (segmental branch)

I II III

Fig. 18.17 Schematic diagram showing three bronchopulmonary segments (I, II, and III).

Characteristic features:

1. It is a subdivision of the lobe of the lung.
2. It is pyramidal in shape with apex directed towards the hilum and base towards the surface of the lung.
3. It is surrounded by the connective tissue.
4. It is aerated by the segmental (tertiary) bronchus.
5. Each segment has its own artery, a segmental branch of the pulmonary artery.
6. Each segment has its own lymphatic drainage and autonomic supply.

Thus, bronchopulmonary segments are the well-defined anatomical, functional, and surgical units of the lungs.

N.B. The segmental veins (the tributaries of pulmonary veins) run in the intersegmental planes of the connective tissue.

NUMBER AND NOMENCLATURE OF BRONCHOPULMONARY SEGMENTS
(Figs 18.18 and 18.19)

The number and terms used to designate the segments vary among different authors, but in this book, the number and terms accepted by the *International Congress of Anatomists*, (1960) has been adopted.

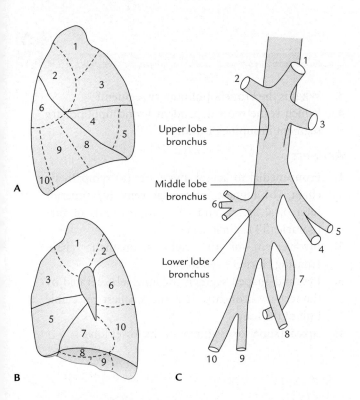

Fig. 18.18 Bronchopulmonary segments of the right lung as seen on: A, lateral aspect; B, medial aspect; C, lobar and segmental bronchi.

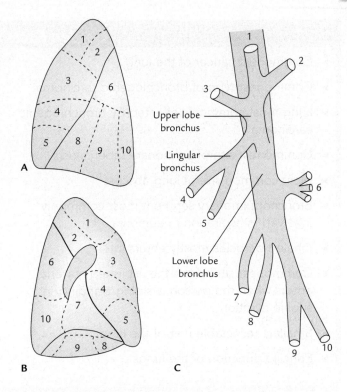

Fig. 18.19 Bronchopulmonary segments of the left lung as seen on: A, lateral aspect; B, medial aspect; C, lobar and segmental bronchi.

There are 10 segments in each lung. They are named and numbered in Table 18.3. The bronchopulmonary segments of right and left lungs are shown in Figures 18.18 and 18.19 respectively.

Clinical correlation

Segmental resection of the lung: The knowledge of the bronchopulmonary segments has led to the advancement in conservation lung surgery. Since each segment is an independent functional unit having its own bronchovascular supply and potential planes of separation exist between the segments. Localized chronic disease, such as tuberculosis, bronchiectasis or benign neoplasm is restricted to one segment; it is, therefore, possible to dissect out and remove the diseased segment leaving the surrounding tissue intact. This procedure is called *segmental resection*.

N.B.
- During segmental dissection, it is important not to ligate intersegmental veins as they will interfere with the venous drainage of the surrounding healthy segments.
- Segmental resection is most often carried out in bronchiectasis.

Golden Facts to Remember

▶ Commonest cancer of the lung	Bronchiogenic carcinoma
▶ Commonest type of bronchiogenic carcinoma	Adenocarcinoma
▶ Lung most commonly affected by bronchiogenic carcinoma	Right lung
▶ Commonest site of pulmonary tuberculosis	Apical regions of the lungs
▶ Most common site of lung abscess	Right lower lobe
▶ Bronchopulmonary segment most commonly involved in aspiration pneumonia	Superior segment of lower lobe of right lung
▶ Inhaled particles mostly enters into	Right principal bronchus
▶ Commonest site where the aspirated material enters when the person is sitting/standing/in supine position	Right lobar bronchus
▶ Smallest resectable unit of the lung	Bronchopulmonary segment
▶ Principal function of the lungs	Exchange of O_2 and CO_2 between inspired air and blood

Clinical Case Study

A heavy smoker, 60-year-old male, visited the hospital and complained that he lost 10 kg of his weight in past 3 months, and has persistent cough with blood-stained sputum. He also noticed loss of sweating on the right side of his face. On physical examination, the doctors found partial ptosis and constriction of pupil in his right eye.

X-Ray chest (PA view) revealed a radiopaque shadow in the apical region of the right lung. Biopsy revealed malignancy. A diagnosis of malignancy of the apex of the lung was made.

Questions

1. Enumerate the posterior relations of the apex of the lung.
2. Mention the anatomical basis of loss of sweating in right half of the face, and partial ptosis and constriction (meiosis) of the right eye.
3. What is the bronchopulmonary segment?
4. Which is the most dependent bronchopulmonary segment in supine position?

Answers

1. From medial to lateral, these are: (a) sympathetic chain, (b) highest intercostal vein, (c) superior intercostal artery, and (d) ventral ramus of first thoracic (T1) spinal nerve.
2. Involvement of the right sympathetic chain (causing Horner's syndrome).
3. Pyramid-shaped segment of lung lobe aerated by the tertiary bronchus. It is the smallest resectable unit of the lung.
4. Apical (superior) segment of the lower lobe.

Mediastinum

The mediastinum (L. middle septum) is the median septum of thoracic cavity between the two pleural cavities. It consists of all the viscera and structures of the thoracic cavity (e.g., heart and its great blood vessels, esophagus, trachea and principal bronchi, aorta, mediastinal lymph nodes, etc.) except the lungs. The mediastinum occupies the central compartment of the thoracic cavity. Thus strictly speaking, it is a broad central partition, which separates the two laterally placed pleural cavities (Fig. 19.1). It is covered on either side by the mediastinal pleura.

BOUNDARIES (Figs 19.2 and 19.4)

Anterior:	Sternum.
Posterior:	Vertebral column (bodies of thoracic vertebrae and intervening intervertebral discs).
Superior:	Superior thoracic aperture.
Inferior:	Diaphragm.
On each side:	Mediastinal pleura.

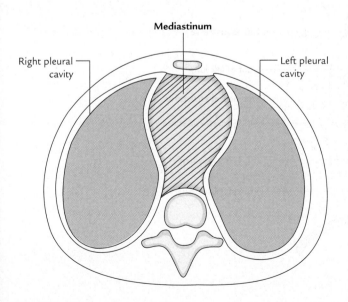

Fig. 19.1 Cross section of the thorax showing the position of the mediastinum.

N.B. The mediastinum is not a rigid structure as observed by the students in the cadaver (embalmed dead body). In a living individual, mediastinum is a highly mobile septum because it consists primarily of hollow visceral structures bound together by loose connective tissue, often infiltrated with fat.

CONTENTS

The major contents of mediastinum are (Fig. 19.2):

1. Thymus.
2. Heart enclosed in the pericardial sac.

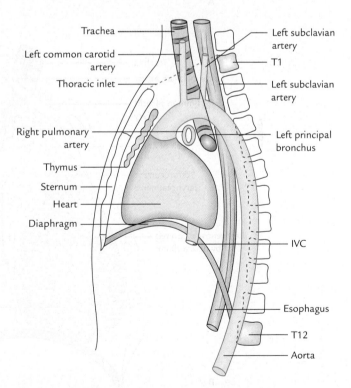

Fig. 19.2 Boundaries and contents of the mediastinum. Note that all the mediastinal structures are not depicted (IVC = inferior vena cava).

3. Major arteries and veins such as thoracic aorta, pulmonary trunk, etc.
4. Trachea.
5. Esophagus.
6. Thoracic duct.

7. Neural structures, such as sympathetic trunks, vagus nerves, phrenic nerve, etc.
8. Lymph nodes.

The structures forming the right and left surfaces of the mediastinum as shown in Figure 19.3.

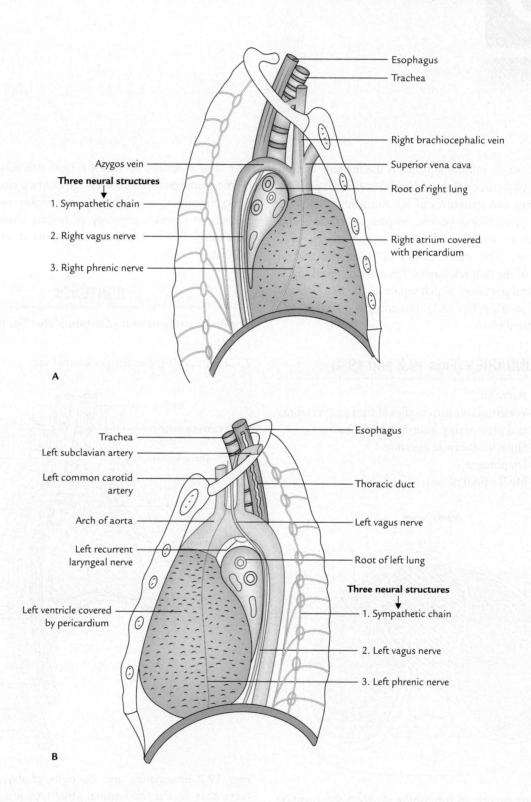

Fig. 19.3 Mediastinal structures as seen from its lateral aspect in sagittal section of the thorax: A, right side; B, left side.

DIVISIONS

For the purpose of description and organization of structures the mediastinum is artificially divided into two parts: (a) **superior mediastinum** and (b) **inferior mediastinum** by an imaginary plane (**transverse thoracic plane**) passing through the sternal angle anteriorly, and lower border of the body of the fourth thoracic (T4) vertebra/intervertebral disc T4 and T5 vertebrae posteriorly.

The inferior mediastinum is further subdivided into three parts by the pericardium (enclosing heart). The part in front of the pericardium is called **anterior mediastinum**, and the part behind the pericardium is called **posterior mediastinum**. The pericardium and its contents (heart and roots of its great vessels) constitute the **middle mediastinum** (Fig. 19.4).

The divisions and subdivisions of the mediastinum are shown in Flowchart 19.1.

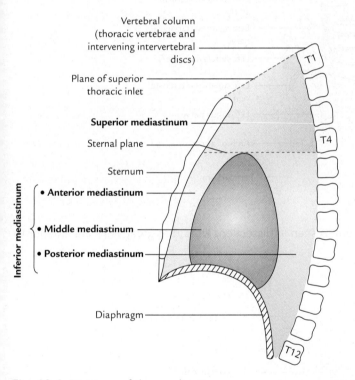

Fig. 19.4 Divisions of the mediastinum.

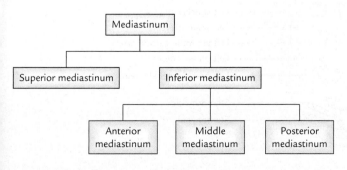

Flowchart 19.1 Divisions and subdivisions of the mediastinum.

Clinical correlation

Visualization of subdivisions of mediastinum in chest radiograph: The subdivisions of mediastinum are well-appreciated in lateral view of X-ray chest (Fig. 19.5).
- The shadow above the sternal plane represents *superior mediastinum*.
- The subdivisions of *inferior mediastinum* are demarcated as under:
(a) cardiac shadow above the anterior part of diaphragm represents the *middle mediastinum*.
(b) retrosternal space/space in the front of cardiac shadow represents the *anterior mediastinum*.
(c) retrocardiac space/space between the cardiac shadow and shadow of vertebral column represents the *posterior mediastinum*.

SUPERIOR MEDIASTINUM

Boundaries (Fig. 19.4)

Anterior:	Manubrium sterni.
Posterior:	Bodies of upper four thoracic vertebrae.
Superior:	Plane of superior thoracic aperture.
Inferior:	An imaginary plane passing through the sternal angle in front and lower border of the body of fourth thoracic vertebra behind (transverse thoracic plane).
On each side (lateral):	Mediastinal pleura.

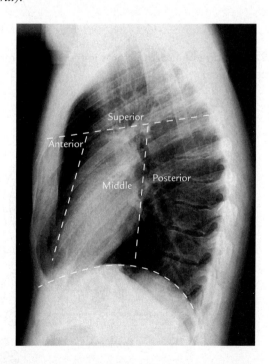

Fig. 19.5 Parts of the mediastinum demonstrated on a chest radiograph (lateral view). (*Source:* Fig. 4.13, Page 99, *Integrated Anatomy*, David JA Heylings, Roy AJ Spence, Barry E Kelly. Copyright Elsevier Limited 2007, All rights reserved.)

Contents (Figs 19.6 and 19.7)

1. Arteries
   (a) Arch of aorta.
   (b) Brachiocephalic artery.
   (c) Left common carotid artery.
   (d) Left subclavian artery.
2. Veins
   (a) Right and left brachiocephalic veins.
   (b) Upper half of the superior vena cava (SVC).
   (c) Left superior intercostal vein.
3. Nerves
   (a) Phrenic nerves (right and left).
   (b) Vagus nerves (right and left).

   (c) Sympathetic trunks and cardiac nerves (right and left).
   (d) Left recurrent laryngeal nerves.
4. Lymphoid organs and lymphatics
   (a) Lymph nodes.
   (b) Thoracic duct.
   (c) Thymus.
5. Tubes
   (a) Trachea.
   (b) Esophagus.
6. Muscles
   (a) Sternohyoid.
   (b) Sternothyroid.
   (c) Longus colli.

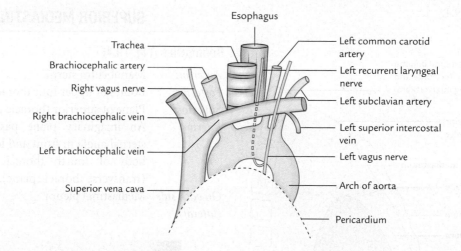

Fig. 19.6 Arrangement of structures in the superior mediastinum as seen in dissection. Note that great veins are anterior to the great arteries.

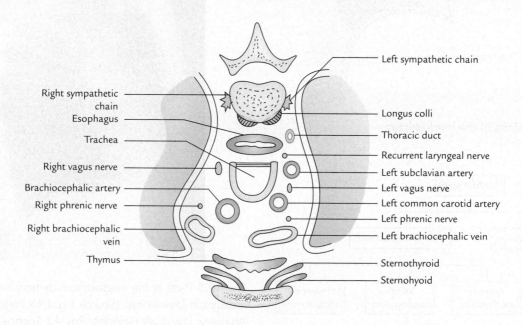

Fig. 19.7 Transverse section of superior mediastinum showing the arrangement of its contents.

N.B. For the purpose of orientation during surgery, the major structures of superior mediastinum are arranged in the following order from anterior to posterior:

- Thymus
- Large veins
- Large arteries
- Trachea
- Esophagus and thoracic duct
- Sympathetic trunks.

Clinical correlation

Potential dead space in superior mediastinum: In superior mediastinum, all large veins (superior vena cava, right and left brachiocephalic veins) are on the right side and all the large arteries (arch of aorta and its three branches) are on the left side. Consequently, during increased blood flow, the large veins expand enormously while the large arteries do not expand at all. This is because there is sufficient dead space on the right side. It is into this space that tumors of mediastinum tend to project.

ANTERIOR MEDIASTINUM

Boundaries (Fig. 19.4)

Anterior: Body of sternum.
Posterior: Pericardium enclosing heart.
Superior: Transverse thoracic plane separating superior and inferior mediastinum.
Inferior: Diaphragm.
On each side: Mediastinal pleura.

Contents

1. Loose areolar tissue.
2. Superior and inferior *sternopericardial ligaments* stretching between sternum and pericardium.
3. Three or four lymph nodes.
4. Mediastinal branches of internal thoracic (mammary) arteries.
5. Lower portion of thymus (in children).

Clinical correlation

The anterior mediastinum is a very narrow space. It is continuous through superior mediastinum with the pretracheal space of the neck. Therefore, neck infection in pretracheal space may spread into the anterior mediastinum.

MIDDLE MEDIASTINUM

Boundaries (Fig. 19.4)

Anterior: Anterior mediastinum.
Posterior: Posterior mediastinum.

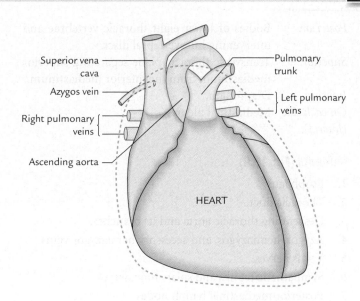

Fig. 19.8 Main contents of the middle mediastinum.

Superior: Superior mediastinum.
Inferior: Diaphragm.

Contents (Fig. 19.8)

1. **Heart**
2. **Pericardium**
3. **Arteries:**
   (a) Ascending aorta
   (b) Pulmonary trunk dividing into two pulmonary arteries
   (c) Pericardiophrenic arteries
4. **Veins:**
   (a) Superior vena cava (lower half)
   (b) Azygos vein (terminal part)
   (c) Pulmonary veins (right and left)
5. **Nerves:**
   (a) Phrenic nerves
   (b) Deep cardiac plexus
6. **Lymph nodes:**
   (a) Tracheobronchial lymph nodes
7. **Tubes:**
   (a) Bifurcation of trachea
   (b) Right and left principal bronchi

N.B. The main contents of middle mediastinum are pericardium and its contents (e.g., the heart and roots of its great vessels).

POSTERIOR MEDIASTINUM

Boundaries (Fig. 19.4)

Anterior: (a) pericardium and its contents, (b) bifurcation of the trachea, and (c) pulmonary vessels.

Posterior: Bodies of lower eight thoracic vertebrae and intervening intervertebral discs.

Superior: Transverse thoracic plane separating superior mediastinum from the inferior mediastinum.

Inferior: Diaphragm.

On each side (lateral): Mediastinal pleura.

Contents (Fig. 19.9)

1. Esophagus.
2. Thoracic duct.
3. Descending thoracic aorta and its branches.
4. Azygos, hemiazygos, and accessory hemiazygos veins.
5. Vagus nerves.
6. Sympathetic trunks and splanchnic nerves.
7. Posterior mediastinal lymph nodes.

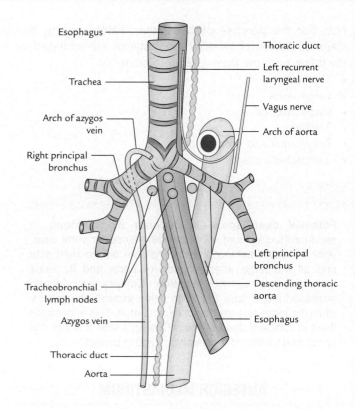

Fig. 19.9 Anterior view of the esophagus trachea bronchi and aorta. Note that the arch of aorta arches over the left bronchus and azygos vein arches over the right bronchus.

Clinical correlation

- **Mediastinitis:** It is the inflammation of the loose connective tissue of the mediastinum. The fascial spaces of the neck (e.g., pretracheal and retropharyngeal spaces) extend below into the mediastinum within the thoracic cavity. Therefore, deep infections of the neck may readily spread into the thoracic cavity causing *mediastinitis*.

- **Subcutaneous emphysema at the root of neck:** The structures that make up mediastinum are embedded in the loose connective tissue which is continuous with the loose connective tissue of the root of the neck. Therefore, in *esophageal perforations* caused by penetrating wounds, air escapes into the connective tissue spaces of mediastinum and may ascend beneath the fascia to the root of the neck producing *subcutaneous emphysema*.

- **Mediastinal syndrome:** The compression of mediastinal structures by any growth such as tumor or cyst gives rise to a group of signs and symptoms, producing a clinical condition called *mediastinal syndrome*.

  The common causes of mediastinal syndrome are bronchiogenic carcinoma, aneurysm of aorta, enlargement of mediastinal lymph nodes in Hodgkin disease.

  The clinical features of mediastinal syndrome are:
  (a) *engorgement of veins* in the upper half of the body: due to obstruction of SVC,
  (b) *dyspnea* (difficulty in breathing): due to compression of trachea,
  (c) *dysphagia* (difficulty in swallowing): due to compression of esophagus,
  (d) *dyspnea* (hoarseness of voice): due to compression of left recurrent laryngeal nerve, and
  (e) *erosion of bodies of thoracic vertebrae:* due to pressure on the vertebral column.

- **Widening of the mediastinum:** The widening of mediastinum is often observed in chest radiographs. It can occur due to a number of reasons, such as
  (a) hemorrhage into the mediastinum from lacerated great vessels (aorta, SVC) following trauma, e.g., head on collision,

  (b) massive enlargement of mediastinal lymph nodes due to cancer of lymphoid tissue, viz. malignant lymphoma, and
  (c) enlargement (hypertrophy) of heart due to congestive heart failure (CHF). It is the common cause of widening of inferior mediastinum.

- **Mediastinal shift:** The mediastinal shift is common in lung and pleural pathology. The mediastinum shifts to the affected (diseased) side due to appreciable reduction in lung volume and decrease in intrapleural pressure—as in *collapse of lung* and *atelectasis*. The mediastinum shifts to the healthy side when the intrapleural pressure is appreciably high on the affected side—as in *pneumothorax* and *hydrothorax*.

  Mediastinal shift indicates lung pathology. The mediastinal shift can be detected by palpating the trachea in the suprasternal notch.

- **Extension of pus into the posterior mediastinum from neck:** The posterior mediastinum is continuous through superior mediastinum with spaces in the neck between pretracheal and prevertebral layers of deep cervical fascia such as retropharyngeal space, etc. Therefore, pus from neck can extend into the posterior mediastinum.

- **Extension of pus into the thighs from posterior mediastinum:** The psoas sheath communicates with the posterior mediastinum by a funnel-shaped orifice. Therefore, pus from posterior mediastinum can easily enter the psoas sheath and tracks down into the thighs in the region of femoral triangle.

Golden Facts to Remember

▶ Mediastinum contains all the thoracic viscera *except*	Lungs
▶ Largest structure of mediastinum	Heart
▶ Commonest cause of widening of inferior mediastinum	Enlargement (hypertrophy) of the heart
▶ Mediastinum is a dynamic, pliable, and movable septum	Because structures forming it are hollow, fluid- or air-filled and bound together by loose connective tissue
▶ Compartment of thoracic cavity occupied by the mediastinum	Central compartment
▶ Common cause of mediastinal shift to the diseased side	Collapse of lung and atelectasis
▶ Common cause of mediastinal shift to the healthy side	Pneumothorax/hydrothorax

Clinical Case Study

A 60-year-old male visited the hospital and complained that he (a) has noticed alternation in his voice, (b) has lost 15 kg weight, and (c) has persistent cough with blood-stained sputum. On asking, he told that he is a chronic smoker and smokes 20–30 cigarettes per day. The X-ray chest revealed a large well-circumscribed radiopaque shadow in the hilar region of his right lung and widening of the mediastinum. A diagnosis of **bronchiogenic carcinoma** was made.

Questions

1. Bronchiogenic carcinoma is common in males or females? Mention the incidence of death.
2. Occurrence of bronchiogenic carcinoma is more common in right lung as compared to the left lung. What is its anatomical basis?
3. What is the cause of hoarseness of the voice?
4. Mention the anatomical basis of metastasis of bronchiogenic carcinoma to brain and bones.

Answers

1. It is common in males and accounts for about one-third of all cancer deaths in men.
2. Because right bronchial tree is more exposed to the carcinogens, e.g., cigarette smoke, tarry particles from roads as right bronchus is wider and lies in line with trachea.
3. The bronchiogenic carcinoma spreads rapidly to tracheobronchial and bronchomediastinal lymph nodes and involves the recurrent laryngeal nerve, leading to the hoarseness of voice.
4. Through blood vessels (i.e., hematogenous spread) (for details please refer *Clinical and Surgical Anatomy*, 2nd edition by Vishram Singh).

CHAPTER

20

Pericardium and Heart

PERICARDIUM

The pericardium (G. around heart) is a fibroserous sac which encloses the heart and the roots of its great blood vessels. The pericardium lies within the middle mediastinum, posterior to the body of the sternum and 2nd–6th costal cartilages and anterior to the middle four thoracic vertebrae (i.e., from T5 to T8).

The functions of the pericardium are:

(a) restricts excessive movements of the heart,
(b) serves as a lubricated container in which heart can contract and relax smoothly, and
(c) limits the cardiac distension.

SUBDIVISIONS

The pericardium consists of two components:

(a) an outer single layered fibrous sac called **fibrous pericardium,** and
(b) inner double layered serous sac called **serous pericardium.**

A little description of embryology makes it easier to understand the formation of different layers of the pericardium.

The heart and great vessels lie inside the fibrous sac and invaginate the serous sac from behind during development. As a result, the external surface of the heart and internal surface of the fibrous pericardium are covered by a layer of serous pericardium. The layer covering the surface of the heart is called **visceral pericardium** or **epicardium** and the layer covering the inner aspect of the fibrous pericardium is called **parietal pericardium.** The intervening potential space between the two serous layers is called **pericardial cavity** (Fig. 20.1).

The pericardium thus consists of three layers (Fig. 20.2). From outside to inwards these are:

1. Fibrous layer of the pericardium.
2. Parietal layer of the serous pericardium.
3. Visceral layer of the serous pericardium (epicardium).

FIBROUS PERICARDIUM

The fibrous pericardium is strong fibrous sac which supports the delicate parietal layer of the serous pericardium with which it is firmly adherent.

Features

The features of fibrous pericardium are as follows:

1. It is conical in shape.

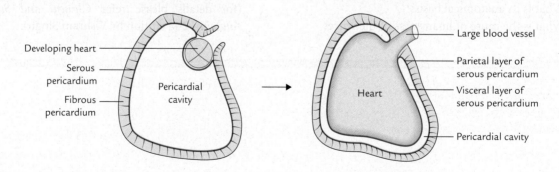

Fig. 20.1 Development of different layers of the pericardium.

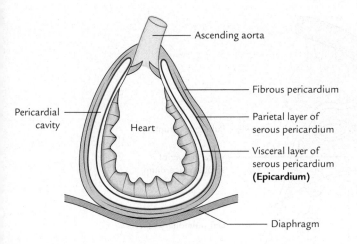

Fig. 20.2 Layers of the pericardium.

2. Its apex is blunt and fused with the outer coats of the roots of great blood vessels (e.g., ascending aorta, pulmonary trunk).
3. Its base is broad and blended with the central tendon of the diaphragm.
4. Anteriorly it is connected to the posterior aspect of the body of sternum by the *superior and inferior sternopericardial ligaments*.
5. Posteriorly it is related to principal bronchi, esophagus, and descending thoracic aorta.
6. On each side it is related to phrenic nerves and pericardiophrenic vessels.

N.B. In quadrupeds the fibrous pericardium is separated from the diaphragm by *serous infracardiac bursa*.

SEROUS PERICARDIUM

The serous pericardium is a thin serous membrane lined by mesothelium. It is double layered, the outer layer is called **parietal layer** and the inner layer is called **visceral layer.**

The outer layer lines the fibrous pericardium and is reflected around the roots of great blood vessels to become continuous with the visceral layer of the pericardium. It is called **parietal pericardium.**

The inner layer is closely applied to the heart except along the cardiac grooves, where it is separated from the heart by blood vessels. It is called **visceral pericardium or epicardium.**

N.B. The two layers of serous pericardium are continuous with each other at the roots of great blood vessels (e.g., ascending aorta, pulmonary trunks, superior and inferior vena cavae), and superior and inferior pulmonary veins where the pericardial sac was invaginated by the developing heart.

The differences between the parietal and serous pericardium are listed in Table 20.1.

Table 20.1 Differences between the parietal and serous pericardium

Parietal pericardium	Visceral pericardium (epicardium)
It is adherent to the fibrous pericardium	It is adherent to the myocardium of the heart
It develops from somatopleuric mesoderm	It develops from splanchnopleuric mesoderm
It is innervated by the somatic nerve fibres	It is innervated by the autonomic nerve fibres
It is sensitive to pain	It is insensitive to pain

PERICARDIAL CAVITY

The slit-like potential space between the parietal and visceral layers of serous pericardium is termed **pericardial cavity.** Normally it contains a thin film of serous fluid (about 50 ml) called **pericardial fluid** which lubricates the opposed surfaces to avoid friction during the movements of the heart.

CONTENTS

The following are the contents of the pericardium:

1. Heart with its vessels and nerves.
2. Ascending aorta.
3. Pulmonary trunk.
4. Superior vena cava (lower half).
5. Inferior vena cava (terminal part).
6. Pulmonary veins (terminal parts).

SINUSES OF PERICARDIUM (Figs 20.3 and 20.4)

There are two sinuses between the parietal and visceral layers of serous pericardium:

1. Transverse sinus.
2. Oblique sinus.

They are formed due to the reflection of visceral layer of serous pericardium around great vessels of the heart.

The visceral pericardium (epicardium) at the roots of great blood vessels is arranged into tubes: (a) arterial tube and (b) venous tube. The *arterial tube* encloses the ascending aorta and pulmonary trunk (*arterial end of the heart tube*). The *venous tube* encloses the superior and inferior vena cava and four pulmonary veins (*venous end of the heart tube*).

Transverse Sinus of Pericardium

It is a transverse recess behind the ascending aorta and pulmonary trunk and in front of superior vena cava and superior pulmonary veins. It develops due to degeneration of *dorsal mesocardium*.

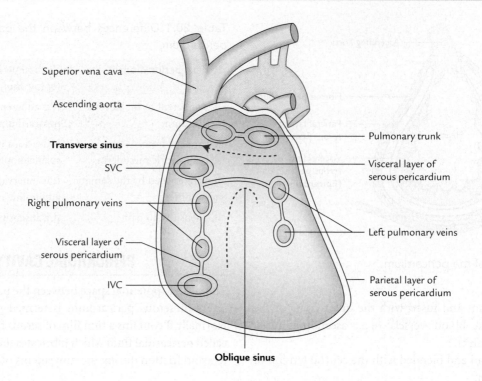

Fig. 20.3 Interior of the serous pericardial sac after section of the large vessels and removal of the heart showing transverse and oblique pericardial sinuses (SVC = superior vena cava, IVC = inferior vena cava).

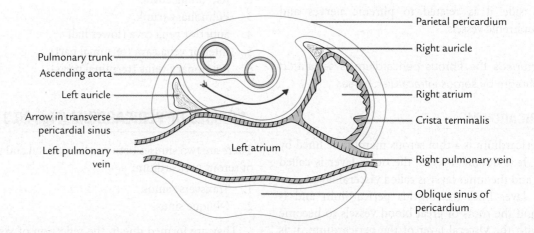

Fig. 20.4 Cross section of heart through the atria showing reflection of pericardium and formation of transverse and oblique pericardial sinuses. Note that the left atrium lies behind the pulmonary trunk and aorta, from which it is separated by transverse sinus of the pericardium.

It is a horizontal passage between the two pericardial tubes. On each side it communicates with the general pericardial cavity.

Oblique Sinus of Pericardium

It is a recess of serous pericardium behind the base of the heart (actually left atrium). It is enclosed by 'J-shaped' sheath of visceral layer of serous pericardium enclosing six veins (i.e., 2 vena cavae and 4 pulmonary veins).

The oblique sinus is akin to lesser sac behind the stomach and develops as a result of absorption of four pulmonary veins into the left atrium. The oblique sinus permits the distension of left atrium during return of oxygenated blood in it from the lungs.

Boundaries

Oblique sinus of pericardium is bounded in the following way:

Anteriorly:	by left atrium.
Posteriorly:	by parietal pericardium.
On right side:	by reflection of visceral pericardium along the right pulmonary veins and inferior vena cava.
On the left side:	by reflection of visceral pericardium along the left pulmonary veins.
Superiorly:	by reflection of visceral pericardium along the right and left superior pulmonary veins.
Inferiorly:	it is open.

Clinical correlation

Surgical significance of transverse pericardial sinus: During cardiac surgery, after the pericardial sac is opened anteriorly, a finger is passed through the transverse sinus of pericardium, posterior to the aorta and pulmonary trunk (Fig. 20.5).

A temporary ligature is passed through the transverse sinus around the aorta and pulmonary trunk. The tubes of heart-lung machine are inserted into these vessels and ligature is tightened.

ARTERIAL SUPPLY

- The *fibrous pericardium* and *parietal layer of visceral pericardium* is supplied by the branches of the following arteries:
  1. Internal thoracic artery.
  2. Musculophrenic arteries.
  3. Descending thoracic aorta.
- The *visceral layer* of serous pericardium is supplied by the coronary arteries.

NERVE SUPPLY

1. The fibrous pericardium and parietal layer of the serous pericardium are supplied by the phrenic nerves (somatic nerve fibres).
2. The visceral layer of the serous pericardium is supplied by the branches of sympathetic trunks and vagus nerves (autonomic nerve fibres). Thus fibrous pericardium and parietal layer of the visceral pericardium are sensitive to pain whereas visceral layer of pericardium is insensitive to pain. Consequently pain of pericarditis originates from parietal pericardium.

Clinical correlation

- **Pericarditis and cardiac tamponade:** The inflammation of the serous pericardium is called *pericarditis* which causes accumulation of serous fluid in the pericardial cavity, the *pericardial effusion*. The excessive accumulation of serous fluid in the pericardial cavity may compress the thin-walled atria and interfere with the filling of the heart during diastole and consequently the cardiac output is diminished. This condition is clinically termed *cardiac tamponade*.

The *pericarditis* is the terminal event in uremia.

- **Pericardiocentesis:** Excessive pericardial fluid can be aspirated from the pericardial cavity by two routes:
  - *Sternal approach:* The needle is inserted through the left 5th or 6th intercostal space immediately adjacent to the sternum.
  - *Subxiphoid approach:* The needle is inserted in the left costoxiphoid angle and passed in an upward and backward direction at an angle of 45° to the skin.
- **Pericardial friction rub:** The roughening of parietal and visceral layers of the serous pericardium by inflammatory exudate can cause friction between the two layers called *pericardial friction rub* which can be felt on palpation and heard through the stethoscope.

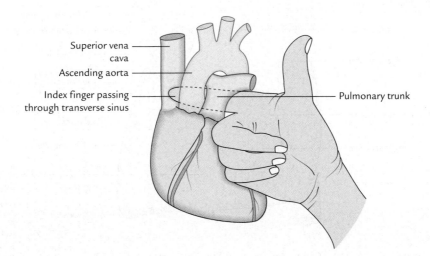

Superior vena cava
Ascending aorta
Index finger passing through transverse sinus
Pulmonary trunk

Fig. 20.5 Finger passing through the transverse pericardial sinus.

HEART

The heart (syn. Gk. *Kardia/Cardia*; L. *Cor/Cordis*) is a hollow muscular organ situated in the mediastinum of the thoracic cavity, enclosed in the pericardium. It is somewhat pyramidal in shape and placed obliquely behind the sternum and adjoining parts of costal cartilages so that one-third of the heart is to the right of median plane and two-third of the heart is to the left of the median plane.

The heart consists of four chambers—right atrium and right ventricle, and left atrium and left ventricle. On the surface the atria are separated from the ventricles by the atrioventricular groove (also called *coronary sulcus*) and ventricles from each other by interventricular grooves.

Shape and Measurements

Shape: Pyramidal or conical.
Measurements: Length = 12 cm.
Width = 9 cm.
Weight = 300 g in males; 250 g in females.

N.B. The heart is slightly larger than one's own clenched fist.

EXTERNAL FEATURES (Figs 20.6 and 20.7)

The heart presents the following external features:

1. Apex.
2. Base.
3. Three surfaces (sternocostal, diaphragmatic, and left)
4. Four borders (right, left, upper, and inferior).

APEX OF THE HEART

The apex of the heart is a conical area formed by left ventricle. It is directed downwards and forwards, and to the left. It lies at the level of the 5th left intercostal space, 3.5 inches (9 cm) from the midline and just medial to the midclavicular line.

Clinical correlation

Apex beat: It is the outermost and lowermost thrust of the cardiac contraction (during ventricular systole) felt on the front of the chest or it is the point of maximum cardiac impulse (**PMCI**). Normally the apex beat is felt as a light tap in left 5th intercostal space in the midclavicular line.

In infants, the heart is positioned more horizontally so that the apex of the heart lies in third or fourth left intercostal space and consequently the apex beat in children up to 7 years of age is felt in the third or fourth intercostal space just lateral to the midclavicular line.

N.B. Normally the apex of the heart is on the left side and apex beat is felt on the left side (left 5th intercostal space) but sometimes the heart is malpositioned with apex on the right side. This condition is called **dextrocardia**. It may be associated with complete reversal of thoracic and abdominal viscera, a condition called *situs inversus*.

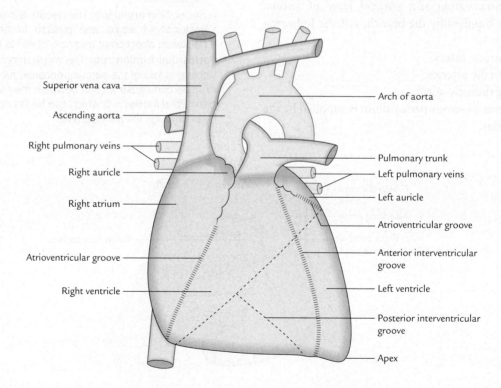

Superior vena cava — Arch of aorta

Ascending aorta — Pulmonary trunk

Right pulmonary veins — Left pulmonary veins

Right auricle — Left auricle

Right atrium — Atrioventricular groove

Atrioventricular groove — Anterior interventricular groove

Right ventricle — Left ventricle

— Posterior interventricular groove

— Apex

Fig. 20.6 Anterior aspect (sternocostal surface) of the heart. Note that the most of the sternocostal surface is formed by the right atrium and the right ventricle.

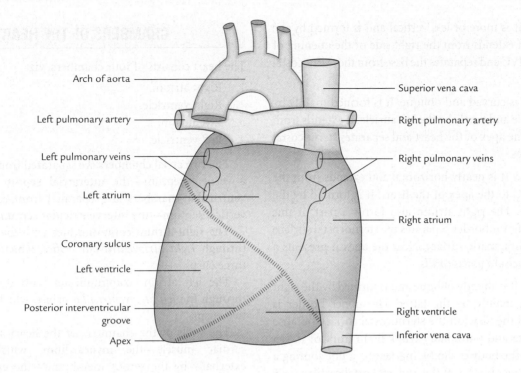

Fig. 20.7 Posterior aspect of the heart.

Labels on figure:
- Arch of aorta
- Left pulmonary artery
- Left pulmonary veins
- Left atrium
- Coronary sulcus
- Left ventricle
- Posterior interventricular groove
- Apex
- Superior vena cava
- Right pulmonary artery
- Right pulmonary veins
- Right atrium
- Right ventricle
- Inferior vena cava

BASE OF THE HEART

The base (or posterior surface) of the heart is formed by two atria, mainly by the left atrium. Strictly speaking two-third of the base is formed by the posterior surface of the left atrium and one-third by the posterior surface of the right atrium. It is directed backwards and to the right (i.e., opposite to the apex).

Characteristic features of the base are as follows:

1. It lies opposite to the apex.
2. It lies in front of the middle four thoracic vertebrae (i.e., T5–T8) in the lying-down position and descends one vertebra in the erect posture (T6–T9).
3. The base is separated from vertebral column by the oblique pericardial sinus, esophagus, and aorta.

N.B. Clinically, base is the upper border of the heart where great blood vessels (superior vena cava, ascending aorta, and pulmonary trunk) are attached.

SURFACES OF THE HEART

The heart has the following three surfaces:

1. Sternocostal (anterior).
2. Diaphragmatic (inferior).
3. Left surface.

Sternocostal surface: It is formed mainly by the right atrium and right ventricle, which are separated from each other by the anterior part of **atrioventricular groove**. The sternocostal surface is also partly formed by the left auricle and left ventricle. The right ventricle is separated from left ventricle by the **anterior interventricular groove**.

N.B.
- The left atrium is hidden on the front by the ascending aorta and pulmonary trunk.
- The part of sternocostal surface is uncovered by the left lung (cardiac notch) forming an *area of superficial cardiac dullness.*

Diaphragmatic surface: This surface is flat and rests on the central tendon of the diaphragm. It is formed by the left and right ventricles which are separated from each other by the posterior interventricular groove. The left ventricles form left two-third of this surface and right ventricle forms only right one-third of this surface.

Left surface: It is formed mainly by the left ventricle and partly by the left atrium and auricle. It is directed upwards, backwards, and to the left.

BORDERS OF THE HEART

The heart has the following four borders:

1. Right border.
2. Left border.
3. Inferior border.
4. Upper border.

Right border: It is more or less vertical and is formed by the right atrium. It extends from the right side of the opening of SVC to that of IVC and separates the base from the sternocostal surface.

Left border: It is curved and oblique. It is formed mainly by the left ventricle and partly by the left auricle. It extends from left auricle to the apex of the heart and separates sternocostal and left surfaces.

Inferior border: It is nearly horizontal and extends from the opening of IVC to the apex of the heart. It is formed by the right ventricle. The right atrium also forms a part of this border. The inferior border separates the sternocostal surface from the diaphragmatic surface. Near the apex it presents a notch called *incisura apicis cordis*.

Upper border: It is slightly oblique and is formed by the right and left atria, mainly by the latter. The upper border is obscured from the view on the sternocostal surface because ascending aorta and pulmonary trunk lie in front of it. On the surface of the body it can be marked by a line joining a point on the lower border of the 2nd left costal cartilage, 1.5 in from the median plane to a point on the upper border of 3rd right costal cartilage, 1 inch away from the median plane.

Clinical correlation

Cardiac shadow in chest radiograph: In X-ray of chest, PA view, the term cardiac-shadow is used for *mediastinal shadow*. The left border of cardiac shadow, from above downwards is formed by: aortic arch, pulmonary trunk, left auricle and left ventricle. The right border from above downwards is formed by SVC and right atrium (Fig. 20.8).

CHAMBERS OF THE HEART

The heart consists of four chambers, viz.

1. Right atrium.
2. Right ventricle.
3. Left atrium.
4. Left ventricle.

The two atrial chambers are separated from each other by a vertical septum—the **interatrial septum** and the two ventricular chambers are separated from each other by a vertical septum—the **interventricular septum**.

The right atrium communicates with the right ventricle through *right atrioventricular orifice*, which is guarded by three cusps.

The left atrium communicates with the left ventricle through the *left atrioventricular orifice*, which is guarded by two cusps.

The walls of the chambers of the heart are made up of cardiac muscle—the **myocardium**, which is covered externally by the serous membrane—the **epicardium** and lined internally by endothelium— the **endocardium**.

The atria are thin walled as compared to the ventricles and have little contractile power.

Demarcation of Chambers of the Heart on the Surface

On the surface the chambers of the heart are demarcated or delineated by the following three sulci/grooves (Figs 20.6 and 20.7):

1. Coronary sulcus (atrioventricular groove).
2. Anterior interventricular sulcus.
3. Posterior interventricular sulcus.

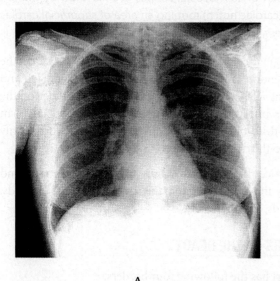

A

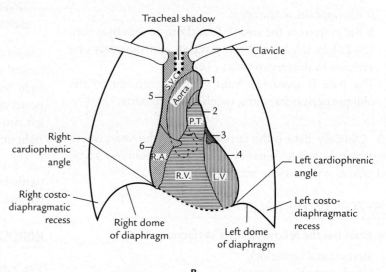

B

Fig. 20.8 X-ray chest PA view; **A**, actual radiograph; **B**, tracing of the cardiac shadow (1 = Aortic knuckle, 2 = Pulmonary conus, 3 = Left auricle, 4 = Left ventricle, 5 = Superior vena cava, 6 = Right atrium). (*Source: **A**, Fig. 4.1, Page 94, Integrated Anatomy, David JA Heylings, Roy AJ Spence, Barry E Kelly. Copyright Elsevier Limited 2007, All rights reserved. **B**; Fig. 3.19, Page 137, Clinical and Surgical Anatomy, 2e, Vishram Singh. Copyright Elsevier 2007, All rights reserved.*)

Coronary sulcus (atrioventricular groove): It encircles the heart and separates the atria from the ventricles. It is deficient anteriorly due to the root of pulmonary trunk.

The atrioventricular groove is divided into anterior and posterior parts.

The **anterior part** consists of right and left halves.

The right half of the anterior part runs downwards and to the right between the right atrium and right ventricle and lodges right coronary artery.

The left anterior part of AV groove intervenes between the left auricle and left ventricle. It lodges circumflex branch of left coronary artery.

The **posterior part of AV groove** intervenes between the base and the diaphragmatic surface of the heart. It lodges coronary sinus.

Anterior and posterior interventricular sulci: They separate the right and left ventricles. The anterior interventricular sulcus is on the sternocostal surface of the heart and lodges anterior interventricular artery and great cardiac vein. The posterior interventricular groove is on the diaphragmatic surface and lodges posterior interventricular artery and middle cardiac vein.

N.B. The meeting point of interatrial groove, posterior interventricular groove, and posterior part of atrioventricular groove is termed **crux of the heart**.

Circulation of Blood

Functionally, the heart is made up of two muscular pumps— the right and left (Fig. 20.9). The **right pump** consists of right atrium and right ventricle while the **left pump** consists of left atrium and left ventricle. The right pump is responsible for **pulmonary circulation** and the left pump is responsible for **systemic circulation** as follows:

- The right atrium receives deoxygenated blood from the whole body through superior and inferior venae cavae. The blood flows from right atrium into right ventricle through *right atrioventricular orifice*. The blood is prevented from regurgitating back to the atrium by means of *right atrioventricular valve*. The right ventricle contracts and propels the blood into the pulmonary trunk, pulmonary arteries, and finally into the lung where blood is oxygenated (*pulmonary circulation*).

- The left atrium receives the oxygenated blood from lungs through four pulmonary veins. The blood from left

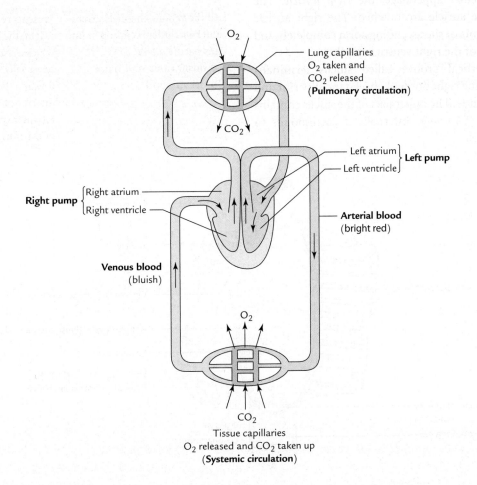

Fig. 20.9 Heart as double pump.

atrium flows into left ventricle through *left atrioventricular orifice*. The blood is prevented from regurgitating back to the atrium by means of *left atrioventricular valve*. The left ventricle strongly contracts and propels the blood into the ascending aorta and then into the systemic circulation.

N.B. The right ventricle is required to pump the blood through a relatively low-resistance vascular bed, whereas the left ventricle is required to pump the blood through a relatively high resistance peripheral vascular bed.

The muscular wall of the left ventricle is, therefore, much thicker than that of the right ventricle.

RIGHT ATRIUM

The right atrium is somewhat quadrilateral chamber situated behind and to the right side of the right ventricle. It consists of a main **cavity** and a small outpouching called **auricle**.

External Features

1. The right atrium is elongated vertically and receives superior vena cava (SVC) at its upper end and the inferior vena cava (IVC) at its lower end.
2. The upper anterior part is prolonged to the left to form the right auricular appendage, the *right auricle*. The margins of the auricle are notched. The right auricle overlaps the roots of the ascending aorta completely and infundibulum of the right ventricle partly.
3. A shallow vertical groove called **sulcus terminalis** extends along the right border between the superior and inferior vena cavae. The upper part of the sulcus contains the *sinuatrial (SA) node*. Internally it corresponds to crista terminalis.

4. The vertical right atrioventricular groove lodges the right coronary artery and the small cardiac vein.

Internal Features (Fig. 20.10)

The interior of the right atrium is divided into two parts: (a) main smooth posterior part – the **sinus venarum**, and (b) rough anterior part – the **atrium proper**. The two parts are separated from each other by **crista terminalis**. The differences between these two parts are enumerated in Table 20.2. The interior of right atrium also presents septal wall of the right atrium.

Septal wall of the right atrium: Developmentally it is derived from septum primum and septum secundum. The septal wall when viewed from within the right atrium presents the following features:

Table 20.2 Differences between the smooth and rough parts of the right atrium

Smooth part (sinus venarum)	Rough part (atrium proper)
Developmentally it is derived from right horn of the sinus venosus	Developmentally it is derived from primitive atrium
All the venous channels *except* anterior cardiac veins open into this part (e.g., SVC, IVC, coronary sinus, and venae cordae minimi)	Presents series of transverse ridges, the musculi pectinati, which arise from the *crista terminalis* and run forwards towards the auricle. The interior of auricle presents reticular sponge-like network of the muscular ridges

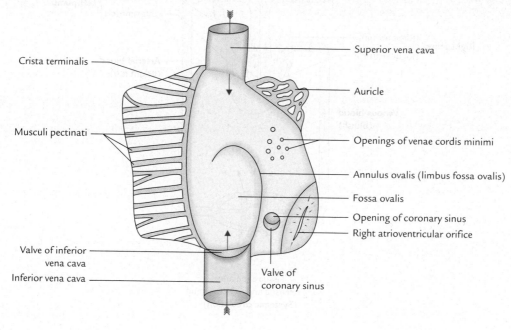

Crista terminalis

Musculi pectinati

Valve of inferior vena cava

Inferior vena cava

Superior vena cava

Auricle

Openings of venae cordis minimi

Annulus ovalis (limbus fossa ovalis)

Fossa ovalis

Opening of coronary sinus

Right atrioventricular orifice

Valve of coronary sinus

Fig. 20.10 Interior of the right atrium.

1. **Fossa ovalis**, a shallow oval/saucer-shaped depression in the lower part, formed by septum primum. It represents the site of **foramen ovale in the foetus.**
2. **Annulus ovalis/limbus fossa ovalis**, forms the distinct upper and lateral margin of the fossa ovalis. It represents the free edge of the *septum secundum*. Inferiorly the annulus ovalis is continuous with the left end of the valve of IVC.
3. **Triangle of Koch**, a triangular area bounded in front by the base of septal leaflet of tricuspid valve, behind by anterior margin of the opening of coronary sinus and above by the tendon of Todaro—a subendocardial ridge. The atrioventricular node lies in this triangle.
4. **Torus aorticus**, an elevation in the anterosuperior part of the septum produced due to bulging of the right posterior (non-coronary) sinus of ascending aorta.

Clinical correlation

The sponge-like interior of right auricle prevents the free flow of blood and thus favors the formation of thrombus. The thrombi may dislodge during auricular fibrillation and may cause pulmonary embolism.

Opening into the Right Atrium

There are number of openings in the right atrium. These are as follows (Fig. 20.10):

1. **Opening of SVC:** The SVC opens at the upper end of the right atrium and has no valve. It returns the blood to the heart from the upper half of the body.
2. **Opening of IVC:** The IVC opens at the lower end of the right atrium close to the interatrial septum. It is guarded by a rudimentary non-functioning semilunar valve called **valve of the inferior vena cava/Eustachian valve.**

N.B. During embryonic life, the Eustachian valve guides the blood of IVC to the left atrium through foramen ovale. The IVC returns the blood to the heart from the lower half of the body. A very small projection called **intervenous tubercle (of Lower)** is scarcely visible on the posterior wall of the right atrium just below the opening of SVC. During embryonic life it directs the blood of SVC to the right ventricle.

3. **Opening of coronary sinus:** The coronary sinus, which drains most of the blood from the heart, opens into the right atrium between the openings of IVC and right atrioventricular orifice. It is also guarded by a rudimentary non-functioning valve, **Thebesian valve.**
4. **Right atrioventricular orifice (largest opening):** It communicates the right atrial chamber with the right ventricular chamber. It lies anterior to the opening of IVC and is guarded by the **tricuspid valve.**
5. **Many small orifices of small veins:** These are the opening of venae cordis minimae (Thebesian veins) and anterior cardiac veins.

RIGHT VENTRICLE

The right ventricle is the thick-walled triangular chamber of the heart which communicates with the right atrium through *right atrioventricular orifice* and with the pulmonary trunk through *pulmonary orifice.*

External Features

1. It forms the most of *sternocostal surface* and small part of the *diaphragmatic surface* of the heart. It also forms the inferior border.
2. It is separated from the right atrium by a more or less vertical anterior part of the coronary sulcus/atrioventricular groove.

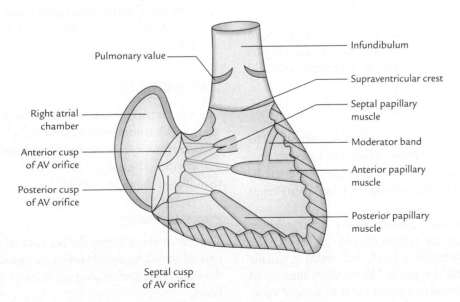

Fig. 20.11 Main features in the interior of right ventricle (AV = atrioventricular).

Labels: Pulmonary value, Right atrial chamber, Anterior cusp of AV orifice, Posterior cusp of AV orifice, Septal cusp of AV orifice, Infundibulum, Supraventricular crest, Septal papillary muscle, Moderator band, Anterior papillary muscle, Posterior papillary muscle.

Table 20.3 Differences of inflowing and outflowing parts of the right ventricle

Inflowing lower part	Outflowing upper part
It develops from primitive ventricle	It develops from bulbus cordis
It is large in size and lies below the supraventricular crest	It is small in size and lies above the supraventricular crest
It is rough due to presence of the muscular ridges—the *trabeculae carneae*. It forms most of the right ventricular chamber	It is smooth and forms upper 1 inch conical part of the right ventricular chamber—the infundibulum, which gives rise to pulmonary trunk

Internal Features (Fig. 20.11)

1. The interior of right ventricle consists of two parts: (a) a large, lower rough inflowing part, and (b) a small upper outflowing part, the **infundibulum**. The two parts are separated from each other by a muscular ridge, the **supraventricular crest** (**infundibuloventricular crest**). The differences of two parts are enumerated in Table 20.3.
2. The cavity of right ventricle is flattened by the forward bulge of the interventricular septum. In transverse section it is crescent shaped (Fig. 20.13).
3. The wall of the right ventricle is thinner than that of the left ventricle (ratio 1:3).

Trabeculae Carneae of Right Ventricular Chamber

These are muscular projections which give the ventricular chamber a sponge-like appearance.

Types of Trabeculae Carneae

Trabeculae carneae are of three types: (a) *ridges* (fixed elevations), (b) *bridges* (only ends are fixed, the central part is free), and (c) *pillars* (base is fixed to ventricular wall and apex is free).

Papillary muscles

These represent the pillars of trabeculae carneae. The papillary muscles project inwards. Their bases are attached to the ventricular wall and their apices are connected by thread-like fibrous cords (the **chordae tendinae**) to the cusps of the tricuspid valve.

There are three papillary muscles in the right ventricle: (a) anterior, (b) posterior (inferior), and (c) septal. The anterior is largest, posterior is small, and septal is usually divided into two or three nipples. The papillary muscles of right ventricle are attached to the cusps of the tricuspid valve.

Moderator band (septomarginal trabeculum)

It is thick muscular ridge extending from ventricular septum to the base of the anterior papillary muscle, across the ventricular cavity. It conveys the *right branch of the atrioventricular bundle* (*bundle of His*), a part of conducting system of the heart. It prevents the over distension of right ventricle.

LEFT ATRIUM

External Features

1. It is a thin-walled quadrangular chamber situated posteriorly behind and to the left side of right atrium. It forms greater part (left 2/3rd) of the base of the heart.
2. Its upper end is prolonged anteriorly to form the left auricle, which overlaps the infundibulum of right ventricle.
3. Behind the left atrium lies: (a) oblique sinus of serous pericardium and (b) fibrous pericardium, which separates it from the esophagus.

Internal Features

1. The interior of left atrium is smooth, but the left auricle possesses muscular ridges in the form of reticulum.
2. The anterior wall of left atrial cavity presents **fossa lunata**, which corresponds to the **fossa ovalis** of the right atrium.

Openings in the Left Atrium

Openings in the left atrium are as follows:

1. Openings of four pulmonary veins in its posterior wall, two on each side. They have no valves.
2. Number of small openings of venae cordis minimae.
3. Left atrioventricular orifice. It is guarded by the mitral valve.

LEFT VENTRICLE

The left ventricle is thick-walled triangular chamber of the heart which communicates with the left atrium through *left atrioventricular orifice* and with the ascending aorta through *aortic orifice*. The walls of left ventricle are three times thicker than that of the right ventricle.

External Features

The left ventricle forms the (a) apex of the heart, (b) small part of the sternocostal surface, (c) most of the (left 2/3rd) diaphragmatic surface, and (d) most of the left border of the heart.

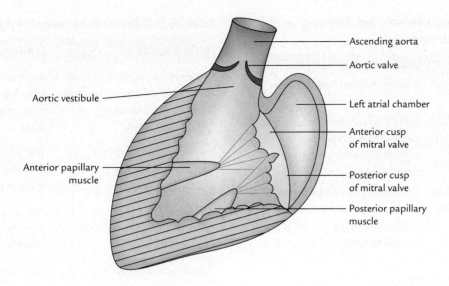

Fig. 20.12 Main features in the interior of left ventricle.

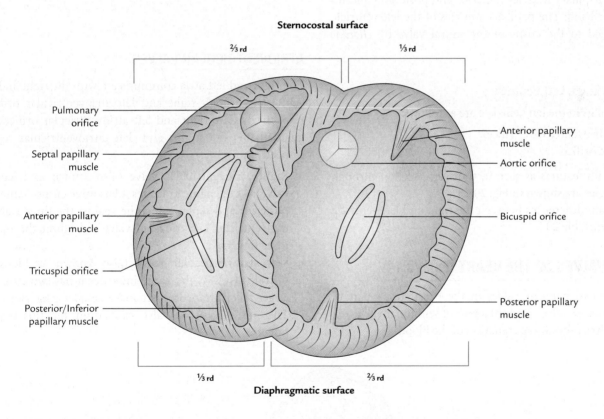

Fig. 20.13 Transverse section across the ventricles of the heart. Note the difference in the thickness of the wall and shape of the right and left ventricular cavities.

Internal Features (Fig. 20.12)

The interior of the left ventricle is divided into two parts: (a) a large lower rough inflowing part, and (b) a small upper smooth outflowing part—the **aortic vestibule**.

The differences between these two parts are enumerated in Table 20.4.

The cavity of the left ventricle is circular in cross section because the interventricular septum bulges into the right ventricle.

Table 20.4 Differences between the inflowing and outflowing parts of the left ventricle

Inflowing part	Outflowing part
It develops from primitive ventricle	It develops from bulbus cordis
It lies below the aortic vestibule	It lies between the membranous part of the interventricular septum and anterior cusp of the mitral valve
It is rough due to presence of trabeculae carneae and forms most of the left ventricular chamber	It is smooth and forms smooth small upper part—the aortic vestibule, which gives rise to the ascending aorta

Trabeculae Carneae of Left Ventricle

The trabeculae carneae of the left ventricle are similar to those of the right ventricle but are well developed and present two large papillary muscles (anterior and posterior) and no moderator band. The papillary muscles of the left ventricle are attached to the cusps of the mitral valve by *chordae tendinae*.

Openings in the Left Ventricle

The openings in the left ventricle are as follows:

1. Left atrioventricular orifice.
2. Aortic orifice.

The main features as seen in transverse section through the ventricles are shown in Fig. 20.13.

The main differences between the right and left ventricle are listed in Table 20.5.

VALVES OF THE HEART (Fig. 20.14)

There are two pairs of valves in the heart: (a) a pair of atrioventricular valves, and (b) a pair of semilunar valves.

The valves prevent regurgitation of the blood.

Table 20.5 Differences between the right and left ventricles

Right ventricle	Left ventricle
Receives deoxygenated blood from right atrium and pumps it to the lungs through pulmonary trunk	Receives oxygenated blood from left atrium and pumps it to the whole body through aorta
Wall of right ventricle is thinner than that of left ventricle (ratio 1:3)	Wall of left ventricle is thicker than that of right ventricle (ratio 3:1)
Possesses three papillary muscles (anterior, posterior, and septal)	Possesses two papillary muscles (anterior and posterior)
Moderator band present	Moderator band absent
Cavity of right ventricle is crescentic in shape in cross section	Cavity of left ventricle is circular in shape in cross section

ATRIOVENTRICULAR VALVES

The right and left atria communicate with the right and left ventricles through right and left atrioventricular orifices, respectively. The right and left atrioventricular orifices are guarded by the right and left atrioventricular valves respectively.

- **Right atrioventricular valve** (also known as **tricuspid valve**): As the name indicates it has three cusps—anterior, posterior and septal, which lie against the three walls of the ventricle. The tricuspid valve can admit the tips of three fingers.
- **Left atrioventricular valve** (also known as **bicuspid/mitral valve**). As the name indicates it has two cusps—a larger anterior/aortic cusp and a smaller posterior cusp. The mitral/bicuspid valve can admit the tips of two fingers.

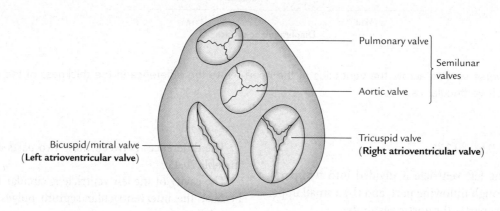

Fig. 20.14 The valves of the heart.

Structure

The atrioventricular valves are made up of two components (Fig. 20.15):

1. A fibrous ring.
2. Cusps.

The fibrous rings surround the orifice. The cusps are formed by the fold of the endocardium enclosing some connective tissue within it. Each cusp has an attached and free margin and atrial and ventricular surfaces. The atrial surfaces are smooth. The ventricular surfaces and free margins are rough and provide attachment to the chordae tendinae. As discussed earlier, the chordae tendinae connect the apices of papillary muscles with margins and ventricular surfaces of the cusps. *The chordae tendinae of each papillary muscle are attached to the contiguous halves of the two cusps.*

The valves are closed during ventricular systole. The papillary muscles shorten and chordae tendinae are pulled upon to prevent the eversion of the cusps of tricuspid valve due to increased intraventricular pressure.

N.B.

- The nutrition to the fibrous ring and basal one-third of cusps is provided by the blood vessels.
- The nutrition to the distal two-third of the cusps is provided directly by the blood within the chambers of the heart.
- The cusps of mitral valve are smaller but thicker than those of tricuspid valve.

Clinical correlation

Role of papillary muscle in acute cardiac failure: The papillary muscles prevent the prolapse of atrio-ventricular valves into the atria during ventricular systole. The rupture of a papillary muscle, following an adjacent myocardial infarction, will allow the prolapse of the affected cusp to occur into the atrium at each systole. This will consequently lead to **acute cardiac failure**.

SEMILUNAR VALVES (Fig. 20.16)

The right and left ventricles pump out blood through pulmonary and aortic orifices, respectively. Each of these orifices is guarded by three semilunar cusps hence they are called *semilunar valves*. Both aortic and pulmonary valves are similar to each other in structure and functions.

Each valve has three cusps which are attached directly to the wall of aorta/pulmonary trunk. (Note that they do not have fibrous ring similar to tricuspid and mitral valves.)

The cusps form small pockets with their mouths directed upwards towards the lumen of great vessels. Each cusp has a **fibrous nodule** at the midpoint of its free edge. On each side of the **nodule** the thickened crescentic edge is called **lunule**, which extends up to the base. When the valve is closed, the nodules meet in the center.

The cusps of semilunar valves are open and stretched during ventricular systole and closed during ventricular diastole to prevent regurgitation of the blood into the ventricle.

N.B.

- No chordae tendinae or papillary muscles are associated with semilunar valves. The attachment of the sides of cusps to the atrial wall prevents regurgitation of blood.
- Opposite to the cusps, the roots of pulmonary trunk and ascending aorta present three dilatations called sinuses. The blood in these sinuses prevents the cusps from sticking to the wall of great vessels. The anterior aortic sinus gives origin to the right coronary artery and left posterior aortic sinus gives origin to the left coronary artery.

Positions of Cusps in the Pulmonary and Aortic Valves

The positions of cusps of pulmonary valves are: (a) right anterior, (b) left anterior, and (c) posterior.

The positions of cusps of aortic valve are just opposite to those of the pulmonary valve. They are: (a) right posterior, (b) left posterior, and (c) anterior.

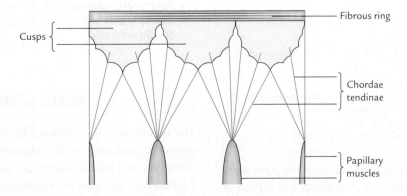

Fig. 20.15 Right atrioventricular (tricuspid) valve spread out to show its structure.

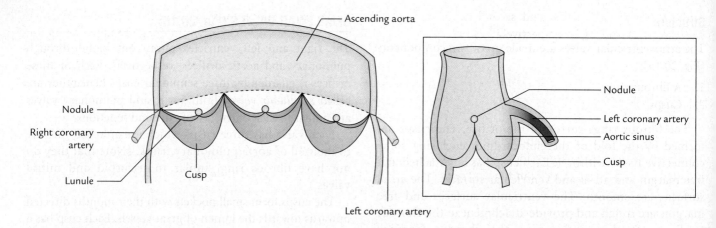

Fig. 20.16 Structure of aortic valve. Note that it consists of three semilunar cusps. Each cusp has a fibrous nodule at the midpoint of its free edge. The thickened crescentic edge on each side of nodule is the lunule (L. luna = moon). Inset figure on right side shows aortic sinus and origin of coronary artery.

The aortic sinuses are also named accordingly, i.e., right posterior aortic sinus, left posterior aortic sinus, and anterior aortic sinus. The right coronary artery arises from anterior aortic sinus and left coronary from left posterior aortic sinus. Since no coronary artery arises from right posterior aortic sinus, it is referred to by some anatomists as *non-coronary sinus.*

N.B. Embryologically, pulmonary valve has anterior, right and left cusps whereas aortic valve has posterior, right and left cusps (Fig. 20.17). Thus the left coronary artery arises from the left aortic sinus, the right coronary artery from the right aortic sinus and no artery arises from the posterior aortic sinus (**non-coronary sinus**).

Clinical correlation

- **Murmurs:** The abnormal heart sounds are called murmurs. They are produced due to regurgitation of blood heard when the valves are either stenosed or when the valves are not closed properly (leading to regurgitation).

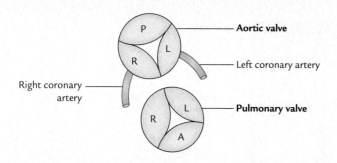

Fig. 20.17 Embryological position of cusps in the pulmonary and aortic valves (P = posterior, A = anterior, R = right, L = left).

- In aortic and pulmonary stenosis the murmur is heard during systole and in insufficiency of these valves they are heard during diastole.
- In stenosis of mitral and tricuspid valves, the murmurs are heard during diastole and in their insufficiency during systole.
- **Mitral stenosis (narrowing of mitral orifice):** It is most common in young age. Usually there is *history* of rheumatic fever in the childhood in these cases. This leads to rise in the left atrial pressure and enlargement of left atrium which may press on the esophagus.

Clinically features of mitral stenosis will be as follows:

1. Shortness of breath (dyspnea).
2. Dysphagia (difficulty in swallowing).
3. Hoarseness of voice (Ortner's syndrome).

- **Tricuspid stenosis:** In tricuspid stenosis blood flow from right atrium to right ventricle is reduced. *The* elevation of right atrial pressure leads to systemic venous congestion and right heart failure.
- **Aortic stenosis:** In aortic stenosis there accumulation of blood in left ventricle, causing its *dilatation* and hypertrophy. There is low cardiac output which may manifest as syncope (fainting) on exertion.
- **Pulmonary stenosis:** It is almost always congenital, usually a part of Fallot's tetralogy. It leads to *hypertrophy* of right ventricle.

HEART SOUNDS

The two sounds are produced by the heart—the **first heart sound** is produced by the closure of the atrioventricular (tricuspid and mitral) valves and the **second heart sound** is produced by the closure of semilunar (aortic and pulmonary) valves. These sounds are heard by the clinician by auscultation with stethoscope. The first and second heart sounds are heard as 'LUB' and 'DUB', respectively.

SURFACE MARKINGS OF THE CARDIAC VALVES AND AUSCULTATORY AREAS (Fig. 20.18)

The sounds produced by closure of valves of the heart are best heard not directly over the location of valve but at areas situated some distance away from the valve in the direction of blood flow through them.

The pulmonary, aortic, mitral, and tricuspid valves are located posterior to the sternum on an oblique line joining the 3rd left costal cartilage to the 6th right costal cartilage.

The position of valves on the surface of the chest and sites of their auscultatory areas are given in Table 20.6 and shown in Figure 20.19.

N.B. Blood tends to carry the sound in the direction of its flow, consequently auscultatory area is located superficial to the vessel or chamber through which the blood passes and is in direct line with the valve orifice.

Table 20.6 Surface markings of the cardiac valves and the sites of their auscultatory areas

Valve	Surface marking	Site of auscultator area
Pulmonary valve	A horizontal line (2.5 cm long) behind the medial end left 3rd costal cartilage and adjoining part of the sternum	Second left intercostal space near the sternum
Aortic valve	A lightly oblique line (2.5 cm long) behind the left half of the sternum opposite the 3rd intercostal space	Second right intercostal space near the sternum
Mitral valve	An oblique line (3 cm long) behind the left half of the sternum opposite the left 4th costal cartilage	Left 5th intercostal space 3½ inches (9 cm) from midline, i.e., over apex beat
Tricuspid valve	Nearly vertical oblique line (4 cm long) behind the right half of the sternum opposite the 4th and 5th intercostal spaces	Right half of the lower end of the body of the sternum

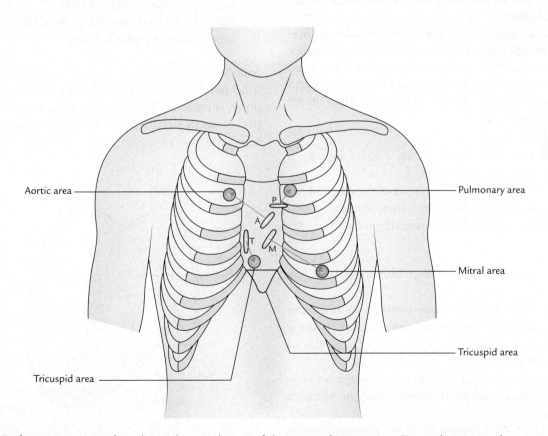

Fig. 20.18 Surface projection of cardiac valves and sites of their auscultatory areas (P = pulmonary valve, A = aortic valve, T = tricuspid valve, M = mitral valve).

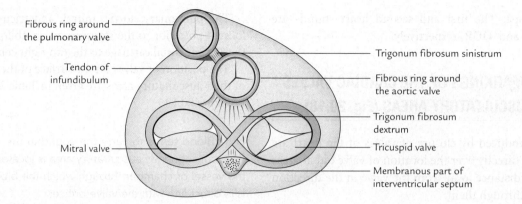

Fig. 20.19 Skeleton of the heart.

Labels in figure:
- Fibrous ring around the pulmonary valve
- Tendon of infundibulum
- Mitral valve
- Trigonum fibrosum sinistrum
- Fibrous ring around the aortic valve
- Trigonum fibrosum dextrum
- Tricuspid valve
- Membranous part of interventricular septum

SKELETON OF THE HEART (Fig. 20.19)

The so called '*skeleton of the heart*' is composed of fibrous tissue and forms the central support of the heart. It consists of fibrous rings that surround the atrioventricular, pulmonary, and aortic orifices. These rings provide circular form and rigidity to the atrioventricular orifices and roots of the aorta and pulmonary trunk. They also provide attachment to the valves and prevent dilatation of these orifices. The cardiac valves are firmly attached to this skeleton. The cardiac skeleton along with membranous part of interventricular septum also provides attachments to the cardiac muscle fibres.

The fibrous rings around the atrioventricular orifices separate the muscle fibres of atria from those of the ventricles, but provide attachment to these fibres. Thus there is no muscular continuity between the atria and ventricles, except for the atria ventricular bundle (**bundle of His**) of the conducting system.

Functional significance:

1. The skeleton of the heart allows cardiac muscle to contract against the rigid base.
2. The fibrous rings support the bases of the cusps of the valves and prevent the valves from stretching and becoming incompetent. The aortic ring is the strongest.

N.B.

- The atrioventricular fibrous rings (AV rings) form the figure of '8'.
- The large mass of fibrous tissue between AV rings and aortic ring is called *trigonum fibrosum dextrum*. In some mammals such as sheep, elephant, etc. a bone—the *os cordis* develops in it.
- The small mass of fibrous tissue between the fibrous rings around semilunar valves is called *trigonum fibrosum sinistrum*.
- The tendon of infundibulum binds the posterior surface of the infundibulum to the aortic ring.

CONDUCTING SYSTEM OF THE HEART (Fig. 20.20)

COMPONENTS

The conducting system of the heart is made up of specialized cardiac muscle fibres (not nervous tissue) and is responsible for initiation and conduction of **cardiac impulse.**

The conducting system of the heart consists of the following five components:

1. Sinuatrial node (SA node).
2. Atrioventricular node (AV node).
3. Atrioventricular bundle (of His).
4. Right and left branches of bundle of His.
5. Subendocardial Purkinje fibres.

Sinuatrial node (SA node or node of Keith Flack): It is a small horseshoe-shaped mass having specialized myocardial fibres, situated in the wall of the right atrium in the upper part of sulcus terminalis just below the opening of superior vena cava.

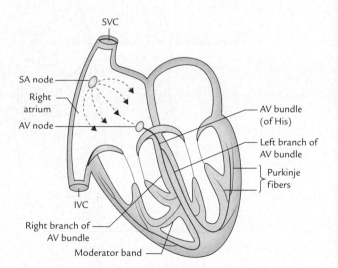

Labels in figure:
- SVC
- SA node
- Right atrium
- AV node
- IVC
- Right branch of AV bundle
- Moderator band
- AV bundle (of His)
- Left branch of AV bundle
- Purkinje fibers

Fig. 20.20 Conducting system of the heart (SA = sinuatrial, AV = atrioventricular).

It is known as **pacemaker of the heart** because it generates impulses (about 70/minute) and initiates the contraction of cardiac muscle producing heart beat.

Atrioventricular node (AV node/node of Tawara): It is smaller than the SA node and is located in the lower part of the atrial septum, just above the attachment of septal cusp of the tricuspid valve/opening of the coronary sinus. It conducts the *cardiac impulse* to the ventricle by the *atrioventricular bundle*. The AV node is capable of generating impulses at the rate of about 60/min. The speed of conduction of cardiac impulse (about 0.11 sec) provides sufficient time to the atria to empty their blood into the ventricle before ventricles start contracting.

Atrioventricular bundle (of His): It begins from AV node, crosses the AV ring and runs along the inferior part of the membranous part of the interventricular septum where it divides into the left and right branches.

N.B. Since the skeleton (fibrous framework) of the heart separates the muscles of atria from the muscles of *the ventricles, the bundle of His is the only means of conducting impulses from the atria to the ventricles.*

Right and left branches of the bundle (of His): The *right branch* passes down the right side of the interventricular septum and then becomes subendocardial on the right side of the septum. A large part of it continues in the septomarginal trabeculum (**moderator band**) to reach the anterior papillary muscle and anterior wall of the ventricle. Its Purkinje fibres then spread out beneath the endocardium.

The *left branch* descends on the left side of the ventricular septum, divides into Purkinje fibres which are distributed to the septum and left ventricle.

Purkinje fibres: They are the terminal branches of right and left branches of the bundle of His and spread subendocardially over the septum and the rest of the ventricular wall.

The conducting system and mode of contraction of cardiac muscle is summarized as follows:

The SA node (a spontaneous source of cardiac impulse) initiates an impulse which rapidly spreads to the muscle fibres of the atria, making them to contract. The AV node picks up the cardiac impulse from atria and conducts it through atrioventricular bundle and its branches to the papillary muscles and the walls of the ventricles. The papillary muscles contract first, to tighten the chordae tendinae and then the contraction of ventricular muscle occurs.

Arterial Supply of the Conducting System

The whole of the conducting system of the heart is supplied by the right coronary artery except a part of the left branch of the AV bundle which is supplied by the left coronary artery.

Clinical correlation

Conducting system defects: The defect/damage of conducting system causes cardiac arrhythmias.

The SA node is the spontaneous source of generation of cardiac impulses. The AV node picks up these impulses from atria and sends them to the ventricles through AV bundle, the only means through which impulses can spread from the atria to ventricles.

If the AV bundle fails to conduct normal impulses, there occurs alteration in the rhythmic contraction of the ventricles (arrhythmias). If complete bundle block occurs there is complete dissociation in the rate of contraction of atria and ventricles. The commonest cause of defective conduction through AV bundle is atherosclerosis of the coronary arteries which leads to diminished blood supply to the conducting system.

N.B. The rapid pulse is called *tachycardia*, the slow pulse is called *bradycardia* whereas irregular pulse is called *arrhythmia*.

ARTERIAL SUPPLY OF THE HEART (Fig. 20.21)

The heart is mostly supplied by the two coronary arteries, which arise from the ascending aorta immediately above the aortic valve.

The coronary arteries and their branches run on the surface of heart lying within the subpericardial fibrofatty tissue.

N.B.

- Coronary arteries are *vasa vasorum* of the ascending aorta.
- Anatomically coronary arteries are not end-arteries but functionally they behave like end-arteries.

RIGHT CORONARY ARTERY

Origin

The right coronary artery arises from the *anterior aortic sinus* of the ascending aorta, immediately above the aortic valve.

Course

After arising from the ascending aorta, the right coronary artery first runs forwards between the pulmonary trunk and the right auricle, and then it descends almost vertically in the right atrioventricular groove (right anterior coronary sulcus) up to the junction of the right and the inferior borders of the heart. At the inferior border of the heart, it turns posteriorly and runs in the posterior atrioventricular groove (right posterior coronary sulcus) up to the posterior interventricular

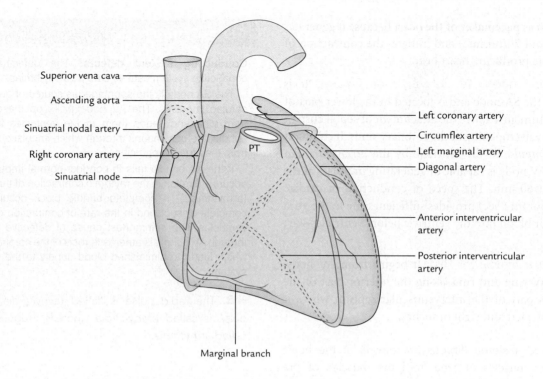

Superior vena cava

Ascending aorta

Sinuatrial nodal artery

Right coronary artery

Sinuatrial node

PT

Left coronary artery

Circumflex artery

Left marginal artery

Diagonal artery

Anterior interventricular artery

Posterior interventricular artery

Marginal branch

Fig. 20.21 Arterial supply of the heart (PT = pulmonary trunk).

groove where it terminates by anastomosing with the left coronary artery.

Branches and Distribution

1. **Right conus artery:** It supplies the anterior surface of the pulmonary conus (infundibulum of the right ventricle).
2. **Atrial branches:** They supply the atria. One of the atrial branches—the *artery of sinuatrial node* (also called *sinuatrial nodal artery*) supplies the SA node in 60% cases. In 40% of individuals it arises from the left coronary artery.
3. **Anterior ventricular branches:** They are two or three and supply the anterior surface of the right ventricle. The *marginal branch* is the largest and runs along the lower margin of the sternocostal surface to reach the apex.
4. **Posterior ventricular branches:** They are usually two and supply the diaphragmatic surface of the right ventricle.
5. **Posterior interventricular artery:** It runs in the posterior interventricular groove up to the apex. It supplies the:
   (a) posterior part of the interventricular septum,
   (b) atrioventricular node (AV node) in 60% of the cases, and
   (c) right and left ventricles.

N.B. In 10% individuals, the posterior interventricular artery arises from the left coronary artery.

LEFT CORONARY ARTERY

Origin
The left coronary artery arises from the *left posterior aortic sinus* of the ascending aorta, immediately above the aortic valve.

Course
After arising from ascending aorta, the left coronary artery runs forwards and to the left between the pulmonary trunk and the left auricle. It then divides into an anterior interventricular and circumflex artery. The **anterior interventricular artery** (left anterior descending/LAD) runs downwards in the anterior interventricular groove to the apex of the heart. It then passes posteriorly around the apex of the heart to enter the posterior interventricular groove to terminate by anastomosing with the **posterior interventricular artery**—a branch of the right coronary artery.

The **circumflex artery** winds around the left margin of the heart and continues in the left posterior coronary sulcus up to the posterior interventricular groove where it terminates by anastomosing with the right coronary artery.

Branches and Distribution

1. **Anterior interventricular artery/left anterior descending (LAD) artery:** It supplies (a) anterior part of interventricular septum, (b) greater part of the left ventricle and part of right ventricle, and (c) a part of left bundle branch (of His).

Table 20.7 Major branches of the right and left coronary arteries

Right coronary artery	Left coronary artery
Right marginal artery	Anterior interventricular artery
Posterior interventricular artery	Circumflex artery
Sinuatrial nodal artery	Diagonal artery

2. **Circumflex artery:** It gives a *left marginal artery* that supplies the left margin of the left ventricle up to the apex of the heart.
3. **Diagonal artery:** It may arise directly from the trunk of the left coronary artery.
4. **Conus artery:** It supplies the pulmonary conus.
5. **Atrial branches:** They supply the left atrium.

The major branches of the right and left coronary arteries are summarized in Table 20.7.

VARIATIONS IN THE CORONARY ARTERIES/ CORONARY DOMINANCE

The origin, course, and distribution of the posterior interventricular artery are variable.

In **right coronary dominance**, the posterior interventricular artery is a branch of the right coronary artery. It is found in 90% of the individuals.

In **left coronary dominance**, the posterior interventricular artery arises from circumflex branch of the left coronary artery. It is found in 10% of the individuals.

ANASTOMOSES OF THE CORONARY ARTERIES

Anastomoses exist between the terminal branches of the coronary arteries at the arteriolar level (collateral circulation). The time factor in occlusion of an artery is very important. If occlusion occurs slowly, there is time for the healthy arterioles to open up and collateral circulation is established, i.e., the anastomoses become functional. But if sudden occlusion of one of the large branches (coronary artery) occurs, the arterioles do not get time to open up to provide collateral circulation.

Clinical correlation

- **Angina pectoris:** If the coronary arteries are narrowed, the blood supply to the cardiac muscles is reduced. As a result, on exertion, the patient feels moderately severe pain in the region of left precordium that may last as long as 20 minutes. The pain is often referred to the left shoulder and medial side of the arm and forearm.

  In angina pectoris pain occurs on exertion and relieved by rest. This is because the coronary arteries are so narrowed that the ischemia of cardiac muscle occurs only on exertion.

- **Myocardial infarction (MI):** A sudden block of one of the larger branches of either coronary artery usually leads to myocardial ischemia followed by the myocardial necrosis (myocardial infarction). The part of heart suffering from MI stops functioning and often causes death. This condition is termed *heart attack* or *coronary attack*.

  The clinical features of MI are as follows:
  1. A sensation of pressure/sinking and pain in the chest that lasts longer than 30 minutes.
  2. Nausea or vomiting, sweating, shortness of breath, and tachycardia.
  3. Pain radiates to the medial side of the arm, forearm, and hand. Sometimes, it may be referred to jaw or neck.

- **Sites of coronary artery occlusion:** The three most common sites of the coronary artery occlusion are as under:
  (a) Anterior interventricular artery/left anterior descending (LAD) artery = 40–50%.
  (b) Right coronary artery = 30–40%.
  (c) Circumflex branch of the left coronary artery = 15–20%.

  Note:
  – The MI mostly occurs at rest whereas angina occurs on exertion.
  – Anterior interventricular artery/left anterior descending (LAD) artery is most commonly blocked.

- **Coronary angiography:** The coronary angiography is a radiological procedure to visualize the coronary arteries after injecting contrast medium in their lumen (Fig. 20.22). The coronary angiography is useful in localizing the sites of the blocks in the coronary arteries.

- **Coronary bypass surgery:** The coronary bypass surgery has become common in recent times in patients with unstable/severe angina due to obstruction of the coronary artery. A segment of a vein or an artery is connected to the ascending aorta (or to the proximal part of the coronary artery) and then to coronary artery distal to the obstruction (Fig. 20.23). A coronary bypass graft shunts blood from the aorta to coronary artery distal to the blockage to increase the circulation.

N.B.
- The great saphenous vein is commonly used for grafting because (a) it is easily dissected, (b) it has diameter equal to or greater than that of coronary artery, and (c) it provides lengthy portions with a minimum occurrence of valves or branching.
- The use of left internal mammary artery graft (**LIMA graft**) and radial artery graft (**RA graft**) have also become increasingly common.

- **Coronary angioplasty:** In this process the cardiologists pass a small catheter with a small inflatable balloon attached to its tip into the obstructed coronary artery. As the catheter reaches the obstruction, the balloon in inflated. As a result atherosclerotic plaque is flattened against the vessel wall and the vessel is stretched to increase the lumen. Consequently the blood flow is increased. Sometimes transluminal instruments with rotating blades and lasers are used to cut the clot. After the artery is dilated, an *intravascular stent* is introduced to maintain the dilatation.

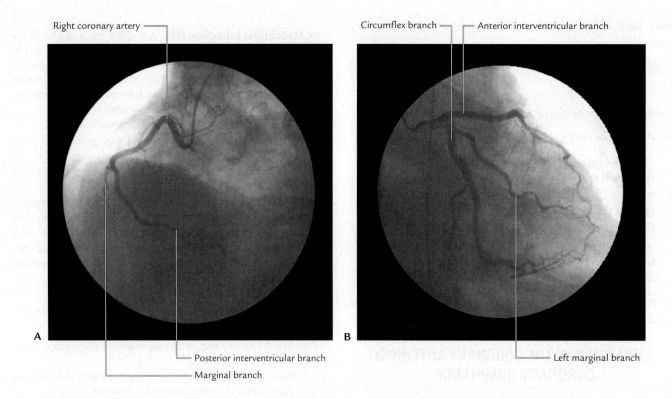

Fig. 20.22 Normal coronary angiogram: **A**, of right coronary artery (left anterior oblique view); **B**, of left coronary artery (right anterior oblique view).

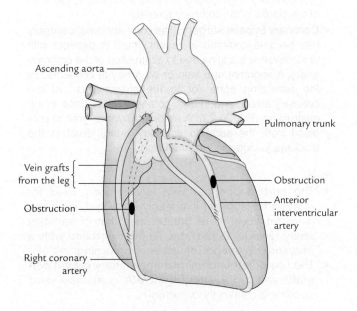

Fig. 20.23 Double coronary artery bypass.

VENOUS DRAINAGE OF THE HEART (Fig. 20.24)

Venous blood from the heart is drained into right atrium by the following:

1. Coronary sinus.
2. Anterior cardiac veins.
3. Venae cordis minimae (Thebesian veins).

Coronary sinus: It is the principal vein of the heart. Most of the venous blood from the walls of the heart is drained into the right atrium through coronary sinus. The coronary sinus is the largest vein of the heart and lies in the posterior part of the atrioventricular groove (left posterior coronary sulcus). *It develops from the left horn of the sinus venosus and a part of the left common cardinal vein.*

Tributaries: The coronary sinus receives the following tributaries (Fig. 20.24A, B, and C):

1. **Great cardiac vein:** It accompanies anterior interventricular and circumflex arteries to join the left end of the coronary sinus.
2. **Middle cardiac vein:** It accompanies the posterior interventricular artery and joins the coronary sinus near its termination.
3. **Small cardiac vein:** It accompanies the right ventricular artery in the right posterior coronary sulcus and the right end of the coronary sinus.
4. **Posterior vein of the left ventricle:** It runs on the diaphragmatic surface of the left ventricle and joins the sinus to the left of the middle cardiac vein.
5. **Oblique vein of the left atrium (vein of Marshall):** It is a small vein which runs downwards on the posterior surface of the left atrium to enter the left end of the coronary sinus. It develops from the left common cardinal vein (**duct of Cuvier**).

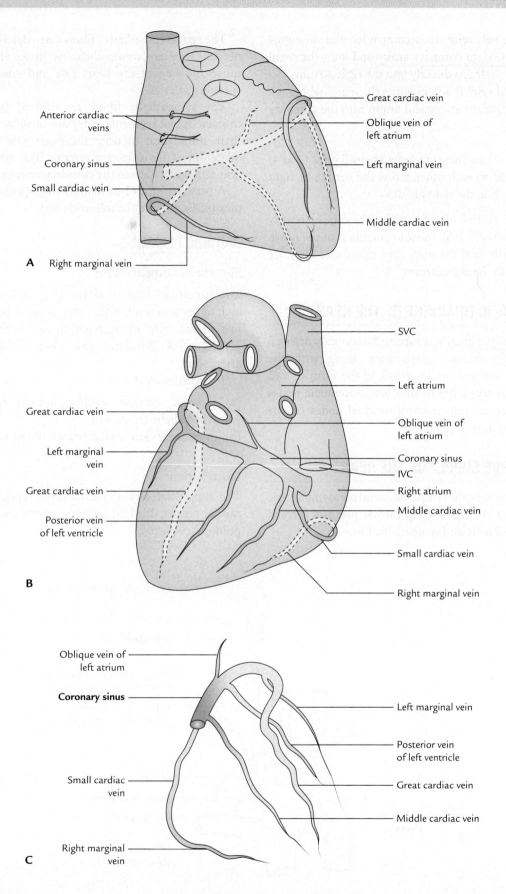

Fig. 20.24 Veins of the heart: **A,** anterior view of the heart showing cardiac veins; **B,** posteroinferior view of the heart showing the cardiac veins; **C,** tributaries of the coronary sinus viewed form the front.

6. **Right marginal vein:** It accompanies the marginal branch of the right coronary artery and joins the small cardiac vein or drains directly into the right atrium.

7. **Left marginal vein:** It accompanies the marginal branch of the left coronary artery and drains into the coronary sinus.

Anterior cardiac veins: These are series of small veins (3 or 4) which run parallel to each other across the surface of right ventricle to open into the right atrium.

Venae cordis minimae (Thebesian veins): These are extremely small veins in the walls of all the four chambers of the heart. They open directly into the respective chambers. They are most numerous in the right atrium.

LYMPHATIC DRAINAGE OF THE HEART

The lymphatics of the heart accompany the coronary arteries, emerge from the fibrous pericardium along with the ascending aorta and pulmonary trunk in the form of two trunks. The **right trunk** drains into **brachiocephalic nodes** and **left trunk** drains into **tracheobronchial nodes** (at the bifurcation of the aorta).

NERVE SUPPLY OF THE HEART

The heart is supplied by the sympathetic and parasympathetic fibres via the superficial and deep **cardiac plexuses** formed by the parasympathetic and sympathetic fibres.

The **parasympathetic fibres** are derived from vagus nerves. They are *cardioinhibitory;* hence their stimulation causes slowing of the heart rate and constriction of the coronary arteries.

The **sympathetic fibres** are derived from upper 3–5 thoracic spinal segments. They are *cardioacceleratory,* hence their stimulation increase the heart rate and causes the dilatation of the coronary arteries. The sympathetic fibres also cause dilatation of the coronary arteries.

A brief account of formation and distribution of cardiac plexuses is given in the following text.

CARDIAC PLEXUSES

Superficial Cardiac Plexus

The **superficial cardiac plexus** (Fig. 20.25) lies below the arch of aorta in front of the bifurcation of pulmonary trunk, just to the right of ligamentum arteriosum. The cardiac ganglion (of Wrisberg) lies close to the ligamentum arteriosum.

It is formed by the:

(a) superior cervical cardiac branch of left cervical sympathetic trunk, and
(b) inferior cervical cardiac branch of left vagus nerve.

Distribution

The superficial cardiac plexus gives branches to (a) deep cardiac plexus, (b) right coronary artery, and (c) left anterior pulmonary plexus.

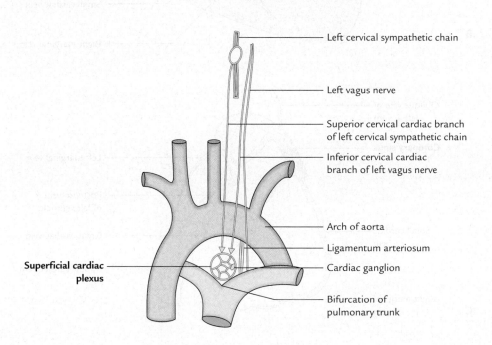

Left cervical sympathetic chain

Left vagus nerve

Superior cervical cardiac branch of left cervical sympathetic chain

Inferior cervical cardiac branch of left vagus nerve

Arch of aorta

Ligamentum arteriosum

Cardiac ganglion

Bifurcation of pulmonary trunk

Superficial cardiac plexus

Fig. 20.25 Superficial cardiac plexus.

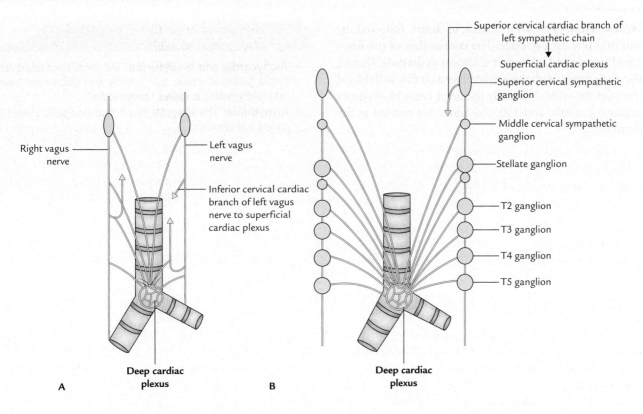

Fig. 20.26 Deep cardiac plexus: **A,** parasympathetic contribution; **B,** sympathetic contribution.

Deep Cardiac Plexus (Fig. 20.26)

The deep cardiac plexus lies in front of the bifurcation of the trachea, behind the arch of the aorta.

It is formed by:

(a) all the cardiac branches derived from three cervical and upper 4 or 5 thoracic ganglia of the sympathetic chains except the *superior cervical cardiac branch* of left cervical sympathetic chain, and

(b) all the cardiac branches of vagus and recurrent laryngeal nerves except the *inferior cervical cardiac branch* of the left vagus nerve.

Distribution

The right and left halves of the plexus distributes branches to (a) corresponding coronary arteries and pulmonary plexus, and (b) separate branches to the atria.

PAIN AND REFLEX PATHWAYS OF THE HEART

Pain Pathways

The sensations of pain arising due to the ischemia of the heart pass through the sympathetic fibres to reach the upper five thoracic spinal segments (T1–T5) through cervical and thoracic sympathetic ganglia and follow the usual somatosensory pathway to the central nervous system. The pain fibres pass from thoracic ganglia to the spinal nerves via white rami communicantes. The cell bodies of the first order sensory neurons are located in the dorsal root ganglia of T1–T5 spinal nerves. Hence cardiac pain is referred mainly in the area of distribution of these nerves, i.e., pectoral region and medial aspect of the arm and forearm.

N.B. Sometimes cardiac pain is referred to the neck and mandible. It is because of the connection of sympathetic fibres with the cervical nerves.

Pathways for Cardiovascular Reflexes

The afferent fibres from heart subserving the cardiovascular reflexes pass by the parasympathetic fibres of vagal nerves to the reticular formation.

ACTION OF THE HEART

The heart is actually a double muscular pump. The right side pumps blood to the lungs and left side pumps blood to all the parts of the body. Each pump is made up of an atrium and a ventricle.

Cardiac cycle: The contraction of heart followed by relaxation is one cardiac cycle. The contraction of the heart is termed **systole** and relaxation is known as **diastole**. During cardiac cycle series of changes take place as it fills with blood and empties the same. Normally the heart beats 70–90 times per minute in adults and 130–150 times per minute in the newborn baby.

Clinical correlation

- **Tachycardia and bradycardia:** The increased heart rate (rapid pulse) is called *tachycardia* and decreased heart rate (slow pulse) is called *bradycardia*.
- **Arrhythmia:** The irregular heart rate (irregular pulse) is called arrhythmia.

Golden Facts to Remember

▶ Most fixed part of the heart	Base of the heart
▶ Most common stenosis of the heart valves	Mitral stenosis
▶ Strongest fibrous ring of the skeleton of the heart	Fibrous ring around the aortic orifice of the heart
▶ Pacemaker of the heart	Sinuatrial node (SA node)
▶ Most commonly blocked artery leading to myocardial infarction (MI)	Anterior interventricular artery (left anterior descending [LAD] artery)
▶ Largest/widest/principal vein of the heart	Coronary sinus
▶ Unique feature of coronary arteries	They fill during ventricular diastole as a result of aortic recoil
▶ Whole of the conducting system of the heart is supplied by the right coronary artery except	A part of left branch of AV bundle which is supplied by the left coronary artery
▶ Third coronary artery	Right conus artery arising directly from the aortic sinus
▶ Kugel's artery	An arterial channel formed by the anastomosis of atrial branch of circumflex artery and similar atrial branch of right coronary artery
▶ Annulus of Vieussens	Circular anastomotic channel around the infundibulum between right and left conus arteries
▶ Triangle of Koch	Small triangular area in the lower part of interatrial septum bounded in front by the septal cusp of tricuspid valve, behind by anteromedial margin of the coronary sinus and above by the tendon of Todaro (a subendocardial ridge)
▶ Heart attack	Acute myocardial infarction

Clinical Case Study

A 60-year-old man visited a cardiologist and complained that he was feeling pressure/tightness within his chest, accompanied by profuse sweating and pain in the left precordium which is radiating along the medial side of the arm and forearm. On questioning he told that earlier also he suffered from such symptoms which always occurred on exertion, e.g., when climbing stairs or digging in the garden. He also told that these symptoms disappear after resting. He was diagnosed as a case of **angina pectoris**.

Questions

1. What is angina pectoris?
2. Mention the anatomical basis of pain felt in the region of left precordium and medial side of the arm and forearm.
3. Name the arteries which supply the cardiac muscle and mention their origin.
4. What is the difference between the angina pectoris and myocardial infarction (MI)?

Answers

1. It is cardiac pain which occurs on exertion due to the narrowing of the coronary artery/arteries or their major branches. The pain is relieved by resting.

2. The afferent pain fibres from heart reach the upper four or five thoracic spinal segments through the cardiac branches of the sympathetic trunks usually on the left side. Pain is referred in the left pericardium—T4 and T3 dermatomes and medial side of the arm (T2 dermatome) and medial side of the forearm (T1 dermatome).

3. Right and left coronary arteries. The right coronary artery arises from anterior aortic sinus at the root of ascending aorta while left coronary artery arises from left posterior aortic sinus at the root of ascending aorta.

4. The differences between angina pectoris and myocardial infarction are follows:

Angina pectoris	Myocardial infarction (MI) (heart attack)
Occurs due to narrowing of the coronary artery/ arteries causing myocardial ischemia	Occurs due to complete block of the coronary artery/arteries causing myocardial ischemia that induces myocardial necrosis
Occurs on exertion and is relieved on rest	Occurs on rest
Sensation of pressure or burning in chest that may last as long as 20 minutes	Sensation of pressure or burning in the chest that lasts longer than 30 minutes

Superior Vena Cava, Aorta, Pulmonary Trunk, and Thymus

The knowledge of anatomy of superior vena cava, aorta, and pulmonary trunk is clinically important because of their involvement in various disease processes such as obstruction of superior vena cava, aortic aneurysm, pulmonary embolism, etc.

SUPERIOR VENA CAVA (Fig. 21.1)

The superior vena cava (SVC) is about 7 cm long and 1.25 cm in diameter. It lies in the superior and middle mediastina. Its extrapericardial part lies in the superior mediastinum and its intrapericardial part lies in the middle mediastinum. It collects blood from the upper half of the body (i.e., head and neck, upper limbs, thoracic wall, and upper abdomen) and drains it into the right atrium. Depending upon the site of obstruction, different collateral pathways develop. In mediastinal syndrome, the signs of obstruction of superior vena cava appear first.

Formation, Course, and Termination

The superior vena cava is formed at the lower border of the right 1st costal cartilage by the union of right and left brachiocephalic (innominate) veins. It passes vertically downwards behind the right border of the sternum and pierces the pericardium at the level of the right 2nd costal cartilage, and opens/terminates into the upper part of the right atrium at the lower border of the right 3rd costal cartilage. It has no valves in its lumen because gravity facilitates the blood flow in it.

Subdivisions

The superior vena cava is subdivided into the following two parts:
1. Extrapericardial part (in superior mediastinum).
2. Intrapericardial part (in middle mediastinum).

Relations (Figs 21.1B and 21.2)

Anterior:
1. Right internal thoracic vessels.
2. Margin of right lung and pleura.
3. Chest wall

Posterior:
1. Trachea (posteromedial).
2. Right pulmonary artery and right bronchus.

To the left:
1. Ascending aorta (anteromedial).
2. Brachiocephalic artery.

To the right:
1. Right phrenic nerve and pericardiophrenic vessels.
2. Right lung and pleura.

Tributaries

1. Right and left brachiocephalic veins.
2. Azygos vein, which arches over the root of the right lung and opens into SVC just before it pierces fibrous pericardium.
3. Mediastinal and pericardial veins.

Brachiocephalic Veins

There are two brachiocephalic veins: (a) right and (b) left. Each of them is formed behind the sternoclavicular joint by the union of corresponding internal jugular and subclavian veins. They unite to form SVC. Both are devoid of valves. Differences between the right and left brachiocephalic veins are enumerated in Table 21.1.

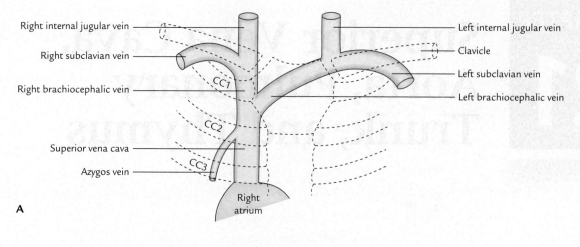

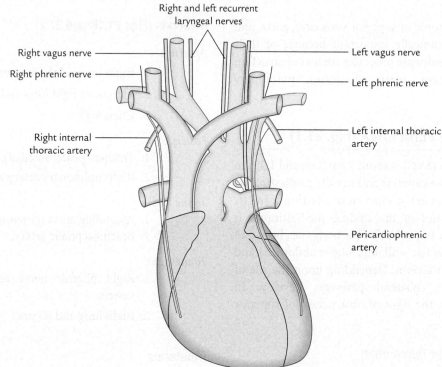

Fig. 21.1 Superior vena cava: **A**, formation, course, and termination; **B**, relations (CC = costal cartilage).

Table 21.1 Differences between right and left brachiocephalic veins

	Right brachiocephalic vein	Left brachiocephalic vein
Length	• Short (2.5 cm)	• Long (6 cm)
Course	• Vertical (runs vertically downwards from right sternoclavicular joint to the lower margin of the right 1st costal cartilage)	• Oblique (runs obliquely across the superior mediastinum from left sternoclavicular joint to the lower margin of the right 1st costal cartilage)
Tributaries	• Right vertebral vein • Right internal thoracic vein • Right inferior thyroid vein • First right posterior intercostal vein	• Left vertebral vein • Left internal thoracic vein • Left inferior thyroid vein • First left posterior intercostal vein • Left superior intercostal vein

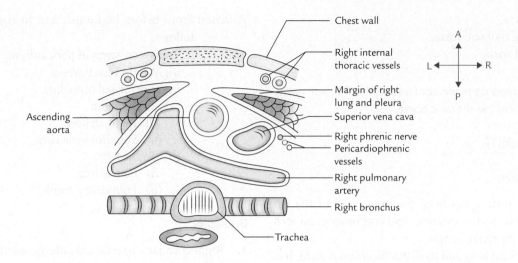

Fig. 21.2 Relations of superior vena cava as seen in the cross section of the thorax.

Clinical correlation

Obstruction of SVC and development of collateral pathways:

The SVC may be obstructed (compressed) at two sites: (a) above the opening of azygos vein (i.e., in superior mediastinum), and (b) below the opening of azygos vein (i.e., in the middle mediastinum).

- *If SVC is obstructed above the opening of azygos vein,* the venous blood from the upper half of the body is shunted to right atrium through azygos vein. The main collateral pathways are provided by the superior intercostal veins. The superficial veins of chest wall do not receive sufficient blood to cause their prominence. If at all they become prominent, the prominence is limited up to the costal margin only (Fig. 21.3).

- *If SVC is obstructed below the opening of the azygos vein,* the venous blood from the upper half of the body is returned to the right atrium through inferior vena cava through the collateral pathways, formed between the tributaries of superior and inferior vena cavae (**caval–caval shunt**). Clinically in this condition, a subcutaneous anastomotic channel between the superficial epigastric vein and lateral thoracic vein (**thoraco-epigastric vein**) is seen on the anterior aspect of the thoraco-abdominal wall (Fig. 20.3).

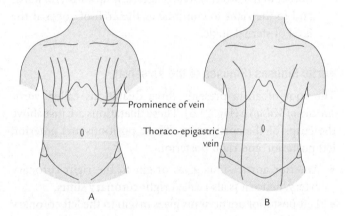

Fig. 21.3 Prominence veins on the front of trunk in obstruction of superior vena cava; **A**, obstruction above the opening of azygos vein; **B**, obstruction below the opening of azygos vein.

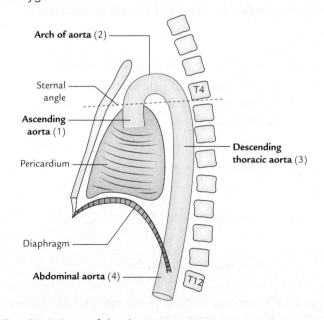

Fig. 21.4 Parts of the thoracic aorta.

AORTA

The aorta is the largest artery (arterial trunk) of the body which carries the oxygenated blood from the left ventricle and distributes it to all the parts of the body.

Parts of the Aorta (Fig. 21.4)

For the convenience of description, the aorta is divided into the following four parts:

1.   Ascending aorta.

2. Arch of aorta.
3. Descending thoracic aorta.
4. Abdominal aorta.

N.B. The first three parts are confined to the thoracic cavity and together form the **thoracic aorta**.

ASCENDING AORTA

Origin and Course

1. Ascending aorta arises from the upper end of the left ventricle (i.e., aortic vestibule) and continues as an arch of aorta at the sternal angle.
2. It is about 5 cm long and its diameter is about 3 cm. It is completely enclosed in the pericardium. It begins behind the left half of the sternum at the level of the lower border of left 3rd costal cartilage, runs upwards, forwards and to the right to continue as the arch of aorta at the level of sternal angle.

Aortic Sinuses (Sinuses of the Valsalva)

The root of aorta presents three dilatations called *aortic sinuses of Valsalva* (Fig. 21.5). These dilatations are just above the cusps of the aortic valve. These positions are: anterior, left posterior, and right posterior.

- Anterior aortic sinus gives origin to the right coronary artery, hence it is also called **right coronary sinus**.
- Left posterior aortic sinus gives origin to the left coronary artery, hence it is also called **left coronary sinus**.
- Right posterior aortic sinus is termed **non-coronary sinus**.

Aortic bulb (Fig. 21.5) is a bulge in the right wall of the ascending aorta at its union with the arch of the aorta.

Relations

Anterior: From below upwards these are as follows:
    1. Infundibulum of right ventricle.
    2. Pulmonary trunk.
    3. Pericardium.

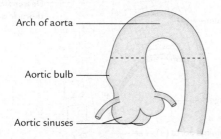

Fig. 21.5 Ascending aorta showing aortic sinuses (sinuses of the Valsalva) and aortic bulb.

Posterior: From before backwards and to right these are as follows:
    1. Transverse sinus of pericardium.
    2. Right pulmonary artery.
    3. Right principal bronchus.
        (a) To the right:
            (i) Right atrium.
            (ii) Superior vena cava.
        (b) To the left:
            (i) Left atrium.
            (ii) Pulmonary trunk.

Branches

1. Right coronary artery from anterior aortic sinus.
2. Left coronary artery from left posterior aortic sinus.

Development

The ascending aorta develops from the truncus arteriosus after its partition by the spiral septum.

Clinical correlation

Aneurysm of ascending aorta: It occurs at the bulb of the ascending aorta. The bulb of aorta is a dilatation in the right wall of ascending aorta which is subjected to constant thrust of the forceful blood current ejected from the left ventricle. It may compress the right atrium, SVC or right principal bronchus. Its rupture (a serious complication) leads to accumulation of blood in the pericardial cavity (hemopericardium).

ARCH OF AORTA

The arch of aorta is the continuation of ascending aorta at the level of sternal angle and continues as descending thoracic aorta at the level of sternal angle. Thus it (both) begins as well as terminates at the level of sternal angle. It is situated in the superior mediastinum. At the beginning the arch is anteriorly located while its termination is posteriorly located, very close to the left side of T4 vertebra. The summit of arch reaches the level of middle of manubrium sterni.

Course

The arch of aorta begins at the level of the right 2nd costal cartilage and runs upwards, backwards, and to the left, in front of the bifurcation of the trachea. Having reached the back of the middle of the manubrium, it turns backwards and downwards behind the left bronchus up to the level of lower border of T4 vertebra where it continues as the descending thoracic aorta.

N.B.

- The arch of aorta arches over the root of left lung.
- It begins and ends at the same level, i.e., at sternal angle.
- It begins anteriorly and ends posteriorly.

Relations (Figs 21.6 and 21.7)

Posterior and to the right:

1. Trachea.
2. Esophagus.
3. Left recurrent laryngeal nerve.
4. Thoracic duct.
5. Vertebral column.

Anterior and to the left:

1. Left lung and pleura.
2. Left phrenic nerve.
3. Left vagus nerve.
4. Left cardiac nerves (i.e., superior cervical cardiac branch of left sympathetic chain and inferior cardiac branch of left vagus nerve).
5. Left superior intercostal vein.

Inferior:

1. Left bronchus.
2. Bifurcation of pulmonary trunk.
3. Ligamentum arteriosum.
4. Left recurrent laryngeal nerve.
5. Superficial cardiac plexus.

Superior:

1. Brachiocephalic trunk.
2. Left common carotid artery.
3. Left subclavian artery.
4. Left brachiocephalic vein.
5. Thymus.

N.B. Arch of aorta is related for 5 structures on each aspect.

Branches

1. Brachiocephalic (innominate) artery.
2. Left common carotid artery.
3. Left subclavian artery.

N.B. Occasionally a fourth branch called *thyroidea ima* artery may arise from the arch of aorta.

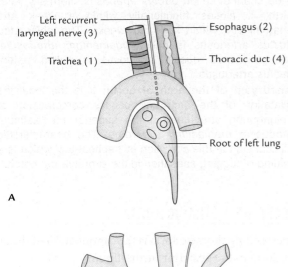

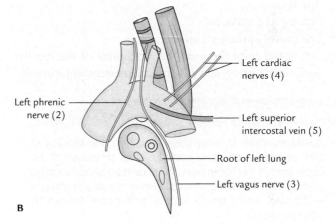

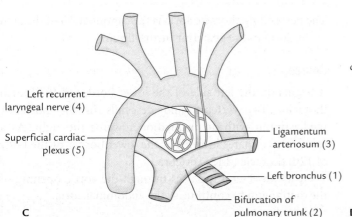

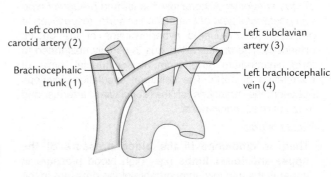

Fig. 21.6 Relations of the arch of aorta: A, posterior and to the right (vertebral column (5) is not shown); B, anterior and to the left (left lung and pleura (1) are not shown); C, inferior; D, superior (thymus (5) is not shown).

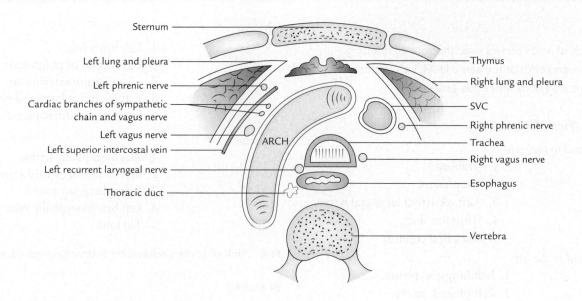

Fig. 21.7 Cross section of superior mediastinum showing relations of arch of aorta (SVC = superior vena cava).

Development

The arch of aorta develops from the following sources:

1. Aortic sac.
2. Left horn of aortic sac.
3. Left fourth aortic arch artery.
4. Left dorsal aorta (between the attachment of the fourth aortic arch (artery) and 7th cervical intersegmental artery.

Clinical correlation

- **Aortic knuckle:** In X-ray chest (PA view), the shadow of arch of aorta appears as small bulb-like projection at the upper end of the left margin of the cardiac shadow called *aortic knuckle*. The aortic knuckle may become prominent in old age due to *undue folding* of the arch caused by atherosclerosis.
- **Coarctation of aorta (Fig. 21.8):** It is congenital narrowing of the aorta just proximal or distal to the entrance of the *ductus arteriosus*. Accordingly it is termed *preductal type* and *postductal type of coarctation of aorta*, respectively. It probably occurs due to hyperinvolution of the ductus arteriosus. The ductus arteriosus is usually obliterated to form ligamentum arteriosum in postductal type of coarctation of aorta. The collateral circulation develops between the branches of the subclavian arteries and those of descending aorta.

Clinical features:

1. There is **difference in the blood pressure of the upper and lower limbs** (i.e., high blood pressure in upper limbs and low unrecordable blood pressure in the lower limbs).
2. **Notching of the lower borders of the ribs** due to dilatation of engorged posterior intercostal arteries.
3. Pulsating scapulae.

- **Patent ductus arteriosus (Fig. 21.9):** In foetal life, pulmonary trunk is connected to the arch of aorta (just distal to the origin of left subclavian artery) by short wide channel called *ductus arteriosus*. Normally, after birth, it closes functionally within a week and anatomically within 4 to 12 weeks. The obliterated ductus arteriosus is called *ligamentum arteriosum*. Non-obliterated ductus arteriosus is called patent ductus arteriosus.
- **Aneurysm of the arch of aorta:** It is the localized dilatation of the arch and causes compression of neighboring structures in the superior mediastinum producing *mediastinal syndrome*. The characteristic clinical sign in this condition is 'tracheal-tug' which is a feeling of tugging sensation in the suprasternal notch.

DESCENDING THORACIC AORTA

The descending thoracic aorta is the continuation of the arch of the aorta in the posterior mediastinum.

Course

It begins on the left side of the lower border of the fourth thoracic (T4) vertebra and descends in the posterior mediastinum with an inclination towards the right. As a result it terminates in front of the lower border of the body of 12th thoracic (T12) vertebra.

At its lower end it passes through the aortic opening of the diaphragm to continue as the abdominal aorta.

Relations

Anterior: From above downwards it is related to:
1. Left lung root.

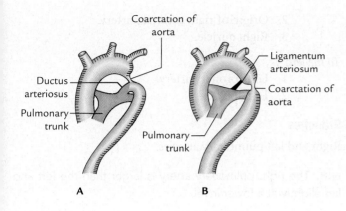

Fig. 21.8 Coarctation of aorta: **A**, preductal type; **B**, postductal type. (*Source*: Fig. 9.24, Page 474, *Clinical and Surgical Anatomy*, 2e, Vishram Singh. Copyright Elsevier 2007, All rights reserved.)

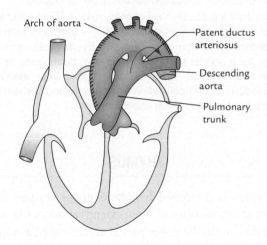

Fig. 21.9 Patent ductus arteriosus. (*Source*: Fig. 9.23, Page 474, *Clinical and Surgical Anatomy*, 2e, Vishram Singh. Copyright Elsevier 2007, All rights reserved.)

2. Pericardium (enclosing heart).
3. Esophagus (in the lower part).
4. Diaphragm.

Posterior:

1. Vertebral column.
2. Hemiazygos and accessory hemiazygos veins.

To the right side:

1. Esophagus (in the upper part).
2. Thoracic duct.
3. Azygos vein.
4. Right lung and pleura.

To the left side: Left lung and pleura.

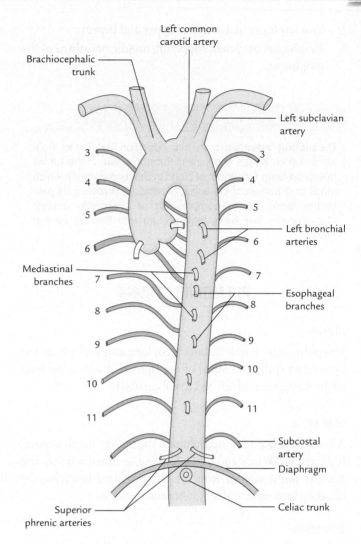

Fig. 21.10 Branches of the thoracic aorta.

(*Note*: Descending thoracic aorta produces a deep vertical groove on the mediastinal surface of the lung posterior to the hilum of the lung.)

Branches (Fig. 21.10)

Parietal branches

1. Nine (3rd–11th) posterior intercostal arteries on each side.
2. Subcostal artery on each side.
3. Superior phrenic artery on each side.

Visceral branches

1. Pericardial branches, to posterior surface of the pericardium.
2. Mediastinal branches, to the lymph nodes and areolar tissue of the posterior mediastinum.

3. Two left bronchial arteries (upper and lower).
4. Esophageal branches, supplying middle one-third of the esophagus.

Clinical correlation

Dissecting aneurysm: In this condition the blood from aortic lumen enters into its wall through a tear in the tunica intima creating a channel of blood in the tunica media which leads to dilatation of the aorta. Clinically, it presents as pain in the back due to compression of intercostal nerves. Occasionally, the aorta may rupture into the left pleural cavity.

PULMONARY TRUNK

Origin

The pulmonary trunk is about 5 cm long and arises from the upper part (infundibulum) of the right ventricle at the level of the sternal end of left 3rd costal cartilage.

Course

After arising from infundibulum in the middle mediastinum, it passes backwards and to the left and terminates below the arch of aorta and in front of left principal bronchus by dividing into right and left pulmonary arteries.

Relations

Anterior:
1. Sternal end of left 2nd intercostal space.
2. Left lung and pleura.

Posterior:
1. Ascending aorta.
2. Commence of left coronary artery.
3. Transverse sinus of pericardium.

To the right:
1. Ascending aorta.

2. Origin of right coronary artery.
3. Right auricle.

To the left:
1. Left coronary artery.
2. Left auricle.

Branches

Right and left pulmonary arteries.

N.B. The right pulmonary artery is larger than the left and lies slightly at a lower level.

Clinical correlation

- **Pulmonary artery catheterization:** Various aspects of cardiopulmonary functions are monitored by the cardiologists by pulmonary artery catheterization.
  The catheter is passed successively as follows:
  Internal jugular vein/subclavian vein → Right atrium → Right ventricle → Pulmonary trunk → Pulmonary artery.
- **Sudden occlusion of pulmonary trunk** by an embolus may be a sequel to the thrombosis of deep veins of the calf (viz. femoral vein) or large pelvic vein following operation or immobilization in the sick-bed. When the block is complete, death ensues rapidly.

THYMUS

The thymus is a bilobed lymphoid organ situated in the superior mediastinum and often extends above in the root of neck and below in the upper part of anterior mediastinum. It is usually prominent in children and gradually increases in size till puberty, when it weighs about 40 g. Thereafter it atrophies and gets infiltrated by fibrous and fatty tissue. It is related anteriorly to sternohyoid and sternothyroid muscles, and sternum; and posteriorly to pericardium, arch of aorta and its branches, left brachiocephalic vein and trachea. It secretes a hormone called **thymosin** which plays an important role in the development of the immunity of the body.

Golden Facts to Remember

► Largest artery of the body	Aorta
► Bulb of aorta	Dilatation in the right wall of ascending aorta at its union with the arch of aorta
► Largest branch of the arch of aorta	Brachiocephalic trunk
► Commonest variation in the origin of great arteries from the arch of aorta	Origin of left common carotid artery from the brachiocephalic trunk
► Aortic knuckle	Projection at the upper end of the left margin of the cardiac shadow in PA view of X-ray chest
► Part of aorta mostly affected by dissecting aneurysm	Descending thoracic aorta
► Smallest part of the aorta	Ascending aorta
► Sinuses of Valsalva	Three dilatations in the ascending aorta above the semilunar valves

Clinical Case Study

A mother took her 12-year-old son to the hospital and complained that he feels weakness even after slight exertion (**reduced exercise tolerance**), leg cramps on walking and shortness of the breath. On examination, the doctors noticed radiofemoral delay. Blood pressure was 126/20 mmHg in upper limbs and 80/60 mmHg in the lower limbs. The X-ray chest showed notching of the lower borders of the ribs. Clinically he was diagnosed as a case of **coarctation of aorta**, which was confirmed later by echocardiography.

Questions

1. What is coarctation of aorta?
2. Why there is delay in radiofemoral pulse?
3. What is the cause of high blood pressure in the upper limbs and low blood pressure in the lower limbs?
4. Mention the reason for notching of the ribs.

Answers

1. It is congenital stenosis of the arch of aorta, usually distal to the origin of left subclavian artery.
2. Because subclavian arteries supplying upper limbs arise proximal to the site of stenosis, whereas femoral arteries supplying lower limbs arise from aorta distal to the site of obstruction.
3. Answer is same as that of question no. 2.
4. Due to dilatation and tortuosity of the posterior intercostal arteries which erode the costal groove of the ribs.

CHAPTER 22

Trachea and Esophagus

TRACHEA

The trachea (syn. windpipe; Fig. 22.1) is a flexible fibrocartilaginous tube forming the beginning of the lower respiratory tract. Its lumen is kept patent by 16–20 C-shaped rings of hyaline cartilage. The gap between the posterior free ends of C-shaped cartilages is bridged by a band of smooth muscle (**trachealis**) and a fibroelastic ligament, which permit expansion of esophagus during the passage of bolus of food.

The arrangement of cartilages and elastic tissue in the tracheal wall prevents its kinking and obstruction during the movements of the head and neck.

LOCATION

The trachea extends from the lower border of cricoid cartilage (corresponding to the lower border of C6 vertebra) in the neck to the lower border of T4 vertebra in the thorax. Thus upper half of the trachea is located in the neck (**cervical part**) and lower half in the superior mediastinum (**thoracic part**).

N.B. The extent of trachea varies as follows:
- C6 to T4 in cadaver placed in supine position.
- C6 to T6 in living individuals in standing position.
- C6 to T3 in newborn.

DIMENSIONS

Length: 10–12 cm.
External diameter: 2 cm in males and 1.5 cm in females.
Internal diameter: 12 mm in adult, 3 mm in newborn.
Lumen of trachea:

1. The lumen of trachea is smaller in living human beings than in the cadavers.
2. It is 3 mm at 1 year of age; during childhood it corresponds to the age in years (i.e., 5-year-old child will have tracheal diameter of 5 mm) with a maximum of

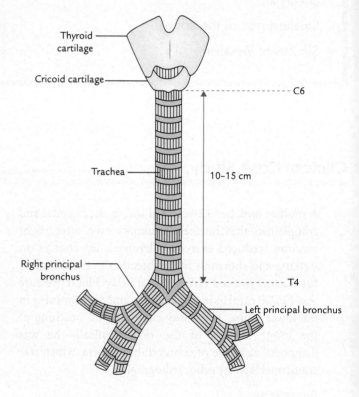

Fig. 22.1 Trachea.

Labels: Thyroid cartilage; Cricoid cartilage; C6; Trachea; 10–15 cm; Right principal bronchus; T4; Left principal bronchus

12 mm in adults. For this reason endotracheal tubes are graduated in mm.

COURSE

The trachea is the continuation of the larynx and begins at the lower border of the cricoid cartilage at the level of C6 vertebra, about 5 cm above the jugular notch.

It enters the thoracic inlet in the midline and passes downwards and backwards behind the manubrium to terminate by bifurcating into two principal bronchi, a little to the right side at the lower border of T4 vertebra corresponding to the sternal angle.

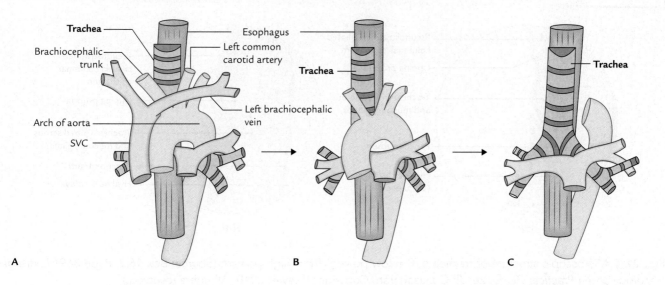

Fig. 22.2 Anterior relations (A–C) of the trachea from superficial to deep (SVC = superior vena cava).

RELATIONS

RELATIONS OF THE CERVICAL PART

The relations of the cervical part of the trachea are described in detail in *Textbook of Anatomy: Head, Neck and Brain, Vol. III* by Vishram Singh.

RELATIONS OF THE THORACIC PART
(Figs 22.2 and 22.3)

Anterior:

1. Arch of aorta.
2. Brachiocephalic trunk and left common carotid artery.
3. Left brachiocephalic vein.
4. Superior vena cava (anterolateral).
5. Deep cardiac plexus.

Posterior:

1. Esophagus.
2. Vertebral column.
3. Left recurrent laryngeal nerve (it ascends up between trachea and esophagus).

To the right:

1. Right lung and pleura.
2. Azygous vein.
3. Right vagus nerve.

To the left:

1. Arch of aorta.
2. Left common carotid artery.
3. Left subclavian vein.

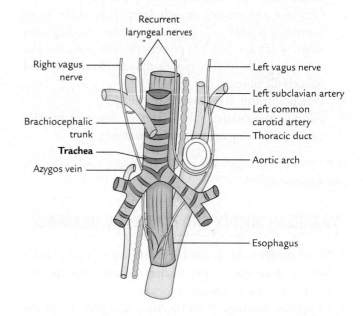

Fig. 22.3 Posterior and lateral relations of the trachea.

4. Left vagus nerve.
5. Left phrenic nerve.

Microscopic structure (Fig. 22.4)

Histologically, tracheal tube from within outward is made up of the following layers:

1. **Mucosa:** It consists of lining epithelium and lamina propria.
   (a) *Lining epithelium* is pseudostratified ciliated columnar with few goblets cells.
   (b) *Lamina propria* consists of longitudinal elastic fibres.

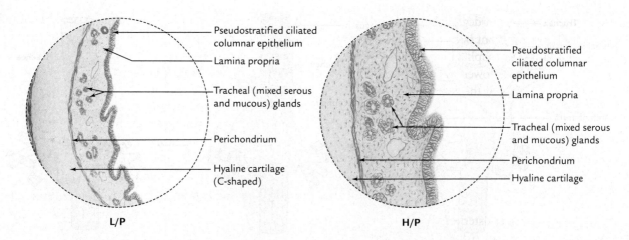

Fig. 22.4 Microscopic structure of trachea (L/P = low power, H/P = high power). (*Source:* Box 16.2, Page 349, *Textbook of Histology and a Practical Guide*, 2e, JP Gunasegaran. Copyright Elsevier 2010, All rights reserved.)

2. **Submucosa:** It consists of loose areolar tissue containing large number of serous and mucous glands.
3. **Cartilage and smooth muscle layer:** It is made up of horseshoe-shaped (C-shaped) hyaline cartilaginous rings, which are deficient posteriorly. The posterior gap is filled chiefly by the smooth muscle (**trachealis**) and fibroelastic fibres.
4. **Perichondrium:** It encloses the cartilage.
5. **Fibrous membrane:** It is a layer of dense connective tissue, containing neurovascular structure.

N.B. There is no clear demarcation between lamina propria and submucosa.

VASCULAR SUPPLY AND LYMPHATIC DRAINAGE

- **Blood supply** to the trachea is by inferior thyroid arteries.
- **Venous drainage** of the trachea occurs into the left brachiocephalic (innominate) vein.
- **Lymphatic drainage** of the trachea is into pretracheal and paratracheal lymph nodes.

NERVE SUPPLY

Nerve supply occurs by the autonomic nerve fibres:

- **Parasympathetic fibres** are sensory and secretomotor to the mucous membrane, and motor to the trachealis muscle.
- Sympathetic fibres are vasomotor.

Clinical correlation

- **Tracheal shadow in radiograph:** It is seen as a vertical translucent shadow in front of cervico-thoracic spine. The translucency is due to the presence of air in the trachea.

- **Palpation of trachea:** Clinically, trachea is palpated in the suprasternal notch. Normally, it is median in position but appreciable shift of trachea to right or left side indicates the *mediastinal shift*.
- **Importance of carina:** It is a keel-like median ridge in the lumen at the bifurcation of trachea. The lowest tracheal ring at the bifurcation of trachea is thick in its central part. From the lower margin of this thick central part a keel-shaped (hook-shaped) process projects downwards and backwards between the right and left principal bronchi. It has both functional and pathological importance.
    - *Functional importance:* The mucosa of trachea over the carina is *most sensitive*. The cough reflex is usually initiated here, which helps to clear the sputum.
    - *Pathological significance:* It is visible as a sharp sagittal ridge at the tracheal bifurcation during *bronchoscopy*, hence serves as a useful landmark. It is located about 25 cm from the incisor teeth and 30 cm from the nostrils. If the tracheobronchial lymph nodes in the angle between the main (principal) bronchi are enlarged due to spread of *bronchiogenic carcinoma*, the carina becomes distorted and flattened.
- **Importance of mucous secretion in tracheal lumen:** It helps to trap the inhaled foreign particles and solid mucous is then expelled during coughing. The *cilia of lining epithelium of mucous membrane* also beat upwards pushing the mucous upwards. The *fibroelastic ligament* prevents overdistension of tracheal lumen while *trachealis muscle* reduces the diameter on contraction during coughing which involves increased velocity of expired air required for cleaning the air passages.

ESOPHAGUS

The esophagus (Fig. 22.5) is a narrow muscular tube extending from pharynx to the stomach. It is about 25 cm long and provides passage for chewed food (bolus) and liquids during the third stage of deglutition. The anatomy of esophagus is clinically important because of its involvement in various diseases such as esophagitis, esophageal varices and cancer. It begins with lower part of the neck and terminates in the upper part of the abdomen by joining the upper end of the stomach.

DIMENSIONS AND LUMEN

Length: 25 cm (10 inches).
Width: 2 cm.
Lumen: It is flattened anteroposteriorly. Normally it is kept closed (collapsed) and opens (dilates) only during the passage of the food.

COURSE

The esophagus begins in the neck at the lower border of the cricoid cartilage (at the lower border of C6 vertebra), descends in front of the vertebral column passes through superior and posterior mediastina, pierces diaphragm at the level of T10 vertebra and ends in the abdomen at the cardiac orifice of the stomach at the level of T11 vertebra (Fig. 22.5).

CURVATURES

The cervical portion of esophagus commences in the midline, then inclines slightly to the left of the midline at the root of neck, enters the thoracic inlet, passes through

superior mediastinum. At the level of T5 vertebra, it returns to the midline, but at T7 it again deviates to the left and inclines forwards to pass in front of the descending thoracic aorta and pierces diaphragm 2.5 cm to the left of the midline (a thumb's breadth from the side of sternum), at the level of 7th left costal cartilage. Here fibres of the right crus of diaphragm sweep around the esophageal opening forming a sling around the esophagus. It enters the abdomen to join the stomach at the level of T11 vertebra. Thus esophagus presents the following curvatures:

1. **Two side-to-side curvatures**, both towards the left.
    (a) First at the root of the neck, before entering the thoracic inlet.
    (b) Second at the level of T7 vertebra, before passing in front of the descending thoracic aorta.
2. **Two anteroposterior curvatures.**
    (a) First corresponding to the curvature of cervical spine.
    (b) Second corresponding to the curvature of thoracic spine.

CONSTRICTIONS

Normally, there are four sites of anatomical constrictions/ narrowings in the esophagus. The distance of each

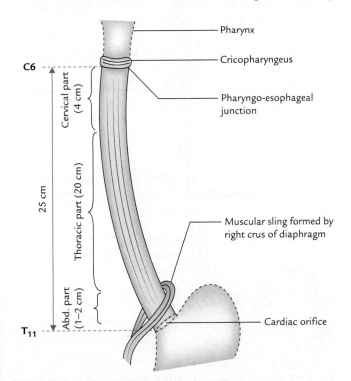

Fig. 22.5 Esophagus (Abd.= abdominal).

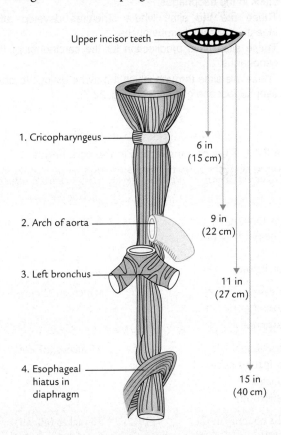

Fig. 22.6 Anatomical sites of constrictions in esophagus. On the right side distances of these sites from the upper incisor teeth are given.

constriction is measured from the upper incisor teeth. The constrictions are as follows (Fig. 22.6):

1. **First constriction**, at the pharyngo-esophageal junction, 9 cm (6 inches) from the incisor teeth.
2. **Second constriction**, where it is crossed by the arch of aorta, 22.5 cm (9 inches) from the incisor teeth.
3. **Third constriction**, where it is crossed by the left principal bronchus, 27.5 cm (11 inches) from the incisor teeth.
4. **Fourth constriction**, where it pierces the diaphragm, 40 cm (15 inches) from the incisor teeth.

The sites of constriction, their respective distances from the upper incisor teeth and their vertebral level are given in Table 22.1.

N.B. The *narrowest part of esophagus* is its commencement at the cricopharyngeal sphincter.

Clinical correlation

Clinical significance of esophageal constrictions: The anatomical constrictions of esophagus are of considerable clinical importance due to the following reasons:

1. These are the sites where swallowed foreign bodies may stuck in the esophagus.
2. These are the sites where strictures develop after ingestion of caustic substances.
3. These sites have predilection for the carcinoma of the esophagus.
4. These are sites through which it may be difficult to pass esophagoscope/gastric tube (Fig. 22.7).

Table 22.1 Sites of constriction in the esophagus

Site of constriction	Vertebral level	Distance from upper incisor teeth
At the pharyngo-esophageal junction (cervical constriction)	C6	6 inches (15 cm)
At crossing of arch of aorta (aortic constriction)	T4	9 inches (22 cm)
At crossing of left principal bronchus (bronchial constriction)	T6	11 inches (27 cm)
At the opening in the diaphragm (diaphragmatic constriction)	T10	15 inches (40 cm)

PARTS OF THE ESOPHAGUS

The esophagus is divided into the following three parts:

1. Cervical part (4 cm in length).
2. Thoracic part (20 cm in length).
3. Abdominal part (1–2 cm in length).

The **cervical part** extends from the lower border of cricoid cartilage to the superior border of manubrium sterni (described in detail in the *Textbook of Anatomy: Head, Neck and Brain, Vol. III* by Vishram Singh.

The **thoracic part** extends from superior border of manubrium sterni to the esophageal opening in the diaphragm.

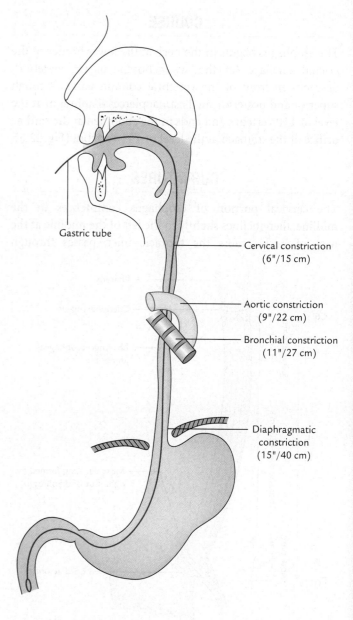

Gastric tube

Cervical constriction (6"/15 cm)

Aortic constriction (9"/22 cm)

Bronchial constriction (11"/27 cm)

Diaphragmatic constriction (15"/40 cm)

Fig. 22.7 Anatomical sites of the esophageal constrictions and passage of the gastric tube.

The **abdominal part** extends form esophageal opening in the diaphragm to the cardiac end of the stomach.

RELATIONS (Figs 22.8 and 22.9)

RELATION OF CERVICAL PART OF THE ESOPHAGUS

For description refer to the *Textbook of Anatomy: Head, Neck and Brain, Vol III* by Vishram Singh, page 181.

RELATIONS OF THORACIC PART OF THE ESOPHAGUS

Anterior: From above downwards these are as follows:
1. Trachea.
2. Arch of aorta.
3. Right pulmonary artery.
4. Left principal bronchus.
5. Left atrium enclosed in the pericardium.
6. Diaphragm.

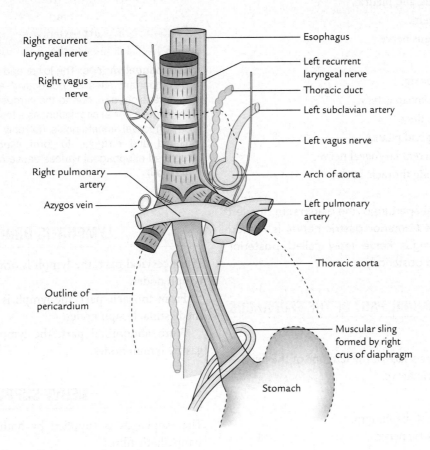

Fig. 22.8 Anterior and lateral relations of esophagus.

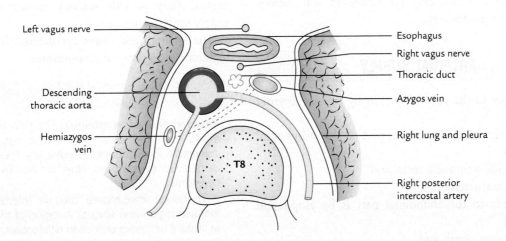

Fig. 22.9 Cross section of posterior mediastinum at the level of T8 vertebra showing posterior relations of the esophagus.

Posterior:
1. Vertebral column.
2. Right posterior intercostal arteries.
3. Thoracic duct.
4. Azygos vein.
5. Hemiazygos veins (terminal parts).
6. Descending thoracic aorta.

To the right:
1. Right lung and pleura.
2. Azygos vein.
3. Right vagus nerve.

To the left:
1. Arch of aorta.
2. Left subclavian artery.
3. Thoracic duct.
4. Left lung and pleura.
5. Left recurrent laryngeal nerve.
6. Descending thoracic aorta.

N.B. In the esophageal aperture of the diaphragm, the left vagus nerve (now called **anterior gastric nerve**) is related anteriorly and right vagus nerve (now called **posterior gastric nerve**) is related posteriorly.

RELATIONS OF ABDOMINAL PART OF THE ESOPHAGUS

Anterior:
1. Posterior surface of the left lobe of the liver.
2. Left gastric nerve.

Posterior:
1. Left crus of diaphragm.
2. Right gastric nerve.

N.B. The abdominal part of esophagus is shortest (1 to 2 cm long) and is the only part covered with serous membrane—the peritoneum.

ARTERIAL SUPPLY

- Blood supply to the cervical part is by inferior thyroid arteries.
- Blood supply to the thoracic part is by esophageal branches of
  (a) descending thoracic aorta, and
  (b) bronchial arteries.
- Blood supply to the abdominal part is by esophageal branches of
  (a) left gastric artery, and
  (b) left inferior phrenic artery.

VENOUS DRAINAGE

- **Cervical part** is drained by inferior thyroid veins.
- **Thoracic part** is drained by azygos and hemiazygos veins.
- **Abdominal part** is drained by two venous channels, viz.
  (a) hemiazygos vein, a tributary of inferior vena cava, and
  (b) left gastric vein, a tributary of portal vein.

Thus abdominal part of esophagus is the site of **portocaval anastomosis**.

Clinical correlation

Esophageal varices: The lower end of esophagus is one of the important sites of *portocaval anastomosis*. In portal hypertension, e.g., due to the cirrhosis of liver there is back pressure in portal circulation. As a result, collateral channels of portocaval anastomosis not only open up but become dilated and tortuous to form *esophageal varices*. The ruptured esophageal varices cause *hematemesis* (vomiting of blood).

LYMPHATIC DRAINAGE

From **cervical part**, the lymph is drained into deep cervical lymph nodes.

From **thoracic part**, the lymph is drained into posterior mediastinal lymph nodes.

From **abdominal part**, the lymph is drained into left gastric lymph nodes.

NERVE SUPPLY

The esophagus is supplied by both parasympathetic and sympathetic fibres.

The **parasympathetic fibres** are derived from recurrent laryngeal nerves and esophageal plexuses formed by vagus nerves. They provide sensory, motor, and secretomotor supply to the esophagus.

The **sympathetic fibres** are derived from T5–T9 spinal segments are sensory and vasomotor.

Clinical correlation

Referred pain of esophagus: The pain sensations mostly arises from the lower part of the esophagus as it is vulnerable to acid-peptic esophagitis. Pain sensations are carried by sympathetic fibre to the T4 and T5 spinal segments.

Therefore, esophageal pain is referred to the lower thoracic region and epigastric region of the abdomen, and at times it becomes difficult to differentiate esophageal pain from the anginal pain.

MICROSCOPIC STRUCTURE

Histologically, esophageal tube from within outwards is made up of the following four basic layers (Fig. 22.10):

1. **Mucosa:** It is composed of the following components:
   (a) *Epithelium*—highly stratified squamous and non-keratinized.
   (b) *Lamina propria*—contains cardiac esophageal glands in the lower part only.
   (c) *Muscularis mucosa*—very-very thick and made up of only longitudinal layer of smooth muscle fibres.
2. **Submucosa:** It contains mucous esophageal glands.
3. **Muscular layer:**
   (a) In upper one-third, it is made up of skeletal muscle.
   (b) In middle one-third, it is made up of both skeletal and smooth muscles.
   (c) In lower one-third, it is made up of smooth muscle.
4. **Fibrous membrane (adventitia).** It consists of dense connective tissue with many elastic fibres.

N.B. A clinical condition in which the stratified squamous epithelium of esophagus is replaced by the gastric epithelium is called *Barrett esophagus*. It may lead to *esophageal carcinoma*.

DEVELOPMENT OF THE ESOPHAGUS AND TRACHEA

The esophagus develops from foregut. The respiratory tract develops from foregut diverticulum called laryngotracheal diverticulum/tube. The following two important events occur in the development of esophagus:

(a) Separation of laryngotracheal tube by the formation of laryngotracheal septum.
(b) Recanalization of obliterated lumen.

N.B. The failure of canalization of the esophagus leads to *esophageal atresia* and maldevelopment of laryngotracheal septum between the esophagus and trachea leads to *tracheoesophageal fistula*.

Clinical correlation

- **Radiological examination of the esophagus by barium swallow:** *It* is performed to detect (a) enlargement of the left atrium due to mitral stenosis, (b) esophageal strictures, and (c) carcinoma and achalasia cardia.

N.B. In normal case, the barium swallow examination presents 3 indentations in its outline caused by the aortic arch, left principal bronchus, and left atrium.

- **Esophagoscopy:** *It* is performed to visualize the interior of the esophagus; while passing esophagoscope, the sites of normal constrictions should be kept in mind.
- **Achalasia cardia:** It is a clinical condition in which sphincter at the lower end of esophagus fails to relax when the food is swallowed. As a result food accumulates in the esophagus and its regurgitation occurs. This condition occurs due to neuromuscular incoordination, probably due to congenital absence of ganglion cells in the myenteric plexus of nerves in the esophageal wall. A radiographic barium swallow examination of the esophagus reveals a characteristic bird's beak/rat tail appearance.
- **Dysphagia (difficulty in swallowing):** It occurs due to:
   (a) compression of esophagus from outside by aortic arch aneurysm, enlargement of lymph nodes, abnormal right subclavian artery (passing posterior to esophagus), etc. and
   (b) narrowing of lumen due to stricture or carcinoma.
- **Tracheoesophageal fistula (Fig. 22.11):** It is a commonest congenital anomaly of esophagus which occurs due to failure of separation of the *lumen* of *tracheal tube* from

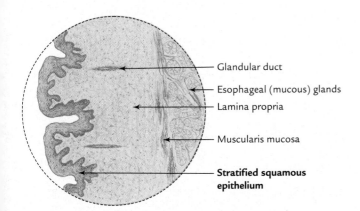

Fig. 22.10 Microscopic structure of esophagus. (*Source:* Box 12.6, Page 223, *Textboook of Histology and a Practical Guide,* JP Gunasegaran. Copyright Elsevier 2010, All rights reserved.)

- Glandular duct
- Esophageal (mucous) glands
- Lamina propria
- Muscularis mucosa
- **Stratified squamous epithelium**

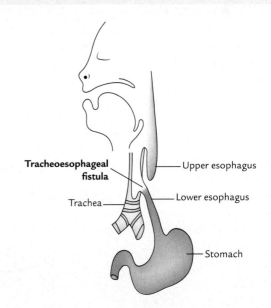

- **Tracheoesophageal fistula**
- Upper esophagus
- Trachea
- Lower esophagus
- Stomach

Fig. 22.11 Tracheoesophageal fistula.

that of *esophagus* by a laryngotracheal septum. In the most commonest type of tracheoesophageal fistula, the upper esophagus ends blindly and lower esophagus communicates with trachea at the level of T4 vertebra. Clinically it presents as: (a) hydramnios because fetus is unable to swallow amniotic fluid, (b) stomach is distended with air, and (c) infant vomit every feed given or may cough up bile. The fistula must be closed surgically to avoid passage of swallowed liquids into the lungs.

• **Malignant tumors of esophagus:** They most commonly occur in its lower one-third.

The lymph vessels from lower one-third of the esophagus descend through the esophageal opening of the diaphragm and drain into the celiac lymph nodes around the celiac trunk. A malignant tumor from lower one-third of esophagus, therefore, spreads below the diaphragm into these lymph nodes. Consequently, surgical resection of the lesion includes not only the primary site (i.e., esophagus) but also celiac lymph nodes and all the regions that drain into these lymph nodes such as stomach, upper half of the duodenum, spleen, and omenta. The continuity of gut is restored by performing an esophagojejunostomy.

Golden Facts to Remember

➤ Most sensitive part of trachea	Carina
➤ Commonest site of malignancy (cancer) in esophagus	Lower one-third
➤ Longest part of esophagus	Thoracic part
➤ Part of GIT having thickest muscularis mucosa in its wall	Esophagus
➤ Most common motility disorder of esophagus	Achalasia cardia
➤ Most common congenital anomaly of esophagus	Tracheoesophageal fistula

Clinical Case Study

A 65-year-old woman visited the hospital and complained of difficulty in swallowing (dysphagia) and marked loss of weight. The barium swallow revealed narrowing of lower end of esophagus. The biopsy was taken from the end of the esophagus and it confirmed the malignancy.

Questions

1. What are extent, length, and functions of esophagus?
2. Name the three factors that can cause dysphagia.
3. Mention the lymphatic drainage of the esophagus.
4. What is the commonest site of malignant tumor in esophagus?

Answers

1. (a) It extends from the lower border of cricoid cartilage in the neck (at the level of C6 vertebra) to the cardiac orifice of stomach in abdomen at the level of T11 vertebra.
   (b) It is 25 cm (10 inches) in length.
   (c) It conducts the chewed food (bolus) from pharynx to the stomach.
2. (a) Aneurysm of the arch of aorta, (b) enlarged lymph nodes, and (c) carcinoma of the esophagus.
3. From the cervical part into deep cervical lymph nodes; from the thoracic part into posterior mediastinal lymph nodes; from abdominal part into the left gastric and celiac lymph nodes.
4. Lower one-third of the esophagus.

Thoracic Duct, Azygos and Hemiazygos Veins, and Thoracic Sympathetic Trunks

THORACIC DUCT

The thoracic duct is the largest lymphatic vessel (trunk or great lymph channel) which drains lymph from most of the body into the bloodstream. The lymph in the thoracic duct is milky-white in appearance because it contains a product of fat digestion (**chyle**) from the intestine. The duct appears beaded due to the presence of numerous valves in its lumen.

Area of drainage: The thoracic duct drains the lymph from all the parts of the body except the (a) right side of the head and neck, (b) right side of the chest wall, (c) right lung, (d) right side of the heart, and (e) right surface of the liver.

N.B. Thoracic duct drains lymph from whole of the body except the right upper quadrant of the body which is drained by the right lymphatic duct (Fig. 23.1).

Extent: The thoracic duct extends to the upper end of cisterna chyli on the posterior abdominal wall at the lower border of T12 vertebra to the junction of left internal jugular and left subclavian veins at the root of the neck.

Measurements: The *measurements* of the thoracic duct are as follows:
Length: 45 cm (18 inches).
Width of lumen: 5 mm (at the ends but narrow in the middle).

FORMATION, COURSE, AND TERMINATION (Fig. 23.2)

The duct begins in the abdomen at the lower border of T12 vertebra, as a continuation of cisterna chyli (lying in front of the bodies of L1 and L2 vertebrae) and enters the thorax through the aortic opening of the diaphragm. It then ascends in the posterior mediastinum to the right of midline on the front of vertebral bodies. On reaching the T5 vertebra, it crosses the midline from right to left side and enters the superior mediastinum to run along the left border of the esophagus and reaches the root of the neck.

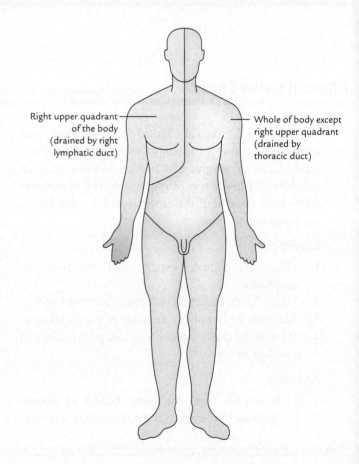

Right upper quadrant of the body (drained by right lymphatic duct)

Whole of body except right upper quadrant (drained by thoracic duct)

Fig. 23.1 Lymphatic drainage of the body. Note that the lymph from right upper quadrant of the body is drained by the right lymphatic duct. The lymph from remaining area of the body is drained by the thoracic duct.

At the root of neck it arches laterally at the level of C7 vertebra—in front of vertebral system (e.g., vertebral artery and vertebral vein) and left cervical sympathetic trunk and behind the carotid system (e.g., left common carotid artery, left internal jugular vein, and left vagus nerve). The summit of arch lies 3–4 cm above the clavicle. Finally, the duct

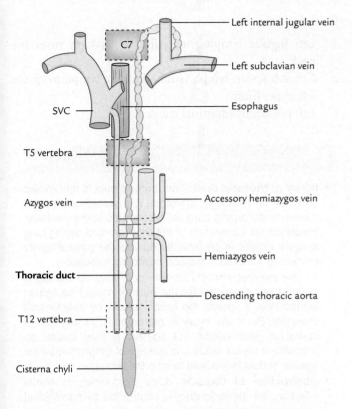

Fig. 23.2 Formation, course, and termination of the thoracic duct.

descends in front of the first part of left subclavian artery and finally terminates by opening into the junction of left subclavian and left internal jugular veins.

N.B. The thoracic duct begins in abdomen, courses through thorax and terminates in the neck.

RELATIONS (Fig. 23.3)

The relations of thoracic duct are as follows:

A. At the aortic orifice of the diaphragm
Anterior: Median arcuate ligament of diaphragm.
Posterior: T12 vertebra.
To the right: Azygos vein.
To the left: Aorta.

B. In the posterior mediastinum
Anterior:
1. Diaphragm.
2. Descending aorta (lower part).
3. Esophagus (upper part).

Posterior:
1. Vertebral column.
2. Anterior longitudinal ligament.
3. Terminal parts of hemiazygos and accessory hemiazygos veins.
4. Right posterior intercostal arteries.

To the right: Azygos vein.
To the left: Descending thoracic aorta.

C. In the superior mediastinum
Anterior:
1. Arch of aorta.
2. Commencement of left subclavian artery.

Posterior: Vertebral column.
To the right: Edge of esophagus.
To the left: Left lung and pleura.

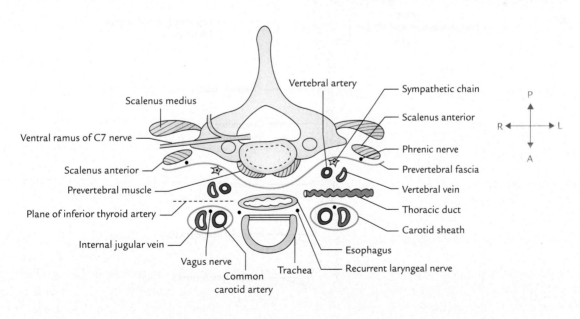

Fig. 23.3 Relations of thoracic duct in the root of the neck.

D. In the root of the neck (Fig. 23.3)

Anterior: Carotid sheath containing left common carotid artery, left internal jugular vein, and left vagus nerve.

Posterior:

1. Vertebral artery and vein.
2. Scalenus anterior muscle (medial border).
3. Phrenic nerve.
4. Thyrocervical trunk and its branches (e.g., suprascapular, transverse cervical, and inferior thyroid arteries).

TRIBUTARIES

The tributaries of the thoracic duct are as follows (Fig. 23.4):

A. In the abdomen

Efferent from lower six intercostal lymph nodes of both sides.

B. In the thorax

1. A pair of the ascending lymph trunks which drains lymph from the upper lumbar lymph nodes (para-aortic lymph nodes).
2. A pair of the descending lymph trunks which drain lymph from the posterior intercostal lymph nodes of upper six spaces.
3. Lymph vessels from the posterior mediastinal lymph nodes.

C. In the neck

1. Left jugular lymph trunk, draining lymph from the neck.
2. Left subclavian lymph trunk, draining lymph from the left upper limb.
3. Left bronchomediastinal trunk.

Clinical correlation

-   **Injury of thoracic duct:** The thoracic duct is thin walled and may be colorless, therefore, it is sometimes injured inadvertently during surgical procedures in the posterior mediastinum. Laceration of the thoracic duct during lung surgery results in chyle entering into the pleural cavity producing a clinical condition called *chylothorax*.

    The cervical part of thoracic duct may be damaged during block dissection of the neck. It should be ligated immediately. If ligated, the lymph returns by anastomotic channels. But if the injury is not detected at the time of operation, and hence not ligated, it may cause an unpleasant *chylus fistula* and leakage of lymph. Immediate ligation of duct is required to stop the leakage.
-   **Obstruction of thoracic duct:** Sometimes in filarial infection, the thoracic duct is obstructed by microfilarial parasites (*Wuchereria bancrofti*) leading to widespread effects, such as *chylothorax, chyloperitoneum, chyluria,* and even the accumulation of chyle in the tunica vaginalis (*chylocele*).

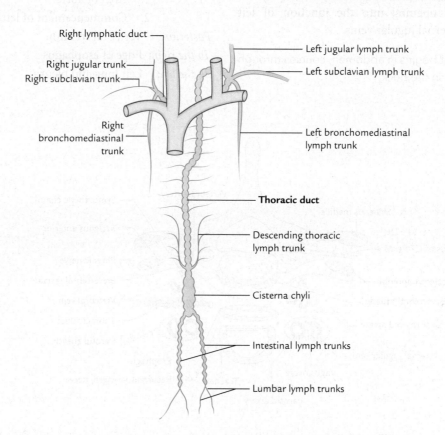

Right lymphatic duct

Right jugular trunk

Right subclavian trunk

Right bronchomediastinal trunk

Left jugular lymph trunk

Left subclavian lymph trunk

Left bronchomediastinal lymph trunk

Thoracic duct

Descending thoracic lymph trunk

Cisterna chyli

Intestinal lymph trunks

Lumbar lymph trunks

Fig. 23.4 Tributaries of the thoracic duct.

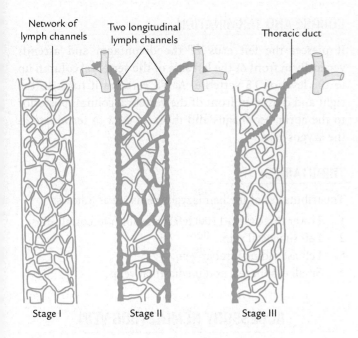

Fig. 23.5 Development of the thoracic duct.

Development

There are three stages in the development of the thoracic duct (Fig. 23.5).

Stage I: In this stage, network of lymph channels is seen in front of the thoracic part of the vertebral column.

Stage II: In this stage, two longitudinal lymph channels appear, in the network of lymph channels, one on the left and another on the right with a number of cross communications.

Stage III: In this stage, the cross communication appears opposite the T5 vertebra, right longitudinal channel below this cross communication and left longitudinal channel above this cross communication persists and form the thoracic duct. All the other parts disappear.

AZYGOS AND HEMIAZYGOS VEINS

The term azygos means single i.e. without a companion. Azygos system of veins consists of azygos, hemiazygos, and accessory hemiazygos veins. These veins lie in front of thoracic part of vertebral column and play an important role in the venous drainage of the thorax.

AZYGOS VEIN (Fig. 23.6)

The azygos vein is present only on the right side in the upper part of the posterior abdominal wall and the posterior mediastinum. It connects the inferior vena cava with the superior vena cava. It is provided with valves and may appear tortuous.

The functions of azygos vein are as follows:

1. It drains venous blood from the thoracic wall and upper lumbar region.
2. It forms an important collateral channel connecting the superior vena cava and inferior vena cava.

FORMATION

The formation of azygos vein is variable. It is formed in one of the following ways:

1. Formed by the union of right subcostal and right ascending lumbar vein at the level of T12 vertebra (common).
2. Arises from the posterior aspect of the inferior vena cava (IVC) near the renal veins.
3. As a continuation of right subcostal vein.
4. Occasionally, it may arise from right renal or right first lumbar vein.

COURSE AND TERMINATION

The azygos vein after formation ascends up and leaves the abdomen by passing through the aortic opening of the diaphragm and enters the posterior mediastinum. There it ascends vertically lying in front of vertebral column up to the level of T4 vertebra, where it arches forwards above the hilum of the right lung to terminate in the superior vena cava at the level of the 2nd costal cartilage.

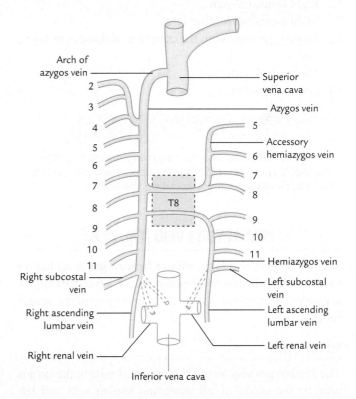

Fig. 23.6 Azygos, hemiazygos, and accessory hemiazygos veins.

RELATIONS

Anterior: Esophagus (right edge).
Posterior:

1. Lower 8th thoracic vertebrae.
2. Right posterior intercostal arteries.

To the right:

1. Right lung and pleura.
2. Greater splanchnic nerves.

To the left:

1. Thoracic duct.
2. Descending thoracic aorta.
3. Esophagus (right border).

The **arch of azygos** vein is related *below* to the root of right lung, on *right side* to the right lung and pleura, and *left side* to the right border of esophagus, trachea, and right vagus nerve.

TRIBUTARIES

The tributaries of the azygos vein are as follows:

1. Lower 7th right posterior intercostal veins except first.
2. Right superior intercostal vein (formed by union of 2nd, 3rd, and 4th right posterior intercostal veins).
3. Hemiazygos vein (at the level of T7 or T8 vertebra).
4. Accessory hemiazygos vein (at the level of T8 or T9 vertebra).
5. Right subcostal vein.
6. Right bronchial vein.
7. Right ascending lumbar vein.
8. Esophageal veins with the exception of those at its lower end.
9. Mediastinal veins.
10. Pericardial veins.

> ### Clinical correlation
>
> In case of obstruction of SVC, it serves as the main collateral channel to shunt the blood from the upper half of the body to IVC (for details see Clinical correlation on p. 285.

HEMIAZYGOS VEIN (Fig. 23.6)

The hemiazygos vein (syn. **inferior hemiazygos vein**) lies on the left side only and corresponds to the lower part of the azygos vein (i.e., mirror image of the lower part of the azygos vein).

FORMATION

The hemiazygos vein formed on the left, similar to the azygos vein, by the union of left ascending lumbar vein and left subcostal vein. It may arise from the posterior surface of the left renal vein.

COURSE AND TERMINATION

It pierces the left crus of the diaphragm and ascends vertically in front of the left side of the vertebral column up to the level of T8 vertebra. At T8 vertebra it turns to the right and crosses in front of the vertebral column posterior to the aorta, esophagus and thoracic duct to terminate in the azygos vein.

TRIBUTARIES

The tributaries of the hemiazygos veins are as follows:

1. Lower three (9th–11th) left posterior intercostal veins.
2. Left subcostal vein.
3. Left ascending lumbar vein.
4. Small esophageal and mediastinal veins.

ACCESSORY HEMIAZYGOS VEIN

The accessory hemiazygos vein (syn. **superior hemiazygos vein**; Fig. 23.6) lies on the left side only and corresponds to the upper part of the azygos vein (i.e., mirror image of the upper part of the azygos vein).

COURSE AND TERMINATION

The accessory hemiazygos vein begins at the medial end of left 4th or 5th intercostal space and descends to the left side of the vertebral column. At the level of T8 vertebra, it turns to the right passes in front of the vertebral column posterior to the aorta, esophagus and thoracic duct to terminate in the azygos vein.

N.B. Sometimes the terminal parts of hemiazygos and accessory hemiazygos veins join together to form a common trunk which crosses across the vertebral column to open into the azygos vein.

TRIBUTARIES

The following are the tributaries of accessory hemiazygos vein:

1. Fifth to eighth (5th–8th) left posterior intercostal veins.
2. Left bronchial veins (sometimes).

THORACIC SYMPATHETIC TRUNKS (Fig. 23.7)

The thoracic sympathetic trunk is a ganglionated chain situated on either side of the vertebral column. Superiorly it is continuous with the cervical sympathetic chain at the thoracic inlet and inferiorly with the lumbar sympathetic chain after passing behind the medial arcuate ligament of the diaphragm.

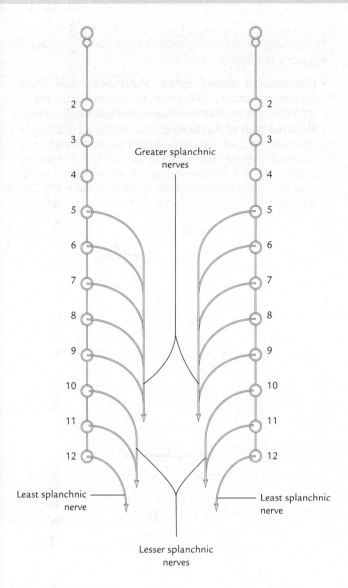

Greater splanchnic nerves

Least splanchnic nerve

Least splanchnic nerve

Lesser splanchnic nerves

Fig. 23.7 Thoracic sympathetic trunks and splanchnic nerves.

COURSE AND RELATIONS

The sympathetic chain descends in front of the neck of the 1st rib, head of 2nd–10th ribs and along the bodies of T11 and T12 vertebrae, in front of posterior intercostal nerve and vessels, passes behind the medial arcuate ligament to become continuous with the lumbar sympathetic trunk.

GANGLIA

Initially, each thoracic sympathetic trunk has 12 ganglia corresponding to the 12 thoracic spinal nerves. The first ganglion commonly fuses with the inferior cervical sympathetic ganglia to form the **cervico-thoracic/stellate ganglion.** The second ganglion also may occasionally fuse with the first ganglion. Thus there are usually 11 ganglia in the thoracic sympathetic trunk; sometimes there may be

only 10 ganglia (*vide supra*). Each ganglion lies at the level of the corresponding intervertebral disc and is connected to the corresponding spinal nerve by white and grey ramus communicans.

BRANCHES

The branches of thoracic sympathetic trunks are divided into two groups: medial and lateral.

A. Medial branches

The medial branches supply the viscera. They are as follows:

1. The medial branches from 1st to 5th ganglia consist of **postganglionic fibres** and are distributed to the heart, great vessels, lungs, and esophagus through the following plexuses:
    (a) Pulmonary plexus.
    (b) Cardiac plexus.
    (c) Aortic plexus.
    (d) Esophageal plexus.
2. Medial branches from 5th to 12th thoracic ganglia consist of **preganglionic fibres** and from three splanchnic nerves as follows:
    (a) *Greater splanchnic nerve*: It is formed by the preganglionic fibres arising from 5th to 9th ganglia. It descends obliquely on the vertebral bodies, pierces the corresponding crus of diaphragm and terminates mainly in the celiac ganglion. Partly it also terminates in the *aorticorenal ganglion* and the *suprarenal gland*.
    (b) *Lesser splanchnic nerve*: It is formed by the preganglionic fibres from 10th and 11th ganglia. It course is obliquely similar to the greater splanchnic nerve, pierces the corresponding crus of diaphragm and terminates in the *celiac ganglion*.
    (c) *Least (lowest) splanchnic nerve*: It is also called *renal nerve*. This tiny nerve arises from the 12th thoracic ganglion and may even be absent. It descends obliquely as greater and lesser splanchnic nerves, pierces either the crus or passes behind the medial arcuate ligament of diaphragm and terminates in the **renal plexus.**

B. Lateral branches

The lateral branches supply limbs and body wall. Their supply is pilomotor, sudomotor, and vasomotor to the skin of these regions.

The preganglionic fibres arise from the lateral horns of spinal segments and enter the sympathetic ganglion via white *rami communicantes* of the spinal nerve. The preganglionic fibres from the ganglion re-enter the spinal nerve via grey rami communicantes and supply the corresponding dermatome of the upper limb and the body wall.

Clinical correlation

- **Thoraco-abdominal sympathectomy:** The bilateral thoraco-abdominal sympathectomy is done to relieve **severe hypertension**. The surgical procedure involves removal of sympathetic trunk from T5 to L2 ganglia and excision of the splanchnic nerves. As a result, there occurs splanchnic vasodilatation and consequent fall in the blood pressure.

    The *upper limb sympathectomy* is used to treat the Raynaud's disease. In this, part of thoracic sympathetic chain is excised below the level of stellate ganglion.

N.B. Injury to stellate ganglion may cause ipsilateral Horner's syndrome.

- **Hypotension during spinal anesthesia:** Sometimes *hypotension* occurs during high spinal anesthesia due to paralysis of sympathetic outflow to the splanchnic nerves.
- **Referred pain of diaphragm:** The irritation of diaphragm secondary to peritonitis causes pain due to stimulation of the phrenic nerve (root value C3, C4, and C5). The pain is referred to the corresponding tip of shoulder, being supplied by the supraclavicular nerve (root value C3, C4, and C5).

Golden Facts to Remember

▶ Largest lymphatic channel in the body   Thoracic duct

▶ Chylothorax   Accumulation of chyle in the pleural cavity

▶ Chylocele   Accumulation of chyle in the tunica vaginalis

▶ Renal nerve   Least splanchnic nerve

▶ Commonest cause of damage of thoracic duct at the root of the neck   Block dissection of the neck

▶ Largest collateral channel connecting superior and inferior vena cavae   Azygos vein

▶ Largest splanchnic nerve   Greater splanchnic nerve

▶ Most posterior intercostal veins drain into   Azygos venous system

Clinical Case Study

A 50-year-old male visited the hospital and complained of swelling of the scrotum associated with periodic fever and passage of milky urine. On examination, the doctor found that scrotum as a whole was enlarged. The scrotal skin was thickened mainly at the bottom. On aspiration of scrotum a milky fluid came out. He was diagnosed as a case of **chylocele** and **chyluria**.

Questions

1. What is chylocele?

2. What is the cause of chylocele?
3. What is the cause of thickening of scrotal skin?

Answers

1. Accumulation of chyle in the tunica vaginalis around the testis.
2. When the thoracic duct is obstructed by the microfilaria (*Wuchereria bancrofti*). It leads to widespread effects such as chylothorax, chyloperitoneum, chyluria.
3. Lymphostasis.

Multiple Choice Questions

CHAPTER 1

1. The most important function of the hand in humans is:
   - (a) Power grip
   - (b) Hook grip
   - (c) Precision grip
   - (d) None of the above

2. Evolutionary changes occurred in human upper limb include all *except:*
   - (a) Appearance of joints permitting rotatory movements of the forearm
   - (b) Addition of clavicle to act as a strut
   - (c) Rotation of thumb to 180° for opposition
   - (d) Rotation of thumb to 90° for opposition

3. Shoulder region includes all of the following regions *except:*
   - (a) Pectoral region
   - (b) Axilla
   - (c) Arm
   - (d) Scapular region

Answers
1. c, 2. c, 3. c

CHAPTER 2

1. Select the incorrect statement about the clavicle:
   - (a) It is only long bone which lies horizontally
   - (b) It has no medullary cavity
   - (c) It ossifies mainly in cartilage
   - (d) It ossifies by two primary centers

2. All the statements about clavicle are correct *except:*
   - (a) It is first bone to start ossifying
   - (b) It acts like a strut to keep upper limb away from the trunk

   - (c) It commonly fractures at the junction of its lateral two-third and medial one-third
   - (d) It can be palpated throughout its extent

3. All the statements about scapula are correct *except:*
   - (a) It has three processes
   - (b) It has head and neck
   - (c) It extends vertically from 1st to 8th rib
   - (d) Its lateral border is thickest

4. All the structures are attached to coracoid process *except:*
   - (a) Coracohumeral ligament
   - (b) Coracoacromial ligament
   - (c) Rhomboid ligament
   - (d) Long head of biceps brachii

5. Select the *incorrect statement* about the surgical neck of humerus:
   - (a) It is commonest site of fracture of humerus
   - (b) It is related to axillary nerve
   - (c) It is a short constriction at the upper end of the shaft below the greater and lesser tubercles
   - (d) It is related to posterior and anterior circumflex humeral arteries

6. Select the *incorrect statement* about the lower end of radius:
   - (a) It is the widest part of the bone
   - (b) Its posterior surface presents Listers's tubercle
   - (c) Groove lateral to Lister's tubercle lodges the tendon of extensor pollicis longus
   - (d) Its medial surface presents the ulnar notch

7. All of the following statements about ulna are correct *except:*
   - (a) It stabilizes the forearm during supination and pronation
   - (b) Its head is directed upwards

(c) Its posterior border provides attachment to three muscles by a common aponeurosis

(d) Its upper end presents two notches

8. Select the *incorrect statement* about carpal bones:

   (a) Scaphoid is the most commonly fractured carpal bone
   (b) Capitate is largest carpal bone
   (c) Pisiform is the first bone to ossify
   (d) Lunate is most commonly dislocated carpal bone

9. All are the peculiar features of first metacarpal bone *except*:

   (a) Its dorsal surface faces laterally
   (b) Its base possesses saddle-shaped articular surface
   (c) Its head is related to two sesamoid bones
   (d) Its epiphysis is at its distal end

10. Select the *incorrect statement* about the phalanges:

    (a) They are 14 in number
    (b) They are short long bones
    (c) All the digits have three phalanges
    (d) Heads of proximal and middle phalanges are pulley-shaped

Answers

1. *c*, 2. *c*, 3. *c*, 4. *d*, 5. *a*, 6. *c*, 7. *b*, 8. *c*, 9. *d*, 10. *c*

CHAPTER 3

1. Muscles of pectoral region include all *except*:

   (a) Pectoralis major
   (b) Serratus anterior
   (c) Pectoralis minor
   (d) Subclavius

2. Select the *incorrect statement* about the pectoralis major muscle:

   (a) It arises from lateral half of the anterior surface of the clavicle
   (b) It is supplied by all the five spinal segments of the brachial plexus
   (c) Its clavicular head flexes the arm
   (d) Its sternocostal head adducts and medially rotates the arm

3. Select the *incorrect statement* about the serratus anterior muscle:

   (a) It arises by 8 digitations from upper eight ribs
   (b) It is inserted into the costal surface of scapula along its lateral border
   (c) Its supplied by long thoracic nerve
   (d) It is the chief protractor of the scapula

4. Regarding clavipectoral fascia, all of the following statements are correct *except*:

   (a) It lies deep to sternocostal head of the pectoralis major
   (b) It encloses subclavius and pectoralis minor muscles
   (c) Vertically it extends from clavicle and axillary fascia
   (d) Its thick upper part is called costoclavicular ligament

5. Clavipectoral fascia is pierced by all of the following structures *except*:

   (a) Cephalic vein
   (b) Thoraco-acromial artery
   (c) Medial pectoral nerve
   (d) Lymph vessels from the breast

6. All of the following statements regarding breast are correct *except*:

   (a) It lies in the superficial fascia of the pectoral region
   (b) It is a modified sebaceous gland
   (c) Vertically, it extends from 2nd to 6th rib
   (d) Horizontally, it extends from sternum to midaxillary line

7. The deep aspect of breast is related to all of the following muscles *except*:

   (a) Pectoralis major
   (b) Pectoralis minor
   (c) Serratus anterior
   (d) Aponeurosis of external oblique muscle of abdomen

8. Regarding breast cancer, which of following statements is *incorrect*:

   (a) It mostly occurs in its superolateral quadrant
   (b) It is immobile and fixed
   (c) It produces retraction of nipple
   (d) Its spread to vertebral column occurs through lymphatics

Answers

1. *b*, 2. *a*, 3. *b*, 4. *a*, 5. *c*, 6. *b*, 7. *b*, 8. *d*

CHAPTER 4

1. The axillary sheath is derived from:

   (a) Investing layer of deep cervical fascia
   (b) Pretracheal fascia
   (c) Prevertebral fascia
   (d) Deep fascia of the axilla

2. The apex of axilla is bounded by all of the following structures *except*:

   (a) Clavicle
   (b) Upper border of scapula

(c) Neck of humerus

(d) Outer border of the 1st rib

3. Which of the following structures is *not* a content of the axilla?

(a) Axillary vessels

(b) Roots of brachial plexus

(c) Axillary tail of the mammary gland

(d) Intercostobrachial nerve

4. Select the *incorrect statement* about the axillary artery:

(a) It extends from outer border of 1st rib to the lower border of teres major muscle

(b) It is divided into three parts of the pectoralis minor muscle

(c) It usually gives rise to five branches

(d) It is the 'key structure' of the axilla

5. Select the *incorrect statement* about the axillary vein:

(a) It is continuation of subclavian vein

(b) It lies medial to the axillary artery

(c) It lies outside the axillary sheath

(d) It receives venae comitantes of the brachial artery

6. Select the *incorrect statement* about the Erb's point:

(a) It is the point on the upper trunk of brachial plexus where six nerves meet

(b) Traction injury of Erb's point involves C5 and C6 fibres

(c) Suprascapular and nerve to subclavius arise at this point

(d) Dorsal scapular and long thoracic nerves arise at this point

7. Which of the following parts of the brachial plexus is involved in Klumpke's paralysis?

(a) Upper trunk

(b) Middle trunk

(c) Lower trunk

(d) None of the above

8. Klumpke's paralysis presents all of the following clinical features *except:*

(a) Claw hand

(b) Sensory loss along the medial border of forearm and hand

(c) Horner's syndrome

(d) Wrist drop

Answers

1. *c,* 2. *c,* 3. *b,* 4. *c,* 5. *a,* 6. *d,* 7. *c,* 8. *d*

CHAPTER 5

1. Which of the following two muscles contract together while climbing a tree?

(a) Latissimus dorsi and trapezius

(b) Teres major and minor

(c) Teres major and pectoralis major

(d) Latissimus dorsi and pectoralis major

2. All of the following muscles are supplied by dorsal scapular nerve *except:*

(a) Supraspinatus

(b) Rhomboideus minor

(c) Rhomboideus major

(d) Levator scapulae

3. All of the following structures form the boundary of triangle of auscultation *except:*

(a) Trapezius

(b) Rhomboideus major

(c) Latissimus dorsi

(d) Medial border of the scapulae

4. All of the following arteries take part in the formation of anastomosis around scapula *except:*

(a) Deep branch of the transverse cervical artery

(b) Suprascapular artery

(c) Lateral thoracic artery

(d) Circumflex scapular artery

5. Select the *incorrect statement* about the deltoid muscle:

(a) It is shaped like an inverted Greek letter delta (∇)

(b) It is supplied by axillary nerve

(c) It abducts the arm from 0° to 90°

(d) Its middle fibres are multipennate

6. All of the following structures pass through quadrangular intermuscular space *except:*

(a) Axillary nerve

(b) Circumflex scapular artery

(c) Posterior circumflex humeral artery

(d) Posterior circumflex humeral vein

7. Which of the following structures pass through the upper triangular intermuscular space?

(a) Anterior circumflex humeral artery

(b) Posterior circumflex humeral artery

(d) Profunda brachii artery

(d) Circumflex scapular artery

8. Which of the following nerves traverse through lower triangular intermuscular space:

(a) Axillary nerve

(b) Thoraco-dorsal nerve

(c) Radial nerve

(d) Median nerve

Answers

1. *d,* 2. *a,* 3. *b,* 4. *c,* 5. *c,* 6. *b,* 7. *d,* 8. *c*

CHAPTER 6

1. All of the following statements about sternoclavicular joint are true *except*:
   - (a) It is a saddle type of synovial joint
   - (b) Its articular surfaces are covered with fibrocartilage
   - (c) It is frequently involved in dislocation
   - (d) Its joint cavity is divided into two parts by an articular disc

2. Musculotendinous cuff is formed by all the muscles *except*:
   - (a) Supraspinatus
   - (b) Teres major
   - (c) Infraspinatus
   - (d) Teres minor

3. Anatomically the shoulder joint is most commonly dislocated:
   - (a) Superiorly
   - (b) Inferiorly
   - (c) Anteriorly
   - (d) Posteriorly

4. The synovial bursa which commonly communicates with the cavity of the shoulder joint is:
   - (a) Subscapular bursa
   - (b) Infraspinatus bursa
   - (c) Subacromial bursa
   - (d) None of the above

5. Which of the following nerves is commonly injured in inferior dislocation of shoulder joint?
   - (a) Radial nerve
   - (b) Ulnar nerve
   - (c) Thoraco-dorsal nerve
   - (d) Axillary nerve

6. Shoulder movements occur at:
   - (a) Glenohumeral joint only
   - (b) Sternoclavicular joint only
   - (c) Acromioclavicular joint only
   - (d) Scapulothoracic joint only
   - (e) All of the above joints

7. Which of the following structures prevent superior dislocation of head of humerus?
   - (a) Coracoclavicular ligament
   - (b) Coracohumeral ligament
   - (c) Coracoacromial arch
   - (d) Transverse humeral ligament

8. Chief articulation of shoulder is:
   - (a) Sternoclavicular joint
   - (b) Acromioclavicular joint
   - (c) Glenohumeral joint
   - (d) Scapulothoracic joint

9. The term *shoulder separation* is used for:
   - (a) Dislocation of shoulder joint
   - (b) Dislocation of acromioclavicular joint
   - (c) Dislocation of sternoclavicular joint
   - (d) None of the above

Answers

1. *c*, 2. *b*, 3. *b*, 4. *a*, 5. *d*, 6. *e*, 7. *c*, 8. *c*, 9. *b*

CHAPTER 7

1. The group of spinal segments supplying cutaneous innervation to upper limb is:
   - (a) C5 to T1
   - (b) C4 to C8
   - (c) C3 to T3
   - (d) C4 to T2

2. The spinal segment providing dermatomal supply to the little finger is:
   - (a) C4
   - (b) T4
   - (c) C8
   - (d) C6

3. All of the following structures are present in the delto-pectoral groove *except*:
   - (a) Cephalic vein
   - (b) Deltopectoral lymph node
   - (c) Basilic vein
   - (d) Deltoid branch of thoraco-acromial artery

4. The lymph vessels from thumb drain into which group of axillary lymph nodes:
   - (a) Anterior
   - (b) Posterior
   - (c) Central
   - (d) Lateral

5. Most commonly used vein for intravenous injection is:
   - (a) Cephalic vein
   - (b) Basilic vein
   - (c) Median cubital vein
   - (d) Median vein of the forearm

6. Which of the following statements about cephalic vein is *incorrect?*
   - (a) Cephalic vein corresponds to the great saphenous vein of the lower limb
   - (b) It is the postaxial vein of the upper limb

(c) It pierces clavipectoral fascia to drain into axillary vein

(d) Greater part of its blood is drained into basilic vein through median cubital vein

7. Select the *incorrect statement* about the basilic vein:

(a) It is the postaxial vein of the upper limb

(b) It begins form the medial end of the dorsal venous plexus

(c) It continues upwards as axillary vein at the upper border of teres major

(d) It is accompanied by medial cutaneous nerve of the forearm

8. All of the following cutaneous nerves are derived from radial nerve *except*:

(a) Lower lateral cutaneous nerve of arm

(b) Upper lateral cutaneous nerve of arm

(c) Superficial terminal branch of radial nerve

(d) Posterior cutaneous nerve of arm

Answers

1. *c*, 2. *c*, 3. *c*, 4. *d*, 5. *c*, 6. *b*, 7. *c*, 8. *b*

CHAPTER 8

1. The all of following muscles are present in the anterior compartment of the arm *except*:

(a) Brachialis

(b) Brachioradialis

(c) Coracobrachialis

(d) Biceps brachii

2. The only muscle of anterior compartment of arm that is inserted into the humerus is:

(a) Biceps brachii

(b) Coracobrachialis

(c) Brachialis

(d) None of the above

3. All transitions which occur at the level of insertion of coracobrachialis are correct *except*:

(a) Median nerve crosses brachial artery from lateral to medial side

(b) Ulnar pierces medial intermuscular septum to enter the posterior compartment of the arm

(c) Cephalic vein pierces the deep fascia

(d) Radial nerve pierces the lateral intermuscular septum to enter the anterior compartment of the arm

4. The nerve that lies in the groove behind the medial epicondyle of humerus is:

(a) Median

(b) Ulnar

(c) Radial

(d) Musculocutaneous

5. Which of the following muscles is innervated by both musculocutaneous and radial nerve?

(a) Biceps brachii

(b) Coracobrachialis

(c) Brachialis

(d) Brachioradialis

6. Select the *incorrect statement* about the coracobrachialis:

(a) It arises from tip of coracoid process of scapula

(b) It has more morphological than functional significance

(c) The ligament of Struthers' represents its third head

(d) It is pierced by ulnar nerve

7. All of the following are branches of brachial artery *except*:

(a) Profunda brachii artery

(b) Main humeral nutrient artery

(c) Radial collateral artery

(d) Superior ulnar collateral artery

8. Select the *incorrect statement* about the biceps brachii muscle:

(a) It normally has two heads

(b) Its long head arises from infraglenoid tubercle of scapula

(c) It is capable of affecting movements at glenohumeral, elbow and superior radio-ulnar joints

(d) It is supplied by musculocutaneous nerve

Answers

1. *b*, 2. *b*, 3. *c*, 4. *b*, 5. *c*, 6. *d*, 7. *c*, 8. *b*

CHAPTER 9

1. All of the following are superficial muscles on the front of forearm *except*:

(a) Flexor carpi radialis

(b) Pronator teres

(c) Palmaris longus

(d) Flexor pollicis longus

2. Select the *incorrect statement* about the pronator teres:

(a) It is the smallest superficial flexor of the forearm

(b) Its medial border forms the medial boundary of cubital fossa

(c) Median nerve passes between its two heads

(d) Ulnar nerve is separated from median nerve by its deep head

3. The radial artery on the front of wrist lies lateral to the tendon of:

    (a) Brachioradialis
    (b) Abductor pollicis longus
    (c) Flexor carpi radialis
    (d) Flexor carpi ulnaris

4. The anterior interosseous nerve is a branch of:

    (a) Superficial branch of radial nerve
    (b) Deep branch of radial nerve
    (c) Median nerve
    (d) Ulnar nerve

5. All of the following deep muscles on the back of the forearm outcrop in the distal third of the forearm *except:*

    (a) Abductor pollicis longus
    (b) Extensor carpi radialis longus
    (c) Extensor pollicis longus
    (d) Extensor pollicis brevis

6. All of the following structures pass through the fourth compartment of extensor retinaculum on the dorsal aspect of wrist *except:*

    (a) Extensor digitorum
    (b) Extensor pollicis longus
    (c) Anterior interosseous artery
    (d) Posterior interosseous nerve

7. The supinator muscle is supplied by

    (a) Ulnar nerve
    (b) Anterior interosseous nerve
    (c) Median nerve
    (d) Posterior interosseous nerve

8. Which of the following statements is *not correct?*

    (a) Ulnar nerve passes between the two heads of flexor carpi ulnaris
    (b) Median nerve passes between the two heads of pronator teres
    (c) Median nerve passes between the two head of flexor digitorum superficialis
    (d) Radial nerve passes between the two heads of flexor digitorum superficialis

Answers

1. *d*, 2. *b*, 3. *c*, 4. *c*, 5. *b*, 6. *b*, 7. *d*, 8. *d*

CHAPTER 10

1. Select the *incorrect statement* about the elbow joint:

    (a) It is a hinge type of synovial joint
    (b) It consists of two articulations, humero-radial and humero-ulnar

    (c) It usually dislocates anteriorly
    (d) Effusion within joint cavity distends elbow posteriorly

2. Medial collateral ligament of elbow joint is closely related to:

    (a) Radial nerve
    (b) Ulnar artery
    (c) Ulnar nerve
    (d) Median nerve

3. Clinically most important synovial bursa around elbow joint is:

    (a) Subtendinous olecranon bursa
    (b) Subcutaneous olecranon bursa
    (c) Bicipitoradial bursa
    (d) Bursa between biceps tendon and oblique cord

4. Select the *incorrect statement* about superior radio-ulnar joint:

    (a) It is a pivot type of synovial joint
    (b) Its cavity does not communicate with the cavity of elbow joint
    (c) It permits movements of supination and pronation
    (d) Its prime stabilizing factor is its annular ligament

5. Nerve entrapments which occur around the elbow include all *except:*

    (a) Median nerve entrapment
    (b) Ulnar nerve entrapment
    (c) Radial nerve entrapment
    (d) Posterior interosseous nerve entrapment

6. Select the *incorrect statement* about the inferior radio-ulnar joint:

    (a) It is a pivot type of synovial joint
    (b) Its cavity communicates with the cavity of wrist joint
    (c) Its prime stability is provided by its articular disc
    (d) It permits supination and pronation of forearm

7. Select the *incorrect statement* about the interosseous membrane of the forearm:

    (a) It is a fibrous membrane which stretches between interosseous border of radius and ulna
    (b) Its fibres run downwards and laterally from ulna to the radius
    (c) Its posterior surface is related to anterior interosseous artery and posterior interosseous nerve
    (d) Its anterior surface is related to anterior interosseous artery and anterior interosseous nerve

8. All are correct statements about oblique cord of forearm *except:*

    (a) It is fibrous band extending between radial and ulnar tuberosities

(b) Its fibres are directed opposite to those of interosseous membrane

(c) Posterior interosseous nerve enters the back of forearm through gap between oblique cord and interosseous membrane

(d) Morphologically it represents the degenerated part of the flexor pollicis longus

Answers

1. *c*, 2. *c*, 3. *b*, 4. *b*, 5. *a*, 6. *b*, 7. *b*, 8. *c*

CHAPTER 11

1. Select the *incorrect statement* about the palmaris brevis muscle:

   (a) It is subcutaneous muscle

   (b) It arises from flexor retinaculum and palmar aponeurosis

   (c) It is innervated by median nerve

   (d) Its contraction causes wrinkling of medial palmar skin

2. All of the following structures pass superficial to the flexor retinaculum *except*:

   (a) Ulnar nerve

   (b) Superficial radial nerve

   (c) Tendon of palmaris longus

   (d) Ulnar artery

3. All the structures pass through carpal tunnel *except*:

   (a) Tendons of flexor digitorum superficialis

   (b) Tendon of flexor digitorum profundus

   (c) Tendon of flexor carpi radialis

   (d) Tendon of flexor pollicis longus

4. Select the *true statement* about the abductor pollicis:

   (a) It is the muscle of thenar eminence

   (b) It is a content of thenar space

   (c) It transmits ulnar artery between its two heads

   (d) It is innervated by ulnar nerve

5. Select the *incorrect statement* about an anatomical snuff-box:

   (a) It is bounded posteromedially by the tendon of flexor pollicis longus

   (b) Its roof is crossed by cephalic vein

   (c) Pulsations of radial artery can be felt in its floor

   (d) Tenderness in the anatomical snuff-box indicates fracture of capitate bone

6. First lumbrical canal is a diverticulum of:

   (a) Thenar space

   (b) Midpalmar space

(c) Space of Parona

(d) None of the above

7. Radial bursa is the synovial sheath enclosing the tendon of:

   (a) Flexor carpi radialis

   (b) Flexor pollicis longus

   (c) Extensor carpi radialis longus

   (d) Extensor carpi radialis brevis

8. All the statements about the palmar interossei are correct *except*:

   (a) They are unipennate

   (b) They take origin from all the five metacarpals

   (c) They are innervated by ulnar nerve

   (d) They adduct the digits

9. All the statements about ulnar bursa are correct *except*:

   (a) It encloses tendons of flexor digitorum superficialis and flexor digitorum profundus

   (b) It communicates with the digital synovial sheath of little finger

   (c) Distally it extends in the palm up to the heads of metacarpals

   (d) Proximally it extends into the forearm about a finger breadth above the flexor retinaculum

10. Select the *incorrect statement* about the superficial palmar arterial arch:

   (a) It is a direct continuation of ulnar artery

   (b) It lies proximal to the deep palmar arch

   (c) It lies deep to the palmar aponeurosis

   (d) It lies superficial to long flexor tendons

Answers

1. *c*, 2. *b*, 3. *c*, 4. *d*, 5. *d*, 6. *a*, 7. *b*, 8. *b*, 9. *c*, 10. *b*

CHAPTER 12

1. Select the *incorrect statement* about the wrist joint:

   (a) It is a synovial joint of saddle variety

   (b) It is a synovial joint of ellipsoid variety

   (c) Ulna does not take part in this articulation

   (d) Its cavity does not communicate with the cavity of inferior radio-ulnar joint

2. Select the *incorrect statement* about the wrist joint:

   (a) Its upper articular surface is formed by radius and ulna

   (b) Its lower articular surface is formed by scaphoid, lunate and triquetral bones

   (c) It is an ellipsoidal joint

   (d) It permits free rotatory movements

3. All of the following bones form the proximal row of carpal bones *except:*

   (a) Lunate
   (b) Pisiform
   (c) Trapezium
   (d) Scaphoid

4. All the carpometacarpal joints are plane type of synovial joint *except:*

   (a) First carpometacarpal
   (b) Second carpometacarpal
   (c) Third carpometacarpal
   (d) Fourth carpometacarpal

5. All are the features of 'position of rest of hand' *except:*

   (a) Forearm is in semiprone position
   (b) Wrist joint is slightly extended
   (c) Fingers are partially flexed
   (d) Plane of thumb-nail lies parallel to the plane of finger-nails

6. Flexion of thumb is produced by all muscles *except:*

   (a) Flexor pollicis longus
   (b) Opponens pollicis
   (c) Flexor carpi radialis
   (d) Flexor pollicis brevis

7. The following muscles cause abduction of wrist *except:*

   (a) Extensor carpi radialis longus
   (b) Extensor carpi radialis brevis
   (c) Abductor pollicis longus
   (d) Abductor pollicis brevis

8. Which finger is *not abducted* by dorsal interossei:

   (a) Second
   (b) Third
   (c) Fourth
   (d) Fifth

Answers

1. *a,* 2. *a,* 3. *c,* 4. *a,* 5. *d,* 6. *c,* 7. *d,* 8. *d*

CHAPTER 13

1. Select the *incorrect statement* about the radial nerve:

   (a) It arises from posterior cord of the brachial plexus
   (b) It gives lateral and posterior cutaneous nerves of arm in spiral groove
   (c) It supplies flexor carpi radialis
   (d) Its lesion in radial groove causes wrist drop

2. Skin over the thenar eminence is supplied by:

   (a) Palmar cutaneous branch of median nerve
   (b) Palmar cutaneous branch of ulnar nerve
   (c) Recurrent branch of ulnar nerve
   (d) None of the above

3. All the statements about superficial radial nerve are true *except:*

   (a) It arises from radial nerve in the spiral groove
   (b) It is entirely sensory
   (c) It arises from radial nerve in cubital fossa
   (d) It provides sensory innervation to skin on the root of thumb

4. Which of the following statements is *incorrect?*

   (a) Median nerve is called 'laborer's nerve'
   (b) Ulnar nerve is called 'musician's nerve'
   (c) Ulnar nerve in the hand is called 'eye of the hand'
   (d) Median nerve in the hand is called 'eye of the hand'

5. Sensory innervation to the skin on the dorsum of hand is provided by:

   (a) Radial nerve
   (b) Median nerve
   (c) Ulnar nerve
   (d) All of the above

6. The 'ape-thumb deformity' occurs due to lesion of:

   (a) Radial nerve
   (b) Median nerve
   (c) Ulnar nerve
   (d) Musculocutaneous nerve

7. All are signs of ulnar nerve lesion *except:*

   (a) Wasting of hypothenar eminence
   (b) Loss of abduction and adduction of fingers
   (c) Absence of flexion of ring and little fingers
   (d) Absence of flexion of index finger

8. A median nerve palsy causes all of the following signs *except:*

   (a) Wasting of thenar eminence
   (b) Loss of opposition of thumb
   (c) Pointing index finger
   (d) Loss of sensation on the palmar aspect of medial 1½ fingers

9. Forearm has all of the following cutaneous nerves *except:*

   (a) Lateral cutaneous nerve of forearm
   (b) Medial cutaneous nerve of forearm
   (c) Anterior cutaneous nerve of forearm
   (d) Posterior cutaneous nerve of the forearm

Answers

1. *c,* 2. *c,* 3. *a,* 4. *c,* 5. *d,* 6. *b,* 7. *d,* 8. *d,* 9. *c*

CHAPTER 14

1. Select the *incorrect statement* about the thoracic inlet:

    (a) It communicates with the root of the neck
    (b) It is roofed on either side by suprapleural membrane
    (c) It is circular in shape
    (d) Its plane slops downwards and forwards

2. All the statements about Sibson's fascia are correct *except*:

    (a) Forms the diaphragm of thoracic inlet
    (b) Its apex is attached to the tip of the transverse process of T1 vertebra
    (c) Its base is attached to the inner border of the 1st rib
    (d) It protects the underlying cervical pleura

3. All of the following nerves pass through thoracic inlet *except*:

    (a) Right and left phrenic nerves
    (b) Right and left first thoracic nerves
    (c) Right and left recurrent laryngeal nerves
    (d) Right and left vagus nerves

4. Which of the following structures does not pass through the aortic orifice of the diaphragm?

    (a) Aorta
    (b) Thoracic duct
    (c) Hemiazygos vein
    (d) Azygos vein

5. Caval opening of diaphragm lies at the level of:

    (a) Body of T6 vertebra
    (b) Body of T8 vertebra
    (c) Body of T10 vertebra
    (d) Body of T12 vertebra

6. Congenital posterolateral defect of diaphragm occurs due to failure of development of:

    (a) Mesoderm of body wall
    (b) Dorsal mesentery of esophagus
    (c) Septum transversum
    (d) Pleuroperitoneal membrane

7. All of the following structures pass through the crura of diaphragm *except*:

    (a) Greater splanchnic nerve
    (b) Lesser splanchnic nerve
    (c) Hemiazygos vein
    (d) Sympathetic chain

8. Sympathetic chain enters the abdomen by passing deep to:

    (a) Median arcuate ligament
    (b) Medial arcuate ligament
    (c) Aortic opening
    (d) Lateral arcuate ligament

Answers

1. *c*, 2. *b*, 3. *c*, 4. *c*, 5. *b*, 6. *d*, 7. *d*, 8. *b*

CHAPTER 15

1. Select the *incorrect statement* about the manubrium sterni:

    (a) It is the thickest and strongest part of the sternum
    (b) It is the commonest site for bone marrow aspiration
    (c) It articulates below with body of sternum to form primary cartilaginous joint
    (d) Upper part of its posterior surface is related to the arch of aorta

2. All the statements about the sternal angle are correct *except*:

    (a) It is formed by the articulation of the manubrium with the body of the sternum
    (b) It lies at the level of 2nd costal cartilage
    (c) It lies opposite the intervertebral disc between the T3 and T4 vertebrae
    (d) Ascending aorta ends at this level

3. All are the atypical ribs *except*:

    (a) 1st rib
    (b) 2nd rib
    (c) 9th rib
    (d) 10th rib

4. Anterior aspect of the neck of 1st rib is related to all structures *except*:

    (a) Sympathetic chain
    (b) Superior intercostal vein
    (c) Superior intercostal artery
    (d) Ventral ramus of first thoracic nerve

5. Select the *incorrect statement* about the 12th thoracic vertebrae:

    (a) It appears like first lumbar vertebra
    (b) Its transverse process presents three tubercles
    (c) Its transverse process has small articular facet
    (d) Its body presents circular articular facet on each side

6. First costosternal/chondrosternal joint is a:

    (a) Synovial joint
    (b) Primary cartilaginous joint
    (c) Secondary cartilaginous joint
    (d) Fibrous joint

7. The rib commonly fractures:

    (a) At its posterior angle

(b) At the middle of its shaft

(c) At its neck

(d) At its anterior angle

8. **All are the atypical features of 1st rib *except*:**

(a) Its shaft has upper and lower surfaces

(b) Its angle and tubercle coincide

(c) Its head bears two articular facets

(d) It is the most curved rib

Answers

1. *c*, 2. *c*, 3. *c*, 4. *b*, 5. *c*, 6. *b*, 7. *a*, 8. *c*

CHAPTER 16

1. **Which of the following muscles is attached on the inner aspects of the ribs?**

(a) External intercostal

(b) Internal intercostal

(c) Intercostalis intimus

(d) None of the above

2. **Anterior intercostal membrane is the continuation of:**

(a) External intercostal muscle

(b) Internal intercostal muscle

(c) Intercostalis intimi muscle

(d) Subcostalis muscle

3. **All of the following are parts of transverse thoracis muscle *except*:**

(a) Intercostalis intimus

(b) Subcostalis

(c) Levatores costarum

(d) Sternocostalis

4. **Typical intercostal nerves are:**

(a) 3rd to 6th intercostal nerves

(b) 7th to 11th intercostal nerves

(c) 7th to 10th intercostal nerves

(d) 1st and 2nd intercostal nerves

5. **The branches of all of the following arteries supply blood to intercostal spaces *except*:**

(a) Descending thoracic aorta

(b) Internal thoracic artery

(c) Superior epigastric artery

(d) Musculophrenic artery

6. **Increase in vertical diameter of thoracic cavity is brought about by:**

(a) Pump-handle movement of the sternum

(b) Bucket-handle movement of the ribs

(c) Contraction of diaphragm

(d) (a) and (b)

7. **During quiet respiration, the elevation of ribs is done mostly by the contraction of:**

(a) Internal intercostal muscles

(b) External intercostal muscles

(c) Intercostalis intimi muscles

(d) Subcostalis muscles

8. **Select the *incorrect statement* about the increase in various diameters of thoracic cavity**

(a) Pump-handle movement of sternum increases its anteroposterior diameter

(b) Contraction of diaphragm increases its vertical diameter

(c) Bucket-handle movement of ribs increases its transverse diameter

(d) Pump-handle movement of sternum increases its vertical diameter

Answers

1. *c*, 2. *a*, 3. *c*, 4. *a*, 5. *c*, 6. *c*, 7. *b*, 8. *d*

CHAPTER 17

1. **Select the *incorrect statement* about the parietal pleura:**

(a) It develops from somatopleuric mesoderm

(b) It is supplied by somatic nerves

(c) It develops from splanchnopleuric mesoderm

(d) It is sensitive to pain and touch

2. **All the statements about visceral pleura are correct *except*:**

(a) It develops from splanchnopleuric mesoderm

(b) It is innervated by autonomic nerves

(c) It lines the thoracic wall

(d) It is insensitive to touch and temperature

3. **Pleura extends beyond the thoracic cage on all of the following sites *except*:**

(a) Root of the neck

(b) Costovertebral angles

(c) Right xiphisternal angle

(d) Left xiphisternal angle

4. **Select the *incorrect statement* about the summit of cervical pleura:**

(a) It lies 2.5 cm above the medial end of the clavicle

(b) It lies 2.5 cm above the 1st costal cartilage

(c) It lies 5 cm above the 1st costal cartilage

(d) It is covered by Sibson's fascia

5. **In the midaxillary line the inferior margin of parietal pleura crosses:**

(a) 6th rib

(b) 8th rib

(c) 10th rib

(d) 12th rib

6. All arteries supply the pleura *except:*

   (a) Internal thoracic
   (b) Intercostal
   (c) Bronchial
   (d) Pulmonary

7. Select the *incorrect statement* about the pulmonary ligament:

   (a) It is a fold of the visceral pleura
   (b) It provides a dead space for expansion of pulmonary veins
   (c) It extends from root of lung as far down as diaphragm
   (d) It extends between mediastinum and the lung

8. Select the *incorrect statement* about the costodiaphragmatic recess:

   (a) It is the lower part of pleural cavity between the diaphragmatic and costal pleura
   (b) It is the least dependent part of the pleural cavity
   (c) It lies 8–9 cm deep in the midaxillary line
   (d) It lies 2.5 cm deep in the midclavicular line

Answers

1. *c*, 2. *c*, 3. *d*, 4. *b*, 5. *c*, 6. *d*, 7. *a*, 8. *b*

CHAPTER 18

1. Mediastinal surface of right lung is related to all *except:*

   (a) Right atrium
   (b) Arch of aorta
   (c) Arch of azygos vein
   (d) Inferior vena cava

2. Mediastinal surface of the left lung is related to all *except:*

   (a) Left ventricle
   (b) Ascending aorta
   (c) Superior vena cava
   (d) Arch of aorta

3. Uppermost structure in the hilum of right lung is:

   (a) Pulmonary artery
   (b) Superior pulmonary vein
   (c) Bronchus
   (d) Bronchial artery

4. During quiet respiration the posterior end of lower border of lung passes across:

   (a) 6th rib
   (b) 8th rib
   (c) 10th rib
   (d) T12 spine

5. Nutrition to the nonrespiratory portions of lung is supplied by:

   (a) Pulmonary artery
   (b) Pulmonary vein
   (c) Bronchial artery
   (d) (a) and (c)

6. All are characteristic features of a bronchopulmonary segment *except:*

   (a) It is pyramidal in shape
   (b) It is aerated by a tertiary bronchus
   (c) It has its own segmental vein
   (d) It is surrounded by the connective tissue

7. Number of bronchopulmonary segments in lower lobe of each lung is:

   (a) Two
   (b) Three
   (c) Four
   (d) Five

8. The lingula is a tongue-shaped projection from:

   (a) Upper lobe of right lung
   (b) Upper lobe of left lung
   (c) Lower lobe of right lung
   (d) Lower lobe of left lung

Answers

1. *b*, 2. *c*, 3. *c*, 4. *c*, 5. *c*, 6. *c*, 7. *d*, 8. *b*

CHAPTER 19

1. All are correct statements about mediastinum *except:*

   (a) It is broad septum within thoracic cavity, which separates two pleural cavities
   (b) It contains all the thoracic viscera and structures except lungs
   (c) Structures forming mediastinum are bound together by loose connective tissue
   (d) It is rigid and nonmovable septum in living people

2. All form the boundaries of superior mediastinum *except:*

   (a) Manubrium sterni
   (b) Upper four thoracic vertebrae
   (c) Diaphragm
   (d) Plane of superior thoracic aperture

3. All are contents of superior mediastinum *except:*

   (a) Arch of aorta
   (b) Pulmonary trunk
   (c) Superior vena cava
   (d) Brachiocephalic trunk

4. All structures traverse the whole length of mediastinum *except:*
   (a) Esophagus
   (b) Trachea
   (c) Thoracic duct
   (d) Sympathetic trunks

5. All are contents of middle mediastinum *except:*
   (a) Heart
   (b) Pulmonary arteries
   (c) Brachiocephalic veins
   (d) Pulmonary veins

6. All the statements regarding posterior mediastinum are correct *except:*
   (a) Pus in the posterior mediastinum can enter the thighs
   (b) Neck infection behind prevertebral layer of deep cervical fascia cannot extend into the posterior mediastinum
   (c) Neck infection in the retropharyngeal space can extend into the posterior mediastinum
   (d) Its superior boundary is formed by superior thoracic aperture

7. Posterior mediastinum provides passage to all structures *except:*
   (a) Esophagus
   (b) Trachea
   (c) Descending thoracic aorta
   (d) Azygos veins

8. The thymus is located in:
   (a) Superior mediastinum
   (b) Middle mediastinum
   (c) Posterior mediastinum
   (d) Anterior mediastinum

Answers

1. *d*, 2. *c*, 3. *b*, 4. *b*, 5. *c*, 6. *d*, 7. *b*, 8. *a*

CHAPTER 20

1. Pericardial cavity lies between:
   (a) Fibrous pericardium and serous pericardium
   (b) Fibrous pericardium and epicardium
   (c) Parietal pericardium and visceral pericardium
   (d) Epicardium and myocardium

2. Select the *correct statement* about the transverse pericardial sinus:
   (a) It lies in front of superior vena cava
   (b) It lies in front of pulmonary veins

   (c) It lies behind the ascending aorta and pulmonary trunk
   (d) It lies in front of ascending aorta and pulmonary trunk

3. Sternocostal surface of the heart is mainly formed by:
   (a) Right atrium
   (b) Right ventricle
   (c) Left ventricle
   (d) (a) and (b)

4. Apex beat in adults is normally felt in the:
   (a) Left 4th intercostal space in the midclavicular line
   (b) Left 5th intercostal space just medial to the midclavicular line
   (c) Left 6th intercostal space just medial to the midclavicular line
   (d) Left 3rd intercostal space just lateral to the midclavicular line

5. Select the *incorrect statement* about the oblique pericardial sinus:
   (a) It is the recess of serous pericardium
   (b) It lies behind the left atrium
   (c) It lies behind the right atrium
   (d) It is closed on all sides except below

6. All the statements are correct about the conducting system of the heart *except:*
   (a) It is made up of specialized cardiac muscle fibres
   (b) It is responsible for initiation and conduction of impulses
   (c) Nearly whole of the conducting system is supplied by left coronary artery
   (d) Its SA node is known as the pacemaker of the heart

7. Select the *incorrect statement* about the area of superficial cardiac dullness:
   (a) It lies in front of right ventricle
   (b) It is related to the left 4th and 5th intercostal spaces
   (c) It is covered by lung and pleura
   (d) It can be used as a site of aspiration of fluid in pericardial effusion

8. The base of the heart is formed by:
   (a) Right and left ventricles
   (b) Right and left atria
   (c) Right atrium and right ventricle
   (d) Left atrium and left ventricle

9. All structures meet at the crux of the heart *except:*
   (a) Posterior interventricular groove
   (b) Posterior atrioventricular groove

(c) Interatrial groove

(d) Sulcus terminalis

10. Most anteriorly located valve of the heart is:

(a) Pulmonary

(b) Aortic

(c) Tricuspid

(d) Bicuspid

11. Conducting system of the heart is a modification of:

(a) Epicardium

(b) Myocardium

(c) Endocardium

(d) None of the above

Answers

1. *c*, 2. *c*, 3. *d*, 4. *b*, 5. *c*, 6. *c*, 7. *c*, 8. *b*, 9. *d*, 10. *a*, 11. *b*

CHAPTER 21

1. All the statements about SVC are correct *except:*

(a) It lies both in superior and middle mediastina

(b) It is devoid of valves

(c) It is formed at the lower border of the right 1st costal cartilage

(d) It pierces pericardium at the level of the right 2nd costal cartilage

2. All are the tributaries of SVC *except:*

(a) Right brachiocephalic vein

(b) Left brachiocephalic vein

(c) Hemiazygos vein

(d) Azygos vein

3. All the statements regarding SVC are correct *except:*

(a) It is 7 cm long and 2 cm wide

(b) It has no valves

(c) Its lower half is covered by pericardium

(d) It is completely enclosed in the pericardium

4. The ascending aorta gives origin to:

(a) Brachiocephalic trunk

(b) Left common carotid artery

(c) Left subclavian artery

(d) Right and left coronary arteries

5. All are the branches of arch of aorta *except:*

(a) Brachiocephalic trunk

(b) Right common carotid artery

(c) Left common carotid artery

(d) Left subclavian artery

6. All are the branches of descending thoracic aorta *except:*

(a) Superior intercostal arteries

(b) Posterior intercostal arteries

(c) Subcostal arteries

(d) Left bronchial arteries

7. All are correct statements about pulmonary trunk *except:*

(a) It is about 5 cm long

(b) It arises from the infundibulum of the right ventricle

(c) Its termination lies in front of the arch of aorta

(d) It is completely enclosed within the fibrous pericardium

8. Select the *incorrect statement* about the pulmonary trunk:

(a) It is completely enclosed within the fibrous pericardium

(b) It along with ascending aorta is enclosed by a common sheath of visceral pericardium

(c) It is intimately related to the two coronary arteries

(d) It lies entirely to the right of ascending aorta

9. Aortic knuckle, a projection in the upper part of left margin of the cardiac shadow in x-ray chest PA view, is cast by:

(a) Ascending aorta

(b) Arch of aorta

(c) Aortic sinuses

(d) Descending aorta

Answers

1. *d*, 2. *c*, 3. *d*, 4. *d*, 5. *b*, 6. *a*, 7. *c*, 8. *d*, 9. *b*

CHAPTER 22

1. Select the *incorrect statement* about the esophagus:

(a) It is narrowest at its commencement

(b) It is about 15 cm long

(c) It ends at the level of T11 vertebra

(d) It pierces diaphragm at the level of T10 vertebra

2. Constrictions of esophagus are present at all sites *except:*

(a) At cricopharyngeal junction

(b) Where it is crossed by the arch of aorta

(c) Where it is surrounded by right crus of diaphragm

(d) Where it is crossed by the left principal bronchus

3. Select the *incorrect statement* about the distances of constrictions in esophagus from upper incisor teeth:

(a) First constriction is 6 inches

(b) Second constriction is 9 inches

(c) Third constriction is 11 inches

(d) Fourth constriction is 17 inches

4. Lymphatics from the lower end of esophagus drains into:

(a) Deep cervical lymph nodes

(b) Pretracheal lymph nodes

(c) Posterior mediastinal lymph nodes

(d) Celiac lymph nodes

5. **Esophagus is supplied by the esophageal branches of all the arteries** *except:*

(a) Inferior thyroid

(b) Descending thoracic aorta

(c) Left gastric

(d) Right gastric

6. **All statements regarding trachea are true** *except:*

(a) It begins in the neck at the lower border of cricoid cartilage

(b) It is about 20 cm long

(c) It is made up of 16–20 C-shaped hyaline cartilages

(d) It terminates in the thorax at the level of sternal angle

7. **Select the** *incorrect statement* **about the trachea:**

(a) It is flexible fibro-elastic tube

(b) It extends from lower border C6 vertebra to the lower border of T4 vertebra

(c) Its external diameter in an adult male is about 2 cm

(d) Its internal diameter in an adult male is 15 mm

8. **Anteriorly the trachea is related to all structures** *except:*

(a) Arch of aorta

(b) Left brachiocephalic vein

(c) Esophagus

(d) Deep cardiac plexus

Answers

1. *b*, 2. *a*, 3. *d*, 4. *d*, 5. *d*, 6. *b*, 7. *d*, 8. *c*

CHAPTER 23

1. **Select the** *incorrect statement* **about the thoracic duct:**

(a) It begins as an upward continuation of cisterna chyli

(b) It enters the thoracic cavity through an aortic opening of the diaphragm

(c) It crosses the vertebral column from right to left side in front of T5 vertebra

(d) It terminates in the external jugular vein

2. **All structures form posterior relations of the thoracic duct in the posterior mediastinum** *except:*

(a) Right posterior intercostal arteries

(b) Terminal parts of hemiazygos and accessory hemiazygos veins

(c) Esophagus

(d) Vertebral column

3. **All structures lie behind the thoracic duct at the root of the neck** *except:*

(a) Vertebral artery and vein

(b) Carotid sheath

(c) Phrenic nerve

(d) Thyrocervical trunk and its branches

4. **All the statements about azygos vein are correct** *except:*

(a) They are paravertebral in position

(b) They are not accompanied by corresponding arteries

(c) They have no valves in their lumen

(d) They may appear tortuous

5. **All are the tributaries of azygos vein** *except:*

(a) Hemiazygos vein

(b) Accessory hemiazygos vein

(c) Right first posterior intercostal vein

(d) Right bronchial vein

6. **The left superior intercostal vein drains into:**

(a) Accessory hemiazygos vein

(b) Hemiazygos vein

(c) Azygos vein

(d) Left brachiocephalic vein

7. **All the statements regarding accessory azygos vein are correct** *except:*

(a) It lies on left side only

(b) It receives left superior intercostal vein

(c) It receives left bronchial veins

(d) It drains into azygos vein

8. **Select the** *incorrect statement* **about the thoracic sympathetic trunk:**

(a) Its upper end lies in front of the neck of the 1st rib

(b) Its lower end passes behind the medial arcuate ligament of diaphragm

(c) It commonly possesses 12 ganglia

(d) It lies in front of posterior intercostal nerve and vessels

9. **Regarding thoracic splanchnic nerves, which is the** *incorrect statement*:

(a) They consist of preganglionic sympathetic fibres

(b) They are three in number

(c) The lower splanchnic nerve is also called renal nerve

(d) Greater splanchnic nerve arises from 1st to 5th thoracic ganglia

Answers

1. *d*, 2. *c*, 3. *b*, 4. *c*, 5. *c*, 6. *d*, 7. *b*, 8. *c*, 9. *d*

Index